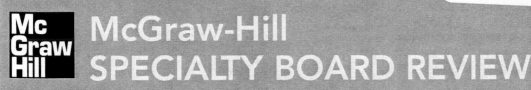

McGraw-Hill SPECIALTY BOARD REVIEW

Tintinalli's Emergency Medicine
Examination & Board Review

Editor

Susan B. Promes, MD, FACEP
Professor of Clinical Emergency Medicine
Residency Program Director
Department of Emergency Medicine
University of California, San Francisco
San Francisco General Hospital
San Francisco, California

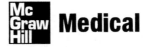

Medical

New York   Chicago   San Francisco   Lisbon   London   Madrid   Mexico City
Milan   New Delhi   San Juan   Seoul   Singapore   Sydney   Toronto

The McGraw·Hill Companies

McGraw-Hill Specialty Board Review:
Tintinalli's Emergency Medicine Examination & Board Review

Copyright © 2013 by The McGraw-Hill Companies, Inc. All rights reserved. Printed in the United States of America. Except as permitted under the United States Copyright Act of 1976, no part of this publication may be reproduced or distributed in any form or by any means, or stored in a data base or retrieval system, without the prior written permission of the publisher.

Previous edition published as *Emergency Medicine: Examination & Board Review* copyright © 2005 by The McGraw-Hill Companies, Inc.

1 2 3 4 5 6 7 8 9 0 QDB/QDB 17 16 15 14 13 12

Set ISBN 978-0-07-160205-1
Set MHID 0-07-160205-4
Book ISBN 978-0-07-160207-5
Book MHID 0-07-160207-0
CD-ROM ISBN 978-0-07-160208-2
CD-ROM MHID 0-07-160208-9

Notice

Medicine is an ever-changing science. As new research and clinical experience broaden our knowledge, changes in treatment and drug therapy are required. The authors and the publisher of this work have checked with sources believed to be reliable in their efforts to provide information that is complete and generally in accord with the standards accepted at the time of publication. However, in view of the possibility of human error or changes in medical sciences, neither the authors nor the publisher nor any other party who has been involved in the preparation or publication of this work warrants that the information contained herein is in every respect accurate or complete, and they disclaim all responsibility for any errors or omissions or for the results obtained from use of the information contained in this work. Readers are encouraged to confirm the information contained herein with other sources. For example and in particular, readers are advised to check the product information sheet included in the package of each drug they plan to administer to be certain that the information contained in this work is accurate and that changes have not been made in the recommended dose or in the contraindications for administration. This recommendation is of particular importance in connection with new or infrequently used drugs.

This book was set in Palatino by Aptara, Inc.
The editors were Anne M. Sydor and Robert Pancotti.
The production supervisor was Sherri Souffrance.
Project management was provided by Indu Jawwad, Aptara, Inc.
Quad/Graphics was printer and binder.

This book is printed on acid-free paper.

McGraw-Hill books are available at special quantity discounts to use as premiums and sales promotions, or for use in corporate training programs. To contact a representative, please e-mail us at bulksales@mcgraw-hill.com.

I would like to dedicate this book to all the emergency medicine residents who I have had the honor working with over the years. You're why I love to teach!

Special thanks to my family for giving me the opportunity to do all the things I do. Mark, Alex, and Aaron, did I tell you? I love you!

Contents

Contributors

Nima Afshar, MD
Assistant Clinical Professor
Medicine and Emergency Medicine
University of California, San Francisco
San Francisco, California
Chapter 12 Nervous System Disorders

G. Patrick Daubert, MD
KPNC Regional Toxicology Service
Department of Emergency Medicine
Kaiser Permanente, South Sacramento Medical
    Center
Sacramento, California
Chapter 21 Toxicologic Emergencies

Elizabeth Magassy Dorn, MD
Clinical Assistant Professor
Department of Emergency Medicine
University of Washington
Seattle, Washington
*Chapter 6 Eye, Ear, Nose, Throat, and Oral
    Emergencies*

Jocelyn Freeman Garrick, MD
EMS Base Director
Emergency Medicine
Alameda County Medical Center – Highland Hospital
Oakland, California
Associate Clinical Professor
Department of Emergency Medicine
University of California,
    San Francisco
San Francisco, California
Chapter 7 Gastrointestinal Emergencies

Cherie A. Hargis, MD
Attending Physician
Emergency Medicine
Alameda County Medical Center – Highland Hospital
Oakland, California
Assistant Clinical Professor
Department of Emergency Medicine
University of California, San Francisco
San Francisco, California
Chapter 2 Cardiovascular Disorders

H. Gene Hern Jr., MD, MS, FACEP, FAAEM
Residency Director
Emergency Medicine
Alameda County Medical Center – Highland Hospital
Oakland, California
Assistant Clinical Professor
Department of Emergency Medicine
University of California, San Francisco
San Francisco, California
Chapter 2 Cardiovascular Disorders

Mark A. Hostetler, MD, MPH
Attending Physician, Pediatrics
Division of Emergency Medicine
Phoenix Children's Hospital
Phoenix, Arizona
Chapter 14 Pediatrics

Christopher Kahn, MD, MPH
Assistant Professor of Clinical Emergency Medicine
Director, Emergency Medical Services and Disaster
    Medicine Fellowship
University of California, San Diego
San Diego, California
*Chapter 15 Prehospital Care and Disaster
    Preparedness*

Michael F. Kamali, MD
Chair
Department of Emergency Medicine
University of Rochester Medical Center
Rochester, New York
Chapter 20 Special Situations

Lucas D. Karaelias, MD
Clinical Instructor (Affiliated) of Surgery
    (Emergency Medicine)
Stanford University School of Medicine
Department of Emergency Medicine
Santa Clara Valley Medical Center
San Jose, California
Chapter 10 Systemic Infectious Disorders

Linda E. Keyes, MD
Assistant Clinical Professor
Emergency Medicine
University of Colorado School of
    Medicine
Aurora, Colorado
Chapter 5 Environmental Disorders

Barbara Kilian, MD
Assistant Professor
Department of Emergency Medicine
University of California, San Francisco
San Francisco, California
Chapter 4 Endocrine and Electrolytes Emergencies

Kristi L. Koenig, MD, FACEP, FIFEM
Professor of Emergency Medicine
Director, Center for Disaster Medical
    Sciences
Director of Public Health Preparedness
Director, International EMS & Disaster Medical
    Sciences Fellowship
University of California, Irvine, School of
    Medicine
Orange, California
*Chapter 15 Prehospital Care and Disaster
    Preparedness*

Ian B. K. Martin, MD
Assistant Professor of Emergency Medicine and
    Internal Medicine
Simmons Scholar
Program Director, UNC EM Global Health and
    Leadership Program
Associate Director, Office of International Activities
Associate Program Director, Emergency Medicine
    Residency
University of North Carolina at Chapel Hill School
    of Medicine
Chapel Hill, North Carolina
Chapter 9 Hematologic Disorders

Daniel C. McGillicuddy, MD
Associate Chair and Director of Clinical Operations
Department of Emergency Medicine
St. Joseph Mercy Hospital
Adjunct Faculty
Emergency Medicine
University of Michigan
Ann Arbor, Michigan
Chapter 22 Trauma

Arun Nagdev, MD
Director, Emergency Ultrasound
Emergency Medicine
Alameda County Medical Center – Highland Hospital
Oakland, California
Clinical Assistant Professor
Department of Emergency Medicine
University of California, San Francisco
San Francisco, California
Chapter 23 Wound Management

Flavia Nobay, MD
Program Director
Department of Emergency Medicine
University of Rochester
Rochester, New York
Chapter 20 Special Situations

Kelly P. O'Keefe, MD, FACEP
Assistant Professor and Program Director
Emergency Medicine Residency
University of South Florida
Tampa, Florida
Chapter 19 Resuscitation

Ronny M. Otero, MD
Division Head, Emergency Medicine
Sterling Heights Medical Center
Henry Ford Hospital
Sterling Heights, Michigan
Associate Professor
Emergency Medicine
Wayne State University
Detroit, Michigan
Chapter 17 Pulmonary Emergencies

Berenice Perez, MD
Clinical Instructor of Medicine
Department of Emergency Medicine
University of California, San Francisco
San Francisco, California
Attending Physician and Co-Medical
   Director
Emergency Department
Alameda County Medical Center – Highland Hospital
Oakland, California
Chapter 7 Gastrointestinal Emergencies

Jennifer V. Pope, MD
Resident
Department of Emergency Medicine
Beth Israel Deaconess Medical Center
Boston, Massachusetts
*Chapter 8 Gynecologic and Obstetric Emergencies
   and Chapter 22 Trauma*

Carlo L. Rosen, MD
Program Director and Vice Chair for
   Education
Department of Emergency Medicine
Beth Israel Deaconess Medical Center
Boston, Massachusetts
Associate Professor
Harvard Medical School
Boston, Massachusetts
Chapter 22 Trauma

Tracy G. Sanson, MD, FACEP
Education Director, Emergency Medicine
   Program
Associate Professor
University of South Florida
Tampa, Florida
Chapter 19 Resuscitation

Mari Siegel, MD
Clinical Instructor
Division of Emergency Medicine
Department of Surgery
Stanford University
Stanford, California
Chapter 18 Renal and Genitourinary Disorders

Barry C. Simon, MD
Chairman
Department of Emergency Medicine
Alameda County Medical Center – Highland Hospital
Oakland, California
Professor
Department of Emergency Medicine
University of California, San Francisco
San Francisco, California
Chapter 16 Psychobehavioral Disorders

Eric R. Snoey, MD
Vice Chair
Department of Emergency Medicine
Alameda County Medical Center – Highland Hospital
Oakland, California
Clinical Professor
Emergency Medicine
University of San Francisco School of Medicine
San Francisco, California
Chapter 16 Psychobehavioral Disorders

Aparajita Sohoni, MD
Faculty/Attending Physician
Emergency Medicine
Alameda County Medical Center – Highland Hospital
Oakland, California
Chapter 23 Wound Management

Colin D. Stack, MD
Attending Physician
Department of Emergency Medicine
Beth Israel Deaconess Medical Center
Boston, Massachusetts
Chapter 22 Trauma

Susan K. Stroud, MD
Clinical Associate Professor of Surgery
Division of Emergency Medicine
University of Utah School of Medicine
Salt Lake City, Utah
Chapter 11 Musculoskeletal Disorders

Suzanne Horine Summer, MD
Attending Physician
Emergency Medicine and Palliative Care
Kaiser Permanente
Oakland, California
*Chapter 1 Analgesia, Anesthesia, and Procedural
    Sedation*

Sukhjit S. Takhar, MD
Attending Physician
Emergency Medicine
Brigham and Women's Hospital
Instructor
Emergency Medicine
Harvard Medical School
Boston, Massachusetts
Chapter 10 Systemic Infectious Disorders

Traci Thoureen, MD, MHS-CL, FACEP
Clinical Assistant Professor
Emergency Medicine
University of Maryland School of Medicine
Baltimore, Maryland
Chapter 3 Cutaneous Disorders

Carrie D. Tibbles, MD
Associate Program Director
Emergency Medicine Residency
Director of Graduate Medical Education
Beth Israel Deaconess Medical Center
Assistant Professor of Medicine
Emergency Medicine
Harvard Medical School
Boston, Massachusetts
Chapter 8 Gynecologic and Obstetric Emergencies

Mercedes Torres, MD
Assistant Professor
Department of Emergency Medicine
University of Maryland School of Medicine
Baltimore, Maryland
Chapter 3 Cutaneous Disorders

Charlotte Page Wills, MD
Associate Residency Director
Department of Emergency Medicine
Alameda County Medical Center – Highland Hospital
Oakland, California
Assistant Clinical Professor of Emergency
    Medicine
Department of Emergency Medicine
University of California, San Francisco School
    of Medicine
San Francisco, California
Chapter 13 Orthopedic Emergencies

Robert D. Yniguez, MD
Attending Physician, Pediatrics
Division of Emergency Medicine
Phoenix Children's Hospital
Phoenix, Arizona
Clinical Assistant Professor
Department of Pediatrics
University of Arizona College of Medicine at
    Phoenix
Phoenix, Arizona
Chapter 14 Pediatrics

Preface

This book was designed as a study tool to complement the popular seventh edition of *Tintinalli's Emergency Medicine: A Comprehensive Study Guide*. This book contains an array of questions to aid in the preparation for the ABEM and AOBEM written examination as well as the annual emergency medicine residency program in-training examination.

This edition of the examination and board review book is slightly different from the previous edition. The explanation of the correct answer for each question is referenced directly to a chapter in the seventh edition of *Tintinalli's Emergency Medicine: A Comprehensive Study Guide*. This new edition of the review book includes an index so that you as a reader can easily find a topic of interest. In addition, there is a CD-ROM associated with this edition, which contains an interactive test bank with a selection of questions from each chapter in the text. I hope that you find these changes valuable.

Susan B. Promes, MD, FACEP

CHAPTER 1

Analgesia, Anesthesia, and Procedural Sedation

Questions

1-1. Which of the following is the recommended treatment for migraines?

(A) Fentanyl (Sublimaze)
(B) Hydrocodone and acetaminophen (Vicodin)
(C) Meperidine hydrochloride (Demerol)
(D) Sumatriptan succinate (Imitrex)
(E) Morphine sulfate

1-2. Which person is most likely to receive adequate pain control in the emergency department?

(A) 2-year-old Caucasian male
(B) 18-year-old African American female college student
(C) 24-year-old Caucasian male athlete
(D) 30-year-old Caucasian male with retardation
(E) 80-year-old Hispanic grandmother

1-3. Which of these should be relied upon in the assessment and treatment of pain?

(A) Health care worker's impression
(B) Patient's position, expression, and movement
(C) Patient's response to a generous dose of an opioid analgesic
(D) Patient's subjective report of pain
(E) Vital signs

1-4. What is an appropriate endpoint for pain management?

(A) Comfortable appearing patient
(B) Normalization of vital signs
(C) Pain score of 2 or less using a 1–10 numeric rating
(D) Sleeping patient
(E) Sufficient pain relief as determined by the patient

1-5. Which of the following is TRUE regarding pain management?

(A) Anxiolytics should not be combined with narcotics due to the increased risk of respiratory depression.
(B) Dosing of opioid analgesics is straightforward and most patients of similar size and age require similar doses.
(C) Opioid agonist–antagonists have no benefit over pure opioid agonists.
(D) Patients of all ages tend to report pain in similar ways.
(E) The proper use of opioids requires consideration of side effects, initial dose, route and timing of onset, and frequency of administration.

1-6. Which of the following side effects is more common when an opioid analgesic is administered intravenously rather than orally?

(A) Constipation

(B) Gastrointestinal bleeding

(C) Nausea

(D) Respiratory depression

(E) Vomiting

1-7. Which of the following statements is TRUE regarding opioids?

(A) Codeine in standard doses of 30–60 mg is significantly better than standard doses of nonsteroidal anti-inflammatory drugs (NSAIDs) or acetaminophen.

(B) Hydrocodone (Vicodin) produces more nausea, vomiting, and dysphoria than other opioids.

(C) Hydromorphone hydrochloride (Dilaudid) can interact with many drugs to precipitate a serotonergic crisis.

(D) Meperidine (Demerol) is metabolized to normeperidine, a neuroexcitatory compound that has a long elimination half-life.

(E) Morphine sulfate should never be given to a patient who reports itching when given fentanyl (Sublimaze) in the past.

1-8. Which of the following is TRUE regarding opioid use in the emergency department?

(A) Fentanyl (Sublimaze) is a good alternative medication in a patient with an allergy to meperidine (Demerol).

(B) A patient on chronic high-dose oxycodone hydrochloride can be safely switched to an opioid agonist–antagonist.

(C) Symptom-targeted use of anxiolytics and antiemetics in addition to opioid analgesics is generally appropriate.

(D) When giving opioids, promethazine or hydroxyzine should routinely be added to enhance analgesic effects and to reduce the amount of opioid required.

(E) When treating acute pain in the emergency department, any existing transdermal opioid patches should be left in place to provide ongoing levels of medication.

1-9. An 80-year-old female arrives in the emergency department with a chief complaint of moderate ankle pain after twisting her ankle. Radiographs are negative for fracture, and she will be discharged home. The patient has a history of mild hepatic impairment and atrial fibrillation. She is on warfarin (Coumadin) and has a history a meperidine (Demerol) allergy. What is the BEST analgesic choice for this patient?

(A) Acetaminophen (Tylenol) 650 mg orally

(B) Fentanyl (Duragesic patch) 25 μg/hour transdermally

(C) Ibuprofen (Motrin) 600 mg orally

(D) Morphine 10 mg intravenously

(E) Propoxyphene hydrochloride (Darvon) 65 mg orally

1-10. Which is NOT generally thought to increase the risk of NSAID-induced acute renal failure?

(A) Loop diuretic use

(B) Preexisting cardiac disease

(C) Preexisting mild hepatic impairment

(D) Preexisting mild renal disease

(E) Volume depletion

1-11. A 60-year-old female presents to the emergency department complaining of pain from postherpetic neuralgia. Acetaminophen (Tylenol) has been ineffective. Which would be the BEST choice for chronic pain control?

(A) Acetaminophen with Codeine No. 3 (Tyco no. 3)

(B) Amitriptyline (Elavil)

(C) Fentanyl (Sublimaze) transmucosal lozenge

(D) Ibuprofen (Motrin)

(E) Ketorolac (Toradol)

1-12. Which of the following is CORRECT regarding addiction, abuse, and dependence?

(A) Addiction is confirmed when stopping a medication results in acute withdrawal symptoms.

(B) Addiction usually requires daily use of narcotics for several weeks.

(C) Fewer than 10% of patients are at risk of prescription medication abuse.

(D) Dependence is the misuse of a medication or drug to the detriment of a patient's well-being.

(E) Dependence may occur after one use of heroin.

1-13. Which of the following methods is NOT an appropriate way to decrease the pain of infiltration from a local anesthetic?

(A) Buffering the anesthetic solution with sodium bicarbonate prior to infiltration

(B) Injecting through the wound margins instead of through intact skin

(C) Rapid injection to minimize the duration of pain

(D) Using 1 mL of sodium bicarbonate 8.4% to buffer 29 mL of bupivacaine 0.25%

(E) Warming the solution to body temperature before injecting

1-14. Which problem is associated with the CORRECT local anesthetic?

(A) Benzocaine: may wear off before long procedures are completed.

(B) Lidocaine: overdose can cause refractory seizures.

(C) Lidocaine: overdose can cause methemoglobinemia.

(D) Lidocaine with epinephrine: may cause ischemia of a digit in an otherwise healthy patient.

(E) Ropivacaine: highest risk of cardiotoxicity.

1-15. Which is TRUE regarding an intracostal nerve block?

(A) Anesthesia duration is generally 24–48 hours.

(B) Pneumothorax occurs in about 25% of patients who have this procedure.

(C) Ribs 1–6 are easiest to block.

(D) This type of block is superior to parenteral analgesia.

(E) 3–5 mL of anesthetic solution should be used for each rib blocked.

1-16. An obese elderly female presents with a head injury and a hip fracture. Her blood pressure is low and she is moaning in pain. You decide to perform a femoral nerve block on this patient, which of the following is correct about that procedure?

(A) Inject after resistance is felt.

(B) Injection should be done 3 cm below the inguinal crease.

(C) Pillow should be placed under the contralateral hip.

(D) Relief is almost immediate.

(E) Ultrasound guidance or a peripheral nerve stimulator should be used if available.

1-17. A 22-year-old female presents to the emergency department on a Tuesday evening with a complaint of kidney stone and blood in her urine. She has no records at your facility as she is visiting from out of town. She forgot to bring a prescription for oxycodone that her urologist gave to her and says she is allergic to ibuprofen (Motrin), which causes itching. The patient appears comfortable and the exam is normal but lab results show hematuria. Which is the BEST choice for treatment among those listed?

(A) An agonist–antagonist opioid should be prescribed.

(B) Give ibuprofen (Motrin); the patient is clearly lying about her allergies.

(C) Obtain a confirmatory test such as a CT scan.

(D) Refuse any pain medicines; the patient is demonstrating drug-seeking behavior.

(E) The stated prescription should be refilled because the hematuria confirms the history of kidney stone.

1-18. A 45-year-old male presents to the emergency department on a Friday night with a complaint of dental pain requesting a refill of his acetaminophen and hydrocodone (Vicodin) prescription. He has had several visits for the same problem over the past 3 months. He states he is allergic to ibuprofen (Motrin), acetaminophen (Tylenol), codeine, and aspirin, all of which cause nausea. His exam shows normal vital signs but multiple dental caries without clear abscess. Which is the MOST appropriate treatment for this patient from among those listed?

(A) Give him an injection of hydromorphone (Dilaudid) if he promises that he will not return to your facility for narcotics in the future.

(B) Offer a dental block with lidocaine and refer him to a dentist in the morning.

(C) Offer a prescription for nabumetone (Relafen).

(D) Refill his prescription for acetaminophen and hydrocodone (Vicodin) as requested.

(E) Refuse any pain medicine; the patient is drug seeking.

1-19. A 90-year-old female presents to the emergency department complaining of pain unrelieved by her home medications. When treating her, which of the following is MOST correct?

(A) Constipation is a minor side effect of opioids.

(B) Her regular doctor need not be involved.

(C) Increasing the dosage of a previously used opioid is inappropriate.

(D) Neuralgia and osteoarthritis are the most common causes of chronic pain in the elderly.

(E) NSAIDs will have fewer side effects than opioids in this population.

1-20. Which is TRUE about chronic pain?

(A) Chronic pain is more common in elderly patients.

(B) Less than 25% of patients whose pain lasts 3 months will continue to have chronic pain for several years.

(C) The goal of emergency treatment should be complete relief of pain.

(D) The head is the most common location of chronic pain.

(E) Patients presenting to the emergency department because of chronic pain are best helped by hospital admission.

1-21. Which of the following is the BEST answer regarding medication for back pain and sciatica?

    (A) Cyclobenzaprine (Flexeril) is an appropriate long-term medication for chronic back pain.

    (B) NSAIDs are an appropriate long-term treatment for chronic low back pain in patients at low risk of side effects.

    (C) Opioids are appropriate long-term agents to use for chronic back pain.

    (D) Steroids are an effective and long-lasting treatment for acute sciatica.

    (E) Tricyclic antidepressants are NOT appropriate long-term medications for use in chronic back pain.

1-22. A 62-year-old man with hypertension, diabetes, and hyperlipidemia complains of symmetric numbness and burning pain to bilateral feet. Pain is provoked by gentle touch. What is the MOST likely diagnosis?

    (A) Complex regional pain syndrome

    (B) Diabetic neuropathy

    (C) Fibromyalgia

    (D) Postherpetic neuralgia

    (E) Sciatica

1-23. For which of the following conditions is a tricyclic antidepressant considered first-line therapy?

    (A) Complex regional pain syndrome, type I, also known as reflex sympathetic dystrophy

    (B) HIV-related neuropathy

    (C) Phantom limb pain

    (D) Postherpetic neuralgia

    (E) Spinal cord injury pain

1-24. An anxious 50-year-old female drug user with a 10-cm thigh abscess from skin-popping is given midazolam (Versed) to facilitate incision and drainage. She remains calm but with her eyes open and cooperative and verbal throughout the procedure. What type of sedation is this called?

    (A) Deep sedation

    (B) Dissociation

    (C) General anesthesia

    (D) Minimal sedation

    (E) Moderate sedation

1-25. Which of these is NOT considered an indication for EMERGENCY procedural sedation?

    (A) Cardioversion for a wide complex tachycardia in a 78-year-old female with chest pain and dizziness

    (B) Intractable pain from a dislocated shoulder in a 34-year-old male

    (C) Obtaining a CT scan in an agitated 15-year-old football player who sustained a head injury

    (D) Reduction of an elbow dislocation in a 65-year-old female with an absent radial pulse

    (E) Sexual assault examination in a 6-year-old girl who was assaulted an hour ago

1-26. Which vital sign is recommended to be continuously monitored for all levels of sedation, from minimal to deep?

    (A) Blood pressure

    (B) End-tidal carbon dioxide (capnography)

    (C) Oxygen saturation

    (D) Pulse

    (E) Respiratory rate

1-27. Which of the following pairs correctly identifies a drug with its associated side effect?

    (A) Etomidate—suppression of the adrenalcortical axis

    (B) Fentanyl—paradoxical agitation

    (C) Ketamine—rigid chest syndrome

    (D) Midazolam—emergence reactions

    (E) Nitrous oxide—myoclonic jerking

1-28. Which of the following physical findings is generally NOT associated with a difficult airway?

(A) Dental caries

(B) Large tongue

(C) Morbid obesity

(D) Short neck

(E) Small jaw

1-29. Which of the following is TRUE about midazolam?

(A) Buffering it will reduce the mucosal irritation with intranasal use.

(B) Hypertension can be a side effect in some patients.

(C) Naloxone will reverse the effects of this drug.

(D) Paradoxical agitation is seen in some patients.

(E) Rectal and intramuscular administration are the preferred methods of administration.

1-30. Which of the following is NOT considered a contraindication to the use of propofol as a sedative in the emergency room for procedural sedation?

(A) Egg allergy

(B) Hypovolemia

(C) Lack of ability to intubate and ventilate the patient

(D) Milk allergy

(E) Soy allergy

1-31. What Mallampati grade is the airway below?

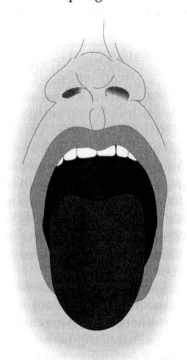

Figure 1-1. Reproduced with permission from Tintinalli JE, Stapczynski JS, Ma OJ, Cline DM, Cydulka RK, Meckler GD: *Tintinalli's Emergency Medicine: A Comprehensive Study Guide,* 7th Edition. Copyright © 2011 The McGraw-Hill Companies, Inc.

(A) Grade I

(B) Grade II

(C) Grade III

(D) Grade IV

Analgesia, Anesthesia, and Procedural Sedation
Answers and Explanations

1-1. **The answer is D** (Chapter 38). Preferred treatment for migraine headaches includes serotonin agonists (triptans such as Imitrex [sumatriptan succinate]) or dopamine antagonists (phenothiazines such as Compazine [prochlorperazine]) rather than opiates. In multiple trials, opiates have demonstrated poor performance.

1-2. **The answer is C** (Chapter 38). Certain patients including minorities, those at the extremes of age, and those with diminished cognitive function are more at risk for inadequate pain control. In addition, there is also a tendency to undertreat pain in women.

1-3. **The answer is D** (Chapter 38). The patient's subjective reporting of pain, not the health care worker's impression, is the basis for pain assessment and treatment. There is poor correlation between vital signs such as tachycardia and tachypnea or changes in patient expression and movement, and the patient's report of pain. The amount of opioids required to treat pain can vary a great deal among different patients. Response to a fixed amount of pain medication does not correlate with the amount of pain an individual is experiencing.

1-4. **The answer is E** (Chapter 38). A value assigned by a patient on a validated pain scale depends on multiple factors including the patient's past personal experiences; therefore, a discrete number cannot be used as an endpoint for acceptable pain management. The endpoint for pain management is the patient's judgment about their pain relief. The interpretation of pain is variable, and the only relevant goal should be that which satisfies the needs of the patient. Vital signs do not correlate well with the subjective rating of a patient's pain.

1-5. **The answer is E** (Chapter 38). Proper use of opioids requires consideration of the following: route and frequency of administration, desired time of onset of action, initial dose, concurrent use of nonopioid analgesics and adjunctive agents, and incidence and severity of side effects. Acute pain is usually accompanied by anxiety and feelings of loss of control. Anxiolytics should be considered if reassurance is insufficient. Patient response to opioid analgesics depends on age, body mass, and previous or chronic exposure to opioids and can vary greatly between individuals. The elderly often report pain very differently than younger patients for various reasons. Unlike pure opioids, opioid agonists–antagonists have a ceiling on respiratory depression despite higher doses.

1-6. **The answer is D** (Chapter 38). Adverse effects of opioids are more common with intravenous, transmucosal, and epidural administration. They include pruritus, urinary retention, confusion, and respiratory depression. Other side effects of opioids include nausea, vomiting, pruritus, constipation, and hypotension. Gastrointestinal bleeding is not generally considered a side effect of opioid analgesics.

1-7. **The answer is D** (Chapter 38). Meperidine (Demerol) interacts with many drugs (such as monoamine oxidase inhibitors) in ways that may precipitate a serotonergic crisis. Meperidine metabolizes to normeperidine, a substance that has neuroexcitatory properties. Codeine in doses from 30 to 60 mg has a similar effect on pain as standard doses of acetaminophen or NSAIDs. Codeine produces more nausea, vomiting, and dysphoria than other opioids. Opioid hypersensitivity is not common; however, true allergic reactions are extremely rare. It is not clear if there is clinical cross sensitivity within opioid classes, but it is reasonable to switch to a drug from a different opioid class if a patient develops a hypersensitivity reaction to an opioid.

1-8. **The answer is C** (Chapter 38). It is recommended that the addition of anxiolytics and antiemetics to opioids should be symptom targeted. Adjuncts can be used as they do enhance the analgesic effect and reduce the amount of opioid required, but since appropriate titration with opioids in the emergency department is highly effective, they should not be routinely given in this setting. When treating patients in the emergency department for acute pain, it is best to remove delayed-release narcotic patches to better titrate opioid dose and to minimize adverse reactions from combining agents. Cross sensitivity has been suggested among the piperidine class of opioids, which includes fentanyl, alfentanil, sufentanil, and meperidine; if a patient reports an allergy to one of these medications, it would be better to try a medication in a different class instead of one of these. Opioid agonist–antagonist agents may precipitate withdrawal symptoms and should be used with caution in patients who are addicted to narcotics.

1-9. **The answer is A** (Chapter 38). Acetaminophen (Tylenol) is effective for mild to moderate pain. No change in dosage is needed for mild hepatic impairment. Elderly patients who are not on opioids regularly are more sensitive to both the analgesic effects and the side effects of these medications.

Propoxyphene (Darvon), in particular, has few analgesic effects and high potential for addiction and overdose. In this elderly patient with moderate pain and a problem that will be treated as an outpatient, 10 mg of IV morphine would be an inappropriate choice as well. Transdermal fentanyl has a slow onset as well as other potential contraindications. Adverse effects of nonsteroidal anti-inflammatory drugs (NSAIDs) include platelet dysfunction and thus increase the risk of bleeding with warfarin (Coumadin), so Ibuprofen (Motrin) would not be a good choice in this case either.

1-10. **The answer is C** (Chapter 38). NSAID-induced acute renal failure is more common in patients who are volume depleted, have preexisting renal or cardiac disease, or are taking loop diuretics. Mild hepatic impairment does not affect the metabolism of most analgesics nor is it known to increase the risk of acute renal failure with this class of medications.

1-11. **The answer is B** (Chapter 38). Patients with neuropathic pain such as postherpetic neuralgia frequently do not respond well to standard analgesics and may be resistant to short-acting opioids. Tricyclics such as amitriptyline (Elavil) as well as some anticonvulsants and long-acting opioids have been found to be effective for neuropathic pain. Most need to be titrated in the outpatient setting.

1-12. **The answer is C** (Chapter 38). Addiction is the misuse of a drug or medication to the patient's detriment and can occur after as little as one use of heroin. Dependence usually requires daily use of a narcotic for 4–6 weeks and is confirmed when the abrupt cessation of the medication results in withdrawal. At most, 10% of patients are at risk of prescription medication abuse.

1-13. **The answer is C** (Chapter 40). There are multiple ways to reduce pain of infiltration of a local anesthetic. They include slow (not fast) injection, warming the solution to body temperature, and injecting through the margins of the wound. Bupivacaine can be buffered as described. Buffering the anesthetic solution with sodium bicarbonate will decrease the pain of injection.

1-14. **The answer is B** (Chapter 40). Lidocaine in high doses can cause refractory seizures. Benzocaine generally has a long duration of action. High doses of benzocaine or prilocaine, not lidocaine, may lead to methemoglobinemia. Ropivacaine is significantly less cardiotoxic than other agents. The use of local anesthetic with epinephrine appears to be safe for use in end-arterial fields (fingers, toes, etc.) in selected healthy patients.

1-15. **The answer is E** (Chapter 40). The correct volume of anesthetic for each intracostal block is 3–5 mL. Pneumothorax occurs in 8–9% of patients or about 1.4% for each individual intercostal block. There are no rigorous controlled trials comparing parental analgesia with intercostal nerve blocks. An intercostal block should provide anesthesia for 8–18 hours. Due to the position of the scapula and rhomboid muscles, ribs 1–6 are difficult to block.

1-16. **The answer is E** (Chapter 40). Femoral nerve blocks are appropriate for hip fractures and are especially useful in the elderly. Femoral nerve blocks are less likely to exacerbate hypotension or alter the patient's mental status if appropriate anesthetic doses are used when compared with parenteral opioid analgesics. The anesthetic should not be injected if resistance is felt, as this indicates the possibility of intraneural injection. Injection should be done at the level of the inguinal crease. In obese patients, placement of a pillow underneath the affected hip can help expose the area. Ten to thirty minutes are required to obtain optimal analgesia. Use of ultrasound or a peripheral nerve stimulator is recommended when available.

1-17. **The answer is C** (Chapter 42). The patient exhibits several features of drug-seeking behavior. Confirming the diagnosis of kidney stones with additional testing is appropriate in this situation. Hematuria can be factitious or menstrual and a witnessed or catheter specimen can be obtained if you are concerned that the patient is trying to obtain narcotics fraudulently. Nonaddictive pain medications should be offered to patients who state they have pain, but ibuprofen (Motrin) would not be the best choice given the patient's stated allergy. Agonist–antagonist opioids should not be given to patients in the emergency department who are suspected of being addicted to opioids, as they may precipitate withdrawal.

1-18. **The answer is C** (Chapter 42). The patient exhibits several features of drug-seeking behavior, but he may have true pain. Offering a nonnarcotic oral medication would be the best thing. A dental block would also be appropriate, but lidocaine is too short acting to be adequate. Refilling a narcotic medication is not the best choice in this type of patient; additionally, the patient states that he is allergic to acetaminophen (a component of Vicodin). One study showed that patients who were refused opioids at one facility were successful in obtaining opioids at another facility 93% of the time and were later successful at obtaining opioids from the same facility 71% of the time; thus, giving a "one time" shot of narcotics is probably not a good strategy.

1-19. **The answer is D** (Chapter 42). Opioids may cause debilitating constipation in the elderly. However, when properly titrated, opioids may produce fewer serious side effects than NSAIDs, as the NSAIDs cause higher rates of gastrointestinal bleeding and renal disease in the elderly. Neuralgia and osteoarthritis are the most common causes of chronic pain in the elderly. The elderly and others are frequently undertreated for pain, and although side effects must be considered, increasing the dosage of a narcotic may be indicated. Follow-up with a regular doctor would be important in this case.

1-20. **The answer is A** (Chapter 42). Chronic pain is more common in elderly patients and the most common site of chronic pain is the back. Complete pain relief is an unrealistic goal for chronic pain patients who present to the emergency department. Chronic pain patients who present to the emergency department may be best helped by referral to a pain clinic or specialists; hospital admission is seldom indicated.

1-21. **The answer is B** (Chapter 42). Administration of steroids for acute sciatica significantly reduces pain scores, but the benefit appears to last only about 24 hours. A systematic meta-analysis of opioids for chronic back pain found no significant long-term benefit. Despite some lack of long-term studies, it is considered reasonable to use NSAIDs in patients with chronic back pain provided that side effects are anticipated when the decision is made to prescribe them. Cyclobenzaprine (Flexeril) appears to have little benefit beyond that of placebo in chronic back pain. Tricyclic antidepressants have been shown to improve mild to moderate chronic back pain.

1-22. **The answer is B** (Chapter 42). The symptoms of diabetic neuropathy are symmetrical pain and abnormal sensation in the legs. Gentle touch may provoke pain in some patients. Postherpetic neuralgia and complex regional pain syndrome are unlikely to be symmetrical as they follow episodes of herpes zoster or injury, respectively. Sciatic is also more commonly unilateral and follows the S1 dermatome. Fibromyalgia is defined by the presence of 11 of 18 specific tender points, none of which are below the knee, nonrestorative sleep, muscle stiffness, and generalized aching pain, with symptom duration of more than 3 months.

1-23. **The answer is D** (Chapter 42). In general, tricyclic antidepressants are an effective therapy in patients with neuropathic pain, which includes postherpetic neuralgia; however, antidepressants are not effective for spinal cord injury pain, phantom limb pain, and HIV-related neuropathy. Intranasal calcitonin (but no other therapy studied) was recommended by a meta-analysis for complex regional pain syndrome, type 1.

1-24. **The answer is D** (Chapter 41). Moderate sedation patients generally have their eyes closed and respond slowly to vocal commands. Dissociative sedation is a type of moderate sedation where cortical centers do not receive sensory stimuli. Deep sedation is characterized by a profoundly depressed level of consciousness, with a purposeful motor response elicited only after repeated or painful stimuli. Minimal sedation is characterized by anxiolysis but with normal arousal to verbal stimuli. With general anesthesia, the patient is unarousable.

1-25. **The answer is E** (Chapter 41). Emergent indications for procedural sedation and analgesia include cardioversion for life-threatening arrhythmias, neuroimaging for head trauma, reduction in fractures or dislocations with soft-tissue or vascular compromise, care of contaminated wounds, or intractable pain. Sexual assault examinations require less urgent sedation.

1-26. **The answer is C** (Chapter 41). It is recommended that oxygenation be monitored continuously for all levels of sedation. Pulse, respiration, and end-tidal carbon dioxide should be monitored continuously for moderate to deep sedation, and blood pressure should be monitored every 5 minutes in these cases. For minimal sedation, heart rate, respiratory rate, and blood pressure be monitored every 15 minutes with blood pressure readings after medication boluses as well.

1-27. **The answer is A** (Chapter 41). Etomidate is associated with suppression of the adrenalcortical axis as well as myoclonic jerking. Ketamine is known for emergence reactions. Fentanyl has been associated with rigid chest syndrome in a small percentage of patients, especially if given as a rapid bolus. Paradoxical agitation has been reported with the use of midazolam. Nitrous oxide may promote expansion of internal gas filled structures.

1-28. **The answer is A** (Chapter 41). A potentially difficult airway should be anticipated when the following are found: short neck, micrognathia, large tongue, and morbid obesity.

1-29.   The answer is D (Chapter 41). Flumazenil will reverse the effects of midazolam; naloxone reverses the effects of opioids. Intranasal midazolam does cause irritation of the mucosa, but buffering the solution does not decrease this irritation. Both the rectal and IM routes have unreliable onset and depth of sedation but may be appropriate in some patients. Hypotension can arise with the use of midazolam in patients who are hypovolemic. Paradoxical agitation has been reported in 1–15% of patients who receive this medication for procedural sedation.

1-30.   The answer is D (Chapter 41). Both egg and soy allergies are contraindications to the use of propofol. Milk allergy is not a contraindication. Hypovolemia increases the risk of hypotension from propofol use and should be corrected before the medicine is given. Additionally, sudden respiratory depression and apnea, are adverse effects seen with this drug, so ventilatory support must be feasible if this medication is used.

1-31.   The answer is B (Chapter 39). This patient has a Mallampati grade II airway. The Mallampati grade (I–IV) predicts the technical ease of intubation. The higher the Mallampati score, the more technically difficult the intubation will likely be.

Cardiovascular Disorders
Questions

2-1. How many hours after a cardiac ischemia event would one expect to reliably find a positive troponin?

(A) 2
(B) 4
(C) 6
(D) 8
(E) 10

2-2. A patient presents with a history of hypertension and epigastric and chest pain for 3 hours with negative biomarkers. His electrocardiogram (ECG) is normal. He responds to antacids and feels better. What is your next appropriate response?

(A) A prescription for the proton pump inhibitor
(B) Admit for cardiac workup
(C) An emergent cardiac catheterization
(D) Nitroglycerin
(E) Repeat biomarkers

2-3. What percentage of patients with a normal ECG will ultimately have a diagnosis of NSTEMI or unstable angina?

(A) 5
(B) 10
(C) 15
(D) 20
(E) 25

2-4. A 64-year-old woman arrives by ambulance with crushing substernal chest pain for the past 40 minutes. She received aspirin and a large bore IV en route. Several tubes of blood are available. Her past medical history includes adult onset diabetes mellitus and hypertension, controlled by metformin and lisinopril, respectively. Vital signs include blood pressure (BP) 90/74, heart rate (HR) 115, respiratory rate (RR) 28, temperature (T) 37°C, room air SaO_2 96%. The patient appears ashen and diaphoretic, with cool, mottled extremities. She is awake but answers questions slowly. Jugular venous distention (JVD) is present. Heart sounds are regular with an S4 gallop but without murmurs or rubs. Lungs sounds are equal bilaterally and clear to auscultation. Her abdomen is soft, nontender, without palpable masses. Femoral pulses are equal. Extremities are cool, but without edema. Peripheral pulses are faint but equal. Despite her slow responses, the patient follows commands and moves all four extremities. The initial ECG showed sinus tachycardia, with ST-segment elevation in leads II, III, and aVF. The second ECG is shown here (Figure 2-1). While arrangements for echocardiography and early revascularization are made with the cardiologist, which of the following is the next MOST appropriate action?

(A) Administer propranolol
(B) Infuse 250–500 mL of normal saline
(C) Initiate thrombolytic therapy
(D) Start a dobutamine drip
(E) Start a phenylephrine drip

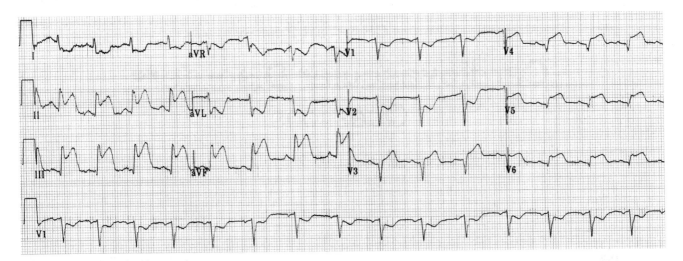

Figure 2-1. Reproduced with permission from Knoop KJ, Stack LB, Storrow AB, Thurman RJ: *The Atlas of Emergency Medicine*, 3rd Edition. Copyright © 2010 The McGraw-Hill Companies, Inc. ECG contributor: Thomas Bottoni, MD.

2-5. What is the MOST common cause of cardiogenic shock?

(A) Acute aortic insufficiency

(B) Aortic stenosis

(C) Hypertrophic cardiomyopathy

(D) Acute myocardial infarction (AMI)

(E) Pericardial tamponade

2-6. A 60-year-old man presents to the ED with acute onset of chest pain and dyspnea for the past 20 minutes. He has a past medical history of adult onset diabetes mellitus. ECG indicates acute STEMI. Vital signs are BP 90/74, HR 123, RR 26, and room air SaO$_2$ 94%. Physical examination shows an ashen, diaphoretic, tachypneic man. He has cool mottled skin, JVD, rales, and a new harsh apical systolic murmur that begins with the first heart sound but ends before the second. Prior medical records do not document any murmurs. Which of the following is the MOST likely diagnosis?

(A) Aortic insufficiency

(B) Aortic stenosis

(C) Mitral regurgitation

(D) Pulmonary embolism

(E) Ventral septal defect

2-7. A patient in acute cardiogenic shock presents with a new soft holosystolic apical murmur that radiates to the axilla. Which of the following is the most likely diagnosis?

(A) Acute aortic insufficiency

(B) Acute aortic stenosis

(C) Acute mitral insufficiency

(D) Acute tricuspid insufficiency

(E) Acute ventral septal defect

2-8. A 63-year-old woman presents to the ED in cardiogenic shock due to an acute STEMI. Symptoms began 2 hours ago. In addition to giving aspirin, what is the BEST management plan?

(A) Support cardiac perfusion, arrange echocardiography, and arrange early revascularization

(B) Support cardiac perfusion, arrange echocardiography, and arrange thrombolytic therapy

(C) Support cardiac perfusion, arrange echocardiography, and transfer to ICU

(D) Support cardiac perfusion, arrange intra-aortic balloon counterpulsation

(E) Support cardiac perfusion, arrange left ventricular assist device (LVAD)

2-9. What percent of women with confirmed cardiac ischemia present without chest pain?

   (A) 5%
   (B) 10%
   (C) 20%
   (D) 25%
   (E) >35%

2-10. What percent of patients with unstable angina present with atypical features?

   (A) 10%
   (B) 20%
   (C) 30%
   (D) 40%
   (E) 50%

2-11. What is the recommended door-to-ECG time in patients presenting with chest pain?

   (A) 1 minute
   (B) 10 minutes
   (C) 15 minutes
   (D) 20 minutes
   (E) 30 minutes

2-12. A 54-year-old man presents with acute substernal chest pain. His ECG has 4 mm acute ST-segment elevation in lead III and 2 mm ST-segment elevation in lead II. Which of the following is the most likely vessel occluded?

   (A) Left anterior descending artery
   (B) Left circumflex artery
   (C) Left main coronary artery
   (D) Right coronary artery
   (E) Sinoatrial node artery

2-13. A 54-year-old man presents with 6 hours of acute substernal chest pain. He has an ECG within the first 10 minutes of arrival. He has 4 mm acute ST-segment elevation in leads V2–V5. What is the American College of Cardiology (ACC) and American Heart Association (AHA) recommended reperfusion strategy?

   (A) Pain control then percutaneous coronary intervention (PCI) once patient is pain free
   (B) Primary PCI in <90 minutes
   (C) Primary PCI in <120 minutes
   (D) Thrombolysis in <90 minutes
   (E) Thrombolysis in <120 minutes

2-14. A 65-year-old male presents with 2 hours of chest pain. He has ST elevations across his precordial leads and is diagnosed with an AMI. He is given thrombolytics in the ED. One hour after administration, he is still having chest pain and his BP is 80/60. The next best course of action would be

   (A) Dopamine infusion
   (B) Nitroglycerin drip
   (C) Placement of an aortic balloon pump
   (D) Repeat thrombolytic administration
   (E) Rescue PCI

2-15. The use of nitroglycerin in AMI patients is associated with what degree of decrease in mortality rates?

   (A) 10%
   (B) 25%
   (C) 35%
   (D) 50%
   (E) No decrease

2-16. In the Framingham Heart Study, which of the following was the MOST common etiology of syncope?

   (A) Cardiac
   (B) Orthostatic
   (C) Seizure
   (D) Vasovagal
   (E) Unknown or indeterminate

2-17. While observing the arrival of a trauma patient with an open tibia fracture, an otherwise healthy 22-year-old male hospital volunteer states he feels lightheaded. He appears pale and diaphoretic and slowly sinks to the floor. Fortunately, an observant nurse prevents him from striking his head. He is unresponsive for 10 seconds, has a brief tonic–clonic movement but spontaneously awakens, and states "That was weird." A brief neurologic exam is nonfocal. Which of the following is the MOST likely cause of his condition?

(A) Dysrhythmia

(B) Grand-mal seizure

(C) Hypoglycemia

(D) Orthostatic hypotension

(E) Vasovagal syncope

2-18. A 68-year-old man presents to the ED after an episode of syncope at home witnessed by his grandson. The patient had allowed his grandson, who was practicing for a first-aid certificate, attempt to locate the "pulse in his neck." The grandson states the patient slumped over after about 5 seconds of neck pressure and was unresponsive. The patient woke up spontaneously after his grandson placed him supine on the floor and 911 was called. The patient has a history of hypertension and takes enalapril. He reports having a similar fainting episode 6 months ago while trimming his sideburns. He denies headache, chest pain, shortness of breath, abdominal pain, or weakness. Vital signs are BP 138/90, HR 70, RR 18, T 98.6, room air saturation 96%. The physical examination, ECG, and bedside transthoracic echocardiogram are unremarkable. Which of the following is the MOST likely etiology of this presentation?

(A) Aortic stenosis

(B) Carotid sinus hypersensitivity

(C) Orthostatic hypotension

(D) Postprandial hypotension

(E) Micturition syncope

2-19. Which of the following causes of syncope decreases in incidence with age?

(A) Cardiac syncope due to dysrhythmia

(B) Cardiac syncope due to structural abnormalities

(C) Neurologic syncope

(D) Orthostatic hypotension

(E) Vasovagal syncope

2-20. A 16-year-old girl presents to the ED with near syncope without antecedent headache, chest pain, shortness of breath, abdominal pain, or weakness. The patient was arguing with a boyfriend and reports feeling her extremities and lips tingling before she "practically passed out." She admits to social stressors but denies suicidal or homicidal ideation. Vital signs are BP 120/80, HR 72, RR 18, T 98.6, room air saturation 100%. Initial physical examination is normal. She had a prior ED visit for anxiety last month. Her urine pregnancy test is negative, her hemoglobin and hematocrit are normal, and an ECG shows normal sinus rhythm. What is the next MOST appropriate step in management?

(A) Admit and arrange inpatient psychiatric consult

(B) Arrange outpatient electrophysiologic (EP) testing

(C) Arrange outpatient tilt-table testing

(D) Ask patient to take slow deep breaths with her mouth open

(E) Discharge immediately

2-21. A 58-year-old man is brought in by paramedics after a witnessed syncopal episode while walking with friends. He denies headache, chest pain, or shortness of breath prior to the event, or now. He has hypertension and takes lisinopril. Vital signs are BP 150/100, HR 78, RR 18, T 98.6, room air saturation 97%. Physical examination is notable for a harsh, systolic murmur at the right base, which radiates into the neck. His lungs are clear to auscultation. A transthoracic echocardiogram is pending. The ECG shows normal sinus rhythm with left atrial enlargement but is otherwise normal. What is the MOST appropriate next step in management?

(A) Admit patient
(B) Arrange computed tomography (CT) of chest
(C) Arrange EEG
(D) Arrange outpatient electrophysiologic testing
(E) Arrange outpatient tilt-table testing

2-22. According to the San Francisco Syncope Rules, which of the following are predictors for an adverse event in a patient with syncope?

(A) Age >65 years
(B) Elevated TSH level
(C) Guaiac positive stool
(D) History of congestive heart failure (CHF)
(E) Positive pregnancy test

2-23. Which of the following is most useful in distinguishing a grand-mal seizure from syncope?

(A) Orofacial trauma
(B) Prodromal symptoms
(C) Tonic–clonic movements
(D) Transitory wide anion gap
(E) Urinary incontinence

2-24. A 65-year-old man with a history of hypertension is brought in by paramedics with 3 hours of dyspnea without chest pain. Paramedics state he became more fatigued and obtunded

on the way into the ED. Vital signs are BP 172/108, HR 114, RR 30, T 98.6, O2 saturation 88% on continuous positive airway pressure (CPAP). The patient is unresponsive to voice, with clammy skin. Physical exam findings include JVD, diffuse rales, an S3 gallop, and mild pitting edema. What is the next most appropriate treatment for this patient?

(A) Begin bioimpedance monitoring
(B) Endotracheal intubation
(C) Furosemide IV
(D) Increase CPAP pressure from 5 to 10 cm of water and readjust mask
(E) Start nitroglycerin IV drip

2-25. What is the significance of a third heart sound (S3) in the diagnosis of CHF?

(A) Absence suggests increased 90-day mortality
(B) Absence suggests worse outcome
(C) Presence suggests an elevated pulmonary capillary wedge pressure
(D) Presence suggests improved outcome
(E) Presence rules out CHF

2-26. A 58-year-old woman presents to the ED with a 4 days of increasing shortness of breath, orthopnea, and dyspnea on exertion. She denies chest pain and claims compliance with her hypertension medication, enalapril. She had Stevens Johnson after taking Septra. Vital signs are BP 160/94, HR 90, RR 24, T 98.8, room air saturation 96%. Physical examination finings include bibasilar rales, JVD, and marked peripheral edema. An IV is established. She received sublingual nitroglycerin. What is the next appropriate step in treatment?

(A) Bumetanide 1 mg IV
(B) Ethacrynic acid 50 mg IV
(C) Furosemide 40 mg IV
(D) Furosemide 40 mg PO
(E) Torsemide 10 mg IV

2-27. Which of the following medications should be avoided in stable patients with a history of heart failure?

(A) Acetaminophen
(B) Angiotensin-converting enzyme (ACE) inhibitors
(C) Angiotensin receptor blockers
(D) Beta-blockers
(E) Nonsteroidal anti-inflammatory agents

2-28. A 62-year-old woman with a history of chronic obstructive pulmonary disease (COPD) and a prior history of inferior MI presents to the ED with 4 days of progressive dyspnea, nonproductive cough, and peripheral edema. She denies chest pain or fever. Vital signs are BP 150/90, HR 115, RR 30, T 100.2, room air saturation 94%. Physical exam findings include JVD, bilateral diffuse rales, wheezing, hepatojugular reflex, and bilateral pitting edema. The ECG shows normal intervals and sinus tachycardia without ST-segment elevation or depression. The chest x-ray shows hyperinflation. The electrolyte panel and first troponin are normal. The brain natriuretic peptide (BNP) is 80 pg/mL. What is the LEAST likely diagnosis for this patient?

(A) Acute coronary syndrome
(B) Congestive heart failure
(C) COPD exacerbation
(D) Pneumonia
(E) Pulmonary embolism (PE)

2-29. Which of the following is the most frequent radiographic finding of left-sided heart failure?

(A) Cardiomegaly
(B) Dilated upper lobe vessels
(C) Enlarged pulmonary artery
(D) Interstitial edema
(E) Pleural effusion

2-30. Which of the following chest radiographic findings is the most sensitive for acute heart failure?

(A) Alveolar edema
(B) Cephalization
(C) Cardiomegaly
(D) Delayed findings of congestion
(E) Interstitial edema

2-31. Which of the following signs or symptoms has the highest specificity in the diagnosis of acute heart failure?

(A) Dyspnea
(B) Edema
(C) Orthopnea
(D) Rales
(E) Weight gain

2-32. Which of the following is the LEAST frequently seen radiographic finding of left-sided heart failure?

(A) Alveolar edema
(B) Enlarged pulmonary artery
(C) Kerley lines
(D) Pleural effusion
(E) Prominent superior vena cava

2-33. Which of the following is the MOST frequent presenting complaint of mitral stenosis?

(A) Atrial fibrillation
(B) Exertional dyspnea
(C) Hemoptysis
(D) Paroxysmal nocturnal dyspnea
(E) Right-sided heart failure

2-34. A 24-year-old woman presents to the ED with acute exertional dyspnea for the past week. Vital signs include HR 130–140, BP 132/80, RR 24, T 37, room air SaO_2 96%. The patient is alert and cooperative. Physical examination is notable for rales, an irregular heart rate, a loud S1, split S2, followed by a high-pitched opening snap heard best to the right of the apex, and a mid-diastolic rumbling murmur, without presystolic accentuation. Peripheral edema, hepatomegaly, and ascites are absent. ECG shows narrow complex atrial fibrillation with a rapid ventricular rate in the 130s. Which of the following ED actions is MOST appropriate?

(A) Aspirin 325 mg orally

(B) Coumadin 5 mg orally

(C) Crystalloid bolus

(D) Echocardiography

(E) Low-molecular-weight heparin

2-35. A 32-year-old woman with known mitral stenosis presents acutely short of breath, with an intermittent cough productive of small amounts of frankly bloody sputum. The ECG shows sinus rhythm with narrow complexes at a rate of 82 without ST or T-wave changes. The patient is placed on a cardiac monitor, and a non-rebreather face mask, and is currently stable, with an SaO_2 of 100%. An IV is started, and multiple tubes of blood are drawn. Cardiology is consulted, and echocardiography is arranged. What is the MOST definitive therapy for this patient?

(A) Beta-blocker therapy to control heart rate below 60

(B) Coumadin therapy to prevent systemic emboli

(C) Furosemide 40 mg intravenously over 2 minutes

(D) Type and screen for blood

(E) Type and screen for blood, emergent bronchoscopy, consult with a thoracic surgeon

2-36. During their ED workups, all of the following patients are found to have murmurs, but each person is asymptomatic at rest and currently stable. Based solely on the information below, which patient MOST warrants admission, cardiology referral, and an echocardiographic study?

(A) 17-year-old boy with fever, pharyngitis, and a systolic ejection murmur

(B) 20-year-old woman, 10 weeks pregnant, with a systolic ejection murmur

(C) 40-year-old woman with fibroids, a hemoglobin of 10, and a systolic ejection murmur

(D) 50-year-old man with syncope and a harsh systolic ejection murmur

(E) 60-year-old man with chronic renal failure, a patent AV shunt, and a systolic ejection murmur

2-37. Which of the following is the MOST accurate way to diagnose acute mitral regurgitation?

(A) Chest x-ray showing pulmonary edema with heart size smaller than expected

(B) Emergent bedside transthoracic echocardiography

(C) History of sudden severe dyspnea

(D) Physical signs of tachycardia, pulmonary edema, and a harsh apical systolic murmur

(E) Transesophageal echocardiography

2-38. Which of the following is the MOST common valvular heart disease in the industrialized world?

(A) Aortic insufficiency

(B) Bicuspid aortic stenosis

(C) Calcific aortic stenosis

(D) Mitral valve prolapse

(E) Tricuspid insufficiency

2-39. Which of the following features have proven association with mitral valve prolapse?

(A) Anxiety

(B) Chest pain

(C) Dyspnea

(D) Obesity

(E) Pectus excavatum

2-40. Which of the following features INCREASES morbidity in a patient with mitral valve prolapse who is otherwise asymptomatic?

(A) Age <45 years at symptom onset

(B) Exercise-induced mitral regurgitation

(C) Female gender

(D) Low body weight

(E) Scoliosis

2-41. What is the leading cause of death in competitive athletes?

(A) Congenital coronary artery anomalies

(B) Commotio cordis

(C) Heat stroke

(D) Hypertrophic cardiomyopathy

(E) Idiopathic dilated cardiomyopathy

2-42. A previously well 25-year-old man presents to the ED with 3 days of dyspnea, and orthopnea, and a recent febrile illness associated with myalgias, dyspnea, and precordial chest pain. Vital signs are BP 124/82, HR 120, RR 26, T 100.6, room air saturation 96%. Physical exam findings include a supple neck, faint bibasilar rales, and a friction rub. His chest x-ray (CXR) is shown here (Figure 2-2). A CBC, serum electrolytes, blood urea nitrogen, and creatinine are normal. The initial troponin is 1 ng/mL and myoglobin is 100 ng/mL. His ECG shows sinus tachycardia with nonspecific ST–T-wave changes. Echocardiography shows a very small pericardial effusion. What is his most likely diagnosis?

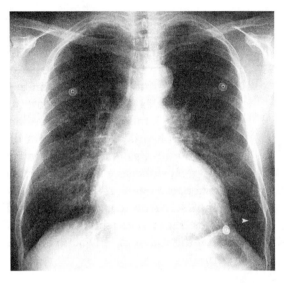

Figure 2-2. Reproduced with permission from Schwartz DT. *Emergency Radiology: Case Studies.* Copyright © 2008 The McGraw-Hill Companies, Inc.

(A) Acute coronary syndrome

(B) Myocarditis

(C) Pericarditis

(D) Pneumonia

(E) Pulmonary embolus

2-43. Which of the following bedside maneuvers increases the systolic ejection murmur of hypertrophic cardiomyopathy (HCM)?

(A) Passive leg raise in supine position

(B) Squatting

(C) Standing

(D) Sustained isometric handgrip

(E) Turning chin toward a stethoscope in the right supraclavicular fossa

2-44. Which of the following can distinguish constrictive pericarditis from restrictive cardiomyopathy?

(A) Early diastolic sound 60–120 milliseconds after second heart sound

(B) Dip and plateau filling pattern

(C) Jugular venous distention

(D) Kussmaul sign

(E) Square root sign

2-45. Which of the following is the most common cause of restrictive cardiomyopathy?

(A) Amyloidosis

(B) Endomyocardial fibrosis

(C) Hemachromatosis

(D) Idiopathic

(E) Sarcoidosis

2-46. A 44-year-old woman presents with dyspnea at rest and with exertion for the past 3 months. Vital signs are BP 1080/80, HR 95, RR 22, T 98.6, room air saturation of 97%. The patient is alert and not in extremis. Physical exam findings include jugular vein distention, soft heart sounds, clear lungs, and a pulsus paradoxus of 25 mm Hg. An ECG shows low-voltage QRS complexes and electrical alternans. While arrangements are made for admission and an echocardiography-guided pericardiocentesis with pigtail catheter insertion, what would be an appropriate temporizing ED treatment.

(A) Furosemide intravenously

(B) Nitroglycerin intravenously

(C) Nitroglycerin sublingual

(D) Nitroprusside intravenously

(E) Volume expansion with 500–1000 mL of NS.

2-47. Which of the following ECG features is indicative of the early stage of acute pericarditis?

(A) Isoelectric ST segment with T-wave inversion

(B) PR segment depression, ST-segment elevation, ST/T amplitude <0.25

(C) PR segment depression, ST-segment elevation, ST/T amplitude >0.25

(D) PR segment elevation, ST-segment elevation, ST/T amplitude <0.25

(E) PR segment elevation, ST-segment elevation, ST/T amplitude >0.25

2-48. What percentage of ambulatory ED patients with a documented PE have a concomitant deep vein thrombosis (DVT)?

(A) 20%

(B) 40%

(C) 60%

(D) 80%

(E) 100%

2-49. Immobilization of which of the following contributes the most risk to the formation of a venous thromboembolism (VTE)?

(A) Ankle

(B) Elbow

(C) Knee and hip

(D) Shoulder

(E) Wrist

2-50. Which kind of immobility confers the greatest risk for VTE?

(A) Limb

(B) Neurologic

(C) Travel >4 hours

(D) Travel >8 hours

(E) Whole body

2-51. What is the average time for presentation with a PE after surgery?

(A) 24 hours

(B) 2–4 days

(C) 4–6 days

(D) 6–8 days

(E) >10 days

2-52. During which period is a pregnant woman at most risk for VTE?

(A) 1st trimester

(B) 2nd trimester

(C) 3rd trimester

(D) 1st week after delivery by cesarean

(E) 1st week after delivery by normal spontaneous vaginal delivery

2-53. What percent of patients who are diagnosed with PE in the ED have a complaint of chest pain?

(A) 25%

(B) 50%

(C) 75%

(D) 90%

(E) 100%

2-54. What is the most common abnormal ECG finding in patients with a PE?

(A) Normal ECG

(B) Right bundle branch block

(C) S1 Q3 T3 (McGinn–White sign)

(D) Sinus tachycardia

(E) T-wave inversions in leads V1–V4

2-55. What is the lifetime risk of a fatal cancer or leukemia after a CT scan of the chest?

(A) 1 in 500

(B) 1 in 1000

(C) 1 in 2000

(D) 1 in 10,000

(E) 1 in 20,000

2-56. A 32-year-old male presents to the ED with chest pain and mild shortness of breath. He has no prior history of VTE, no recent surgery or trauma, no hemoptysis, estrogen use, or leg swelling. His initial vitals are BP 130/80, HR 92, RR 20, T 37.0, and saturation 98%. What is the most appropriate diagnostic test to rule out a PE in this patient?

(A) Angiogram of chest

(B) CT scan of chest

(C) D-dimer

(D) No study is needed

(E) V/Q scan

2-57. The Pulmonary Embolism Rule-Out Criteria (PERC) states that if all the criteria are met, then the risk of PE falls to less than what percent?

(A) 2%

(B) 5%

(C) 10%

(D) 15%

(E) 20%

2-58. A patient with a recent immobilization presents with unilateral swelling of his entire right leg, pitting edema, and calf swelling of greater than 3 cm. His vitals are normal and he has no shortness of breath. It is Sunday morning 4 AM and you do a compression ultrasound of his right leg. It is nondiagnostic showing neither complete compression nor a clot present. There is no on-call vascular tech this weekend. The next most appropriate step in your workup is

(A) A "holding dose" of low-molecular-weight heparin and arrange for a confirmatory ultrasound on Monday

(B) Admission and IV heparin

(C) D-dimer

(D) No treatment and arrangements for a confirmatory ultrasound on Monday

(E) Thrombolysis

2-59. A patient with lung cancer presents with an extremely painful swollen, bluish colored left lower leg (Figure 2-3). What is the next step in management?

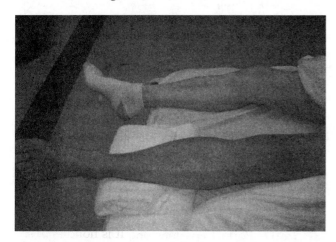

Figure 2-3. Reproduced with permission from Knoop KJ, Stack LB, Storrow AB, Thurman RJ: *The Atlas of Emergency Medicine*, 3rd Edition. Copyright © 2010 The McGraw-Hill Companies, Inc. Photo contributor: Selim Suner, MD.

(A) CT scan of chest with venous runoff study
(B) D-dimer
(C) IV heparin
(D) Low-molecular-weight heparin
(E) Thrombolysis

2-60. A 20-year-old woman presents with palpitations and anxiety 2 hours after smoking crack cocaine for the first time. She denies headache, chest pain, or shortness of breath. Vital signs are BP 224/122, HR 110, RR 22, T 98.9, room air saturation of 100%. The patient is alert and diaphoretic, but otherwise has a normal physical examination. Which of the following medications is the most preferred initial treatment for this patient?

(A) Esmolol
(B) Labetalol
(C) Lorazepam
(D) Nicardipine
(E) Phentolamine

2-61. Which of the following cardiac medications is contraindicated in the treatment of pregnant women?

(A) Angiotensin-converting enzyme inhibitors
(B) Hydralazine
(C) Labetalol
(D) Magnesium sulfate
(E) Nifedipine

2-62. What is the most common first-dose side effect of enalaprilat?

(A) Angioedema
(B) Bradycardia
(C) Cough
(D) Hyperkalemia
(E) Hypotension

2-63. Which of the following is contraindicated in the treatment of aortic dissection?

(A) Clevidipine
(B) Esmolol
(C) Labetalol
(D) Nicardipine
(E) Nitroprusside

2-64. A 45-year-old man with poorly controlled hypertension due to medication noncompliance presents with gradual onset of headache, confusion, and vision changes over the past 2 days. Vital signs include BP 230/132, HR 90, RR 20, T 98.6, room air saturation 98%. Physical examination findings include a supple neck, S4 gallop without murmurs, clear lungs, and a nontender abdomen without masses or bruits. Funduscopy is shown here (Figure 2-4). The neurologic examination is nonfocal, and CT scan of the head is negative for a mass, shift, or bleed. A toxicology screen for cocaine, amphetamines, and phencyclidine is negative. Which of the following is contraindicated in the treatment of this patient?

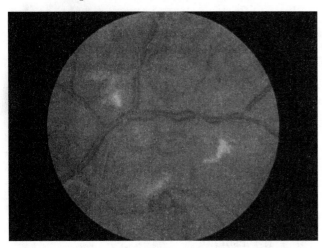

Figure 2-4. Reproduced with permission from Knoop KJ, Stack LB, Storrow AB, Thurman RJ: *The Atlas of Emergency Medicine*, 3rd Edition. Copyright © 2010 The McGraw-Hill Companies, Inc. Photo contributor: Richard E. Wyszynski, MD.

(A) Esmolol
(B) Fenoldopam
(C) Labetalol
(D) Nicardipine
(E) Nifedipine

2-65. Concurrent use of acetaminophen can increase the levels in which of the following medications?

(A) Enalapril
(B) Fenoldopam
(C) Labetalol
(D) Nitroprusside
(E) Phentolamine

2-66. Which of the following conditions is associated with the highest incidence of pulmonary hypertension?

(A) CREST syndrome/limited scleroderma
(B) Hemoglobinopathies
(C) HIV
(D) Portal hypertension
(E) Sleep apnea

2-67. Which of the following conditions would MOST likely to respond well to vasodilator therapy (nitroglycerin or nitroprusside) in standard doses?

(A) Aortic stenosis
(B) Hypertrophic cardiomyopathy
(C) Hypertensive heart failure syndrome
(D) Right-ventricular infarction
(E) Volume depletion

2-68. What is the most important clinical complication of nitroglycerin use?

(A) Headache
(B) Persistent hypotension
(C) Methemoglobinemia
(D) Thiocyanate toxicity
(E) Transient hypotension

2-69. Which of the following best describes the ages of patients who develop aortic dissections?

(A) Bimodal age distribution
(B) Patients between 45 and 65 years
(C) Patients between 65 and 85 years
(D) Patients older than 85 years
(E) Young patients with risk factors

2-70. What is the most common location of pain in patients with aortic dissection?

(A) Abdominal pain

(B) Back pain

(C) Chest pain

(D) Left arm pain

(E) Neck pain

2-71. An 85-year-old male with a history of chronic hypertension presents with 2 hours of chest pain, which radiates to his back. It is the worst pain he has ever had and feels it ripping down his back. His initial BP in the ED is 180/110. He has a widened mediastinum on his chest x-ray, and his ECG is unchanged. In approximately 45 minutes, you notice that he has become altered and his BP is now 75/50. What is the most appropriate diagnostic modality for this patient?

(A) CT scan

(B) Central venous pressure monitoring

(C) Echocardiogram

(D) Repeat chest x-ray

(E) Repeat ECG

2-72. What is the best medication for a patient with a BP of 180/100 and confirmed aortic dissection on CT?

(A) Esmolol

(B) Hydralazine

(C) Lisinopril

(D) Nitroglycerin

(E) Nitroprusside

2-73. What risk factor is highly predictive of developing an abdominal aortic aneurysm (AAA)?

(A) Diabetes

(B) Family history

(C) Hypercholesterolemia

(D) Hypertension

(E) Smoking history

2-74. A 65-year-old man with a history of smoking, hypertension, diabetes mellitus, and a family history of a ruptured AAA presents with abdominal pain, hematuria, and weakness.

His initial vitals are BP 85/60, HR 110, RR 20, T 37.0, and pulse ox 100%. What is the best imaging modality for him?

(A) Cross table lateral radiography

(B) CT scan with IV contrast

(C) CT scan without contrast

(D) Magnetic resonance image (MRI)

(E) Ultrasound

2-75. What is the most common serious complication of a popliteal artery aneurysm?

(A) Acute limb ischemia

(B) Bruising

(C) Deep VTE

(D) Pain

(E) Rupture of aneurysm

2-76. Which of the following are pathophysiologically the most important risk factors for occlusive arterial disease?

(A) Diabetes and hyperlipidemia

(B) Diabetes and hypertension

(C) Diabetes and smoking

(D) Elevated C-reactive protein and hyperhomocysteinemia

(E) Hypertension and hyperlipidemia.

2-77. What is the most common cause of acute limb ischemia?

(A) Atheroemboli

(B) Cardiac emboli

(C) Mural thrombi in arterial aneurysms

(D) Thoracic aortic dissection

(E) Thrombotic occlusion

2-78. Which of the following is considered a late finding of complete arterial obstruction?

(A) Hypoesthesia or hyperesthesia

(B) Muscle weakness

(C) Pain

(D) Pallor

(E) Paralysis

2-79. A 78-year-old man presents with gradual onset of severe pain in his left lower leg over 4 days. His past medical history is peripheral artery disease and intermittent claudication with calf pain, relieved by rest. The patient continues to smoke tobacco. He currently denies chest pain, shortness of breath, or headache. Vital signs include BP 140/85, HR 80, RR 20, T 98.6, room air saturation 97%. Physical exam findings include shiny, hyperpigmented skin and absent hair on both the mid-lower legs. The left lower leg is cool, mottled, and cyanotic, with diminished posterior tibial and dorsalis pedis pulses, and decreased sensation to vibration and proprioception but intact deep sensation. The left ankle-brachial index is 0.20. The right leg is slightly warmer with normal color and faintly palpable pulses and right ankle-brachial index of 0.7. An ECG shows sinus rhythm without ST-segment elevation or depression. An IV has been started and blood is available for laboratory studies. A vascular surgeon has been paged but has not yet responded. What is the next most appropriate action?

(A) Arrange CTA of lower extremities

(B) Arrange transthoracic echocardiogram

(C) Administer unfractionated heparin at 80 units/kg bolus followed by an 18 units/kg/hour infusion

(D) Obtain cardiac markers

(E) Order electrolytes, myoglobin, creatine kinase, and coagulation panel

2-80. Which of the following features distinguishes neurogenic claudication from intermittent vascular claudication?

(A) Leg and buttock pain

(B) Relieved by lumbar flexion

(C) Relieved by rest

(D) Triggered by exercise

(E) Worsened by upright posture

Cardiovascular Disorders
Answers and Explanations

2-1. **The answer is C** (Chapter 52). Troponins leak out of damaged myocardium cells after prolonged ischemia. Thus, it takes 6 hours for cellular death and breakdown for these biomarkers to leak into the bloodstream. Myoglobin elevations may be seen earlier (in the 2–4 hours range). Patients who present soon after symptoms may have NO elevation in biomarkers.

2-2. **The answer is E** (Chapter 52). It is important NOT to be swayed by response to therapy in patients with chest pain. Antacids provide pain relief in 18–45% of patients with acute coronary syndrome. Lack of pain relief with nitroglycerin should also not be convincing. In one study, 65% of patients with acute coronary syndrome did not respond to nitroglycerin. This type of patient, with an atypical story of chest pain and some risk factors, should at least get a second set of biomarkers.

2-3. **The answer is B** (Chapters 52, 53, and 55). Remember that ECG findings alone cannot rule out acute coronary syndrome. Up to 6% of patients with a normal ECG will ultimately be proven to have an NSTEMI. Another 4% will be proven to have unstable angina. Nonspecific changes (T-wave flattening or inversion) can also be concerning if they reverse when the patient is pain free.

2-4. **The answer is B** (Chapter 54). This patient is in cardiogenic shock due to an RV infarction complicating her acute inferior STEMI. This acutely ill patient needs an emergency bedside transthoracic echocardiogram to assess cardiac contractility and to rule out any mechanical cause of shock such as acute pulmonary embolus or pericardial effusion. If she can be stabilized, transesophageal echocardiography would be appropriate. Since the patient does not have signs of pulmonary congestion, a judicious trial of crystalloid is indicated. Patients with RV infarcts may require several boluses of IV fluid. Early revascularization, either by PCI or coronary artery bypass graft (CABG), has been shown to increase survival of cardiogenic shock compared with the use of an intra-aortic balloon pump (IABP) along with thrombolytics or with thrombolytics alone. Mortality remains high (~50%) despite appropriate treatment. Beta-blockers should be avoided in cardiac shock because of their negative inotropy and chronotropy. Pure α_1-adrenergic receptor agonists such as phenylephrine should be avoided since they increase cardiac afterload. If crystalloid therapy does not improve perfusion, vasopressors or inotropes should be considered. Dobutamine is indicated if the patient is not profoundly hypotensive. However, dobutamine should be avoided if the systolic BP remains below 90 mm Hg, due to its vasodilator potential. Dopamine is the preferred single agent if the systolic BP is below 70 mm Hg. Dopamine in combination with dobutamine can be more effective than either agent alone but pharmacologic therapy is only a temporizing measure until early revascularization is arranged.

2-5. **The answer is D** (Chapter 54). Cardiogenic shock is mostly commonly due to extensive MI with suppressed myocardial contractility. Pump failure is the underlying factor in most causes of cardiogenic shock (Table 54-2). Hypoperfusion, with or without hypotension, is the unifying feature of cardiogenic shock, regardless of etiology. During an AMI, several mechanical complications can precipitate cardiogenic shock, including acute myocardial regurgitation due to papillary muscle rupture, ventricular septal defect (VSD), and free-wall rupture. Mechanical complications cause one-fourth of the cardiogenic shock following AMI. Right ventricular infarction can also cause cardiogenic shock due to loss of preload. Cardiac contractility can also be severely depressed due to sepsis, myocarditis, myocardial contusion, and cardiomyopathy. Mechanical obstruction to forward blood flow can also lead to cardiogenic shock, including aortic stenosis, HCM, mitral stenosis, left atrial myxoma, and pericardial tamponade. Regurgitation of LV output due to chordal rupture or aortic insufficiency can cause profound cardiogenic shock.

2-6.   **The answer is C** (Chapter 58). Acute mitral regurgitation due to papillary muscle dysfunction causes a harsh apical systolic murmur that starts with the first heart sound but ends before the second. Acute mitral regurgitation due to chordae tendineae rupture causes a soft apical holosystolic murmur that radiates to the axilla, but is often obscured by rales, or ambient noise in the ED. Acute ventral septal defect is characterized by a new loud holosystolic left parasternal murmur, usually with a palpable thrill that diminishes as the interventricular pressures equilibrate. Acute aortic insufficiency produces a high-pitched blowing diastolic murmur immediately after S2 and heard best at the left parasternal border.

2-7.   **The answer is B** (Chapter 58). Acute mitral regurgitation due to chordae tendineae rupture produces a holosystolic apical murmur, which radiates to the axilla but may be difficult to hear due to rales. Papillary muscle rupture also causes acute mitral regurgitation, but the apical systolic murmur begins with the first heart sound and ends before

the second. Aortic insufficiency produces a soft diastolic murmur heard best at the right base. Acute tricuspid insufficiency causes a soft blowing holosystolic murmur, which increases with inspiration and is heard best along the left parasternal border. Acute ventral septal defect produces a loud holosystolic left parasternal murmur with a palpable thrill that tapers in intensity as intraventricular pressures equilibrate.

2-8.   **The answer is A** (Chapter 54). Early revascularization, whether by PCI or CABG, is the treatment of choice for cardiogenic shock. Early revascularization is associated with the highest survival, followed by IABP combined with thrombolytic therapy. Thrombolytic therapy alone results in the lowest survival rate but still reduces mortality compared with supportive treatment alone. While in the ED, the patient should receive fluids and pressors to support cardiac perfusion. Echocardiography can support the diagnosis of cardiogenic shock by demonstrating impaired LV contractility, mechanical causes of shock such as acute mitral regurgitation, acute VSD, RV infarction, or high pulmonary pressures suggesting acute pulmonary embolus. Echocardiography can also detect pericardial effusion and aortic root dissection. An LVAD may be indicated if cardiogenic shock persists despite revascularization, medical therapy, or intra-aortic balloon support. Although newer LVADs can be inserted percutaneously, the US FDA currently limits placement as a bridge to transplantation, so cardiogenic shock patients are not appropriate candidates. Study trials for LVAD and cardiogenic shock are underway. Transfer to an ICU with medical therapy only would be associated with the lowest rate of survival for cardiogenic shock.

2-9.   **The answer is E** (Chapter 53). It has been reported that as many as 37.5% of women and 27.4% of men presenting with ischemia may present without chest pain. Up to 30% of patients with AMI in longitudinal studies are unrecognized.

2-10. The answer is E (Chapter 53). Women and the elderly are more likely to have atypical symptoms. Up to 50% of patients with atypical symptoms are found to have unstable angina. In addition, the prognosis for patients who present with atypical symptoms is worse.

2-11. The answer is B (Chapter 53). The current recommendations are for ECGs to be performed as soon as possible and preferably within the first 10 minutes. This short door-to-ECG time is an effort by the ACC and AHA to shorten the door to intervention time in patients with an AMI.

2-12. The answer is D (Chapter 53). The presence of ST elevation in lead III greater than in lead II predicts an right coronary artery (RCA) lesion. When this is accompanied by ST elevation in V1 or V4R, it predicts proximal RCA lesions with accompanying right ventricular infarction.

2-13. The answer is B (Chapter 57). Both the AHA and the ACC recommend primary coronary intervention within 90 minutes if possible. If the time is greater than 3 hours from symptom onset, PCI is even more preferred. The door-to-balloon time may be as long as 120 minutes if the patient is transferred to a PCI capable center.

2-14. The answer is E (Chapter 53). Rescue PCI is indicated in patients in the following groups after thrombolysis: patients who are in cardiogenic shock and younger than 75 years, patients with severe heart failure or pulmonary edema, patients with hemodynamically compromising ventricular arrhythmias, patients with a large area of myocardium at risk, and for whom fibrinolytic therapy has failed. There is no role for repeat thrombolytic administration in this type of patient. A balloon pump might help temporarily, but rescue PCI is the procedure of choice. Nitroglycerin is a poor choice as the patient's BP is too low. Dopamine infusion will increase myocardial oxygen demand.

2-15. The answer is C (Chapter 53). A variety of benefits have been shown when nitroglyc-

erin is used in patients with AMI. Several trials have demonstrated a reduced infarct size, improved regional function, and decreased cardiovascular complications. Mortality rate appears to be reduced to 35% with the use of nitrates. IV nitroglycerin was titrated to a mean arterial pressure reduction of 10% in normotensive patients and 30% in hypertensive patients. Nitroglycerin was NOT titrated to symptom resolution. In addition, nitroglycerin should be used VERY cautiously in patients with inferior wall ischemia, as these patients are preload dependent and do not tolerate much of a BP decrease.

2-16. The answer is E (Chapter 56). The longitudinal Framingham study described 822 reports of syncope in the 7814 patients followed for 17 years. The causes of syncope were vasovagal (21%), cardiac (10%), orthostatic (9%), seizure (5%), neurologic (4.1%), and unknown (37%). Other studies also report an unknown cause in about 40% of cases, despite extensive workups. Limited ED evaluations may not determine a specific cause of syncope in 50–60% of cases. The ED focus is to identify patients at increased risk of immediate decompensation or future serious morbidity or sudden death.

2-17. The answer is E (Chapter 56). This patient's report of lightheadedness and the prodrome of pallor and sweating after viewing an intense visual stimulus suggest vasovagal syncope, rather than orthostatic hypotension. Brief, tonic–clonic, or asynchronous movements may occur with any form of syncope. The duration and intensity of movements during grand-mal seizures often causes muscle pain. The patient's rapid recovery also makes the diagnoses of hypoglycemia or seizure unlikely. Although an acute dysrhythmia might not be entirely excluded in this scenario, it was not the most likely cause in a previously healthy young person.

2-18. The answer is B (Chapter 56). The patient's prior history of syncope during head turning and the current scenario suggest carotid sinus hypersensitivity syndrome. Direct pressure on baroreceptors in the carotid body may trigger an abnormal vagal response of bradycardia and asystole or a drop in BP without a decrease in heart rate. Both reactions may also occur simultaneously. This patient's sitting position at the time of syncope precludes a diagnosis of orthostatic hypotension. Neither micturition nor postprandial syncope are suggested by this scenario. Aortic stenosis should always be considered in the differential diagnosis of syncope in an elderly patient, but physical exam findings such as delayed carotid pulse and a harsh systolic murmur would be evident.

2-19.   The answer is E (Chapter 56). The incidence of vasovagal syncope actually decreases with age due to decreased responsiveness of the autonomic nervous system. Orthostatic hypotension is common in the elderly due to a less-sensitive thirst mechanism and a decreased endocrine response to volume depletion. Orthostatic hypotension is also related to increased medication use in older patients. Advancing age increases the risk of syncope but cardiovascular risk is thought to be a better predictor. Cardiac syncope due to dysrhythmias or structural conditions is very common and more likely with increasing age. Neurologic syncope is a rare cause of syncope at any age, since it must be transient and allow a return to baseline neurologic function. Vertebrobasilar insufficiency can transiently affect the reticular activating system and cause a brief loss of consciousness, but other posterior circulation signs and symptoms also occur, such as vertigo or diplopia.

2-20.   The answer is D (Chapter 56). Given her age, normal physical examination, and negative workup, this patient is most likely hyperventilated and had a near syncopal episode. Asking her to take slow deep breaths with her mouth open might reproduce her symptoms and provide her with insight into her breathing pattern in response to stress. This patient does not require admission, although she might benefit from a referral for psychological counseling. In general, patients with recurrent syncope associated with falls should

undergo tilt-table testing. EP testing is indicated for patients with documented dysrhythmia, preexcitation, or underlying heart disease.

2-21.   The answer is A (Chapter 56). This patient has strong evidence of a structural cardiac abnormality, most likely aortic stenosis, and should be admitted for further evaluation of cardiac function. A transthoracic echocardiography is essential. Critical aortic stenosis is associated with a classic triad of chest pain, dyspnea on exertion, and syncope. Older patients with aortic stenosis and syncope who are asymptomatic upon ED presentation should still be admitted due to the increases risk of death. Patients with documented cardiac syncope have a 6-month mortality exceeding 10%. Electrophysiologic testing is done for patients with dysrhythmias, preexcitation, or conduction delays. Tilt-table testing is performed on patients with recurrent unexplained syncope, suspected to have a reflex-mediated etiology. EEGs would be reserved for patients with suspected seizures.

2-22.   The answer is D (Chapter 56). The acronym CHESS summarizes the San Francisco Syncope Rules' five predictors of adverse events, including arrhythmia and mortality: history of CHF, hematocrit less than 30, abnormal ECG, shortness of breath, and systolic BP less than 90. An abnormal ECG would include any non-sinus rhythm, conduction delays, new changes to the QRS, or ST segment not previously seen on prior tracings. A new prolonged QT interval would meet the criteria and would warrant admission, due to risk of torsades des pointes. Patients with a clear cause of syncope, such as vasovagal, hypovolemia, situational (cough or micturition), medication-related events, which improved with treatment, and are stable during an observation period, may be discharged. Unfortunately, the etiology of syncope remains unclear in over half of the patients who presented to the ED.

2-23.   The answer is D (Chapter 56). Distinguishing grand-mal seizures from true syncope is essential yet very challenging. Historical features such a classic aura, prolonged postictal confusion, witnessed head turning, unusual posture or automatisms, and muscle pain suggest seizure. Patients with syncope may have premonitory symptoms of nausea or light headedness if the event is reflex mediated (vasovagal), but a dysrhythmia may occur without prodrome. Brief tonic–clonic movements can occur with syncope yet be mistaken for seizure. Trauma with or without defensive injuries to the hands or knees suggests a sudden event without warning, which could occur with dysrhythmia, noncardiac syncope, or seizure, so trauma is not a distinguishing feature. Urinary incontinence could occur with seizure or syncope. A transitory wide anion gap occurs after a grandmal seizure but not after an uncomplicated syncopal event.

2-24. **The answer is B** (Chapter 57). This patient requires immediate endotracheal intubation because he now has impaired consciousness and severe respiratory distress and has failed a trial of CPAP, a form of noninvasive ventilation. Readjusting his mask or increasing the pressure would be ineffective since he is now hypoxic and has a depressed sensorium. Although treatment with nitroglycerin followed by furosemide is indicated in this patient with probable pulmonary edema, control of airway takes precedence. Bioimpedance monitoring, which can noninvasively provide accurate information about cardiac output and thoracic water content, is a useful bedside adjunct for diagnosing and managing suspected heart failure in the ED and could be implemented after the airway is secured.

2-25. **The answer is C** (Chapter 57). The presence of third heart sound, or ventricular filling gallop, has a specificity of 99% and highly suggests increased pulmonary capillary wedge pressure and helps rule in CHF. Detection by stethoscope can be challenging and has a sensitivity of only 20%. Use of digital microphone detection during ECG testing improves sensitivity to 40.2%; specificity is 88.5%. The presence of an S3 is associated with notably worse outcomes, including a doubling of 90-day mortality. JVD is another excellent physical finding for an elevated pulmonary capillary wedge pressure, with a specificity of 94% and a sensitivity of 39%.

2-26. **The answer is B** (Chapter 57). Ethacrynic acid, a loop-diuretic, is indicated for treatment of CHF, in patients with a significant sulfonamide allergy. Furosemide, bumetanide, and torsemide are all sulfonamide-containing loop-diuretics. Parenteral dosing of furosemide is preferable in fluid-overloaded patients, since bowel wall edema may diminish gastrointestinal absorption of an oral dose.

2-27. **The answer is E** (Chapter 57). Nonsteroidal anti-inflammatory agents inhibit the effects of ACE inhibitors and diuretics and can worsen cardiac and renal function. The emergency physician (EP) should review the medication lists of heart failure patients and also avoid prescribing nonsteroidal anti-inflammatory drugs (NSAIDs) when such patients present for injuries or chronic pain. The main risk of acetaminophen, at excessive levels, is hepatotoxicity. Stable heart failure patients are discharged on ACE inhibitors and beta-blockers because these medications have been conclusively shown to decrease mortality. Angiotensin receptor blockers have fewer side effects than ACE inhibitors but can still cause cough or angioedema.

2-28. **The answer is B** (Chapter 57). Patients with chronic lung disease can have elevated BNP levels due to right ventricular strain. The low and high cutoff points for BNP are 100 and 500 pg/mL, respectively. A BNP below 100 has a high negative likelihood ratio for CHF in patients with lung disease. In this patient, the clinical picture of prior MI, rales, JVD, lower extremity edema, and Q waves raise concern for possible congestive heart failure. However, the BNP of 80 pg/mL makes the diagnosis less likely. Echocardiography would be helpful if clinical suspicion remained high for CHF or PE. This patient should have serial troponins to evaluate possible acute coronary syndrome. Possible pneumonia remains high on the differential for this patient.

2-29. **The answer is B** (Chapter 57). Normally, vascularity in the lower lung fields is more prominent than in the upper lung fields. When this situation is reversed, dilated upper lobe vessels create a pattern called cephalization. The frequency of left-side heart failure radiographic findings are, in decreasing order, dilated upper lobe vessels, cardiomegaly, interstitial edema, enlarged pulmonary artery, pleural effusion, alveolar edema, prominent superior vena cava, and Kerley lines. Pleural effusions can be difficult to detect on a supine chest x-ray. In one study of patients with pleural effusions, the sensitivity of a supine chest x-ray for heart failure was 67% and specificity was 70%.

2-30. **The answer is B** (Chapter 57). Echocardiography is the gold standard for heart failure, but it is not initially obtained in most EDs, possibly due to lack of availability along with cost concerns. Chest radiographs are readily obtainable but findings lack sensitivity for acute heart failure. Cephalization, interstitial edema, and alveolar edema, respectively, have sensitivities of 41%, 27%, and 6%. Up to 18% of patients will not have any findings of congestion on chest x-ray. There may be a time lag up to 6 hours between presentation and appearance of radiographic findings, but treatment should be started immediately. Cardiomegaly is suggestive of heart failure, but sensitivity is considered poor. Intrathoracic cardiac rotation can decrease the apparent cardiothoracic ratio. In one study, 22% of patients with cardiomegaly detected by echocardiography had normal cardiothoracic ratios. A cardiothoracic ratio greater than 60% is associated with an increased 5-year mortality.

2-31. **The answer is C** (Chapter 57). The specificities of orthopnea and dyspnea for heart failure are, respectively, 88%, and 50%. Rales

have a predictive accuracy of 70%. Peripheral edema and weight gain are more likely to occur in normotensive acute decompensated heart failure, which develops over days or weeks. Hypertensive heart failure, which occurs over 48 hours or less, is the most common acute presentation. Hypotensive acute heart failure is the least common presentation of acute decompensated heart failure.

2-32. **The answer is C** (Chapter 57). Kerley lines are thickened interstitial septal markings that can represent pulmonary edema, as well as other interstitial processes. Kerley B lines are short parallel lines that extend from the periphery and intersect the pleura. The frequency of left-side heart failure radiographic findings are, in decreasing order, dilated upper lobe vessels, cardiomegaly, interstitial edema, enlarged pulmonary artery, pleural effusion, alveolar edema, prominent superior vena cava, and Kerley lines.

2-33. **The answer is B** (Chapter 58). Mitral stenosis is characterized by limited mobility and progressive narrowing of the mitral valve leading to loss of normal diastolic filling of the LV. Rheumatic heart disease still remains the principal cause. Postinflammatory changes from rheumatic carditis include fusion of the valvular commissures, matting of the chordae tendineae, calcification, leading to limited valve mobility, and narrowing. Exertional dyspnea is the most frequent presenting complaint. Triggers include anemia, pregnancy infection, tachycardia, atrial fibrillation, or emotional upset. In the past, hemoptysis due to ruptured bronchial vein was a very common presenting complaint. Earlier diagnosis via echocardiography and treatment have decreased the incidence of hemoptysis. Severe mitral stenosis results in rising left atrial pressure, left atrial enlargement, pulmonary congestion, pulmonary hypertension, and, ultimately, right-sided failure. Atrial fibrillation develops from progressive atrial dilatation, and systemic emboli occur in 20–30% of patients.

2-34. **The answer is D** (Chapter 58). This patient has mitral stenosis and atrial fibrillation, which is why there is no presystolic accentuation of the rumbling, mid-diastolic murmur. In this case, the duration of atrial fibrillation is uncertain, but the current rapid ventricular rate has caused increased left atrial pressure and pulmonary congestion. A fluid bolus is contraindicated. Aspirin could be given but does not address the patient's heart rate or valvular condition. Controlling the heart rate in atrial fibrillation is very important, but this patient is at risk for a systemic embolus if she medically cardioverts with diltiazem. Hence, an echocardiogram to assess the presence of a left-ventricular thrombus would be highly appropriate. Transesophageal echocardiography can give a more complete analysis of mitral valve function than a transthoracic study. However, transthoracic echocardiography is usually done first, due to easier availability. If echocardiography demonstrates a thrombus, the patient would then be anticoagulated, initially with heparin and later with coumadin.

2-35. **The answer is E** (Chapter 58). This patient has mild hemoptysis but is at risk for severe hemoptysis due to mitral stenosis-induced pulmonary hypertension. Arrangements should thus be made for possible blood transfusion, emergent bronchoscopy, and consult with a thoracic surgeon. Ideally, patients with symptomatic mitral stenosis should receive a mechanical intervention such a balloon valvotomy, valve repair, or valve replacement before severe pulmonary hypertension develops. Coumadin would be contraindicated in the face of hemoptysis, and beta-blockers are contraindicated in the face of pulmonary hypertension. Judicious use of furosemide might help decrease pulmonary congestion but does not address the patient's hemoptysis and need for mechanical intervention.

2-36. **The answer is D** (Chapter 58). The 55-year-old man with syncope and a harsh systolic ejection murmur should be admitted for suspected aortic stenosis, despite being asymptomatic at rest, since he is at risk for sudden death and heart failure. When assessing a patient with a new cardiac murmur, the EP should always consider the patient's underlying medical condition. Fever, pregnancy, anemia, renal failure with chronic volume overload, thyrotoxicosis, arteriovenous fistula, and sepsis all cause increased cardiac output and systolic murmurs in patients with normal cardiac anatomy. If the new murmur is diastolic, or if symptoms occur at rest, the murmur may be pathologic. Patients with suspected aortic stenosis and syncope, who look well at rest, are the exception to this rule and should be admitted, with cardiology referral and an echocardiographic study.

2-37. **The answer is E** (Chapter 58). Transesophageal echocardiography is considered the gold standard study for acute mitral regurgitation because it provides more information about valvular function than transthoracic echocardiography does. However, bedside transthoracic echocardiography is often more readily available to assess an acutely ill patient and could be done first. Acute mitral regurgitation should be considered in all patients with new onset of pulmonary edema, heralded by sudden severe dyspnea. Classically, the harsh apical systolic murmur ends before the second heart sound, but the murmur may still be obscured by ambient ED noise. Since the left atrium has not had time to adapt to the retrograde flow and resultant steep left atrial pressures that cause pulmonary edema in acute mitral regurgitation, the heart may appear relatively small on chest x-ray.

2-38. **The answer is D** (Chapter 58). Mitral valve prolapse affects about 2.4% of the population in the industrialized world. Rheumatic heart disease is uncommon in the United States but is a major cause of aortic valve disease worldwide. Calcific aortic stenosis is the most common cause of adult aortic stenosis in the United States, while younger adults have a bicuspid aortic valve or underlying congenital heart disease.

2-39. **The answer is E** (Chapter 58). Pectus excavatum, scoliosis, and low body weight have been found to be associated with mitral valve prolapse. Studies have not demonstrated an association of chest pain, dyspnea, or anxiety with the disorder.

2-40. **The answer is B** (Chapter 58). Patients with mitral valve prolapse and exercise-induced mitral regurgitation have an increased risk of morbidity. Patients with mitral valve prolapse (MVP) and mitral regurgitation require endocarditis prophylaxis before invasive procedures. Other factors that place patients at risk for complications include male sex and age older than 45 years. Low body weight and scoliosis are associated with mitral valve prolapse.

2-41. **The answer is D** (Chapter 59). Hypertrophic cardiomyopathy is the leading cause of sudden death in competitive athletes and in adolescents. Commotio cordis and congenital coronary artery anomalies are, respectively, the second and third leading causes of sudden death in adolescents. Commotio cordis is a term used when a physical blow to the chest wall causes ventricular fibrillation or sudden death without evident structural damage to the thorax or heart. Idiopathic dilated cardiomyopathy is the most common cardiomyopathy and the cause of about one-fourth of all cases of congestive heart failure. Heat stroke is a preventable cause of injury or death in athletes.

2-42. **The answer is B** (Chapter 59). This patient, with a pericardial friction rub, elevated cardiac biomarkers, and radiographic and clinical signs of CHF, has myocarditis, a common cause of dilated cardiomyopathy. Etiologies of myocarditis include viral, bacterial, fungal causes, as well as malignant, drug-induced, and systemic diseases. Echocardiography is nonspecific for myocarditis but can show myocardial depression (global hypokinesis) and wall motion abnormalities in severe cases. Diagnosis of myocarditis may require a nuclear scan, heart biopsy, or MRI. Cardiac enzymes are elevated with myocarditis and

should be followed serially. Acute coronary syndrome is unlikely in a young, previously well patient. The pericardium can be inflamed in myopericarditis. Pulmonary embolus belongs to the differential diagnosis for acute dyspnea, but other elements in this presentation suggest myocarditis. Most patients with idiopathic or presumed viral myocarditis respond well to nonsteroidal anti-inflammatory medications and can be treated as outpatients, with echocardiographic follow-up. Patients who require admission may have one or more of the following poor prognostic indicators: temperature $>38°C$, subacute onset over weeks, immunosuppression, oral anticoagulant use, associated myocarditis, and a large pericardial effusion. Pericardial tamponade can occur with very large effusions in acute pericarditis.

2-43. **The answer is C** (Chapter 59). The murmur of HCM intensifies with actions that decrease LV filling and the distending pressure of the LV outflow tract, such as standing, and the Valsalva maneuver (strain phase). The murmur of HCM also intensifies with increased force of myocardial contraction. Hence, the murmur is louder with the first sinus beat after a premature ventricular contraction. The systolic ejection murmur of HCM is heard best at the lower left sternal border or the apex. Maneuvers that increase LV filling (squatting, passive leg raise, and sustained handgrip) decrease the murmur of HCM (see Table 59-5). When a patient turns their chin toward a stethoscope in the right supraclavicular fossa, a venous hum decreases.

2-44. **The answer is A** (Chapter 59). A pericardial knock, an early diastolic sound, that can be heard at the apex 60–120 milliseconds after the second heart sound but before an S3 is associated with constrictive pericarditis but is clinically very challenging to differentiate from an S3. Both conditions share the signs of JVD and Kussmaul, which is an increase in venous pressure with inspiration. The dip and plateau filling pattern, also known as the square root sign, is seen in both conditions. A marked decrease followed by a rapid rise and plateau in early-diastolic ventricular pressure is seen in hemodynamic studies, such as Doppler echocardiography or cardiac catheterization. CT and MRIs of the heart can differentiate constrictive pericarditis from restrictive cardiomyopathy. Pericardial thickening is seen with constrictive pericarditis, but not with restrictive cardiomyopathy. Constrictive pericarditis can be treated surgically. Restrictive cardiomyopathy is symptomatically managed with diuretics and ACE inhibitors and medical therapies specific to the underlying etiology, for example, corticosteroids for sarcoidosis and chelation for hemachromatosis.

2-45. **The answer is D** (Chapter 59). Most cases of restrictive cardiomyopathy are idiopathic, often with an autosomal-dominant familial pattern. The remainder of causes are systemic disorders such as those listed earlier, as well as progressive systemic sclerosis (scleroderma), and hypereosinophilic syndrome. All etiologies affect the heart muscle, either by scarring or infiltration, and cause stiffness that affect diastolic filling and raises end-diastolic pressures. Systolic LV function is normal. The EP should consider restrictive cardiomyopathy in a patient presenting with signs of CHF but without cardiomegaly or systolic dysfunction.

2-46. **The answer is E** (Chapter 59). This patient has cardiac tamponade, as indicated by the narrow pulse pressure, pulsus paradoxus, electrical alternans, and RV collapse in diastole on echocardiogram. However, she is hemodynamically stable. Pericardiocentesis is the definitive therapy for cardiac tamponade and should be performed either emergently or urgently with echocardiographic guidance. Fluid samples should also be sent for studies to rule out malignancy, which is the most common cause of nontraumatic pericardial tamponade. Patients with pericardial tamponade have intrapericardial pressures, which exceed normal filling pressures, as seen by RA and RV diastolic collapse. Preload must be maintained to support filling pressure, so the EP can temporize with a 500–1000 mL of NS. Therapies that would decrease preload, such as diuretics or vasodilators, would worsen cardiac tamponade and should be judiciously avoided.

2-47. **The answer is C** (Chapter 59). Early acute pericarditis can mimic the ST–T-wave changes of early repolarization, a normal variant. The early ECG stage of acute pericarditis is characterized by PR segment depression (especially in II, aVF, and V4–V6), ST-segment elevation (especially in I, V5, and V6), and ST/T amplitude >0.25 (Table 59-7). Using the PR segment baseline as 0 mV, the height in millivolts, of the ST segment at its onset, is divided by the height in millivolts of the T wave, from its baseline to peak. An ST/T ratio >0.25 suggests acute pericarditis, while a ratio <0.25 does not. The ST/T ratio >0.25 has a sensitivity and specificity greater than 85% and 80%, respectively. As acute pericarditis progresses, the ST segment becomes isoelectric with inverted T waves (especially in I, V5, and V6). In the final stage, the T wave normalizes to an upright position.

2-48. **The answer is B** (Chapter 60). Pulmonary emboli form when proximal portions of DVTs break off and lodge in the precapillary pulmonary arteries. In hospitalized patients, 75–80% have image demonstrated DVTs. In ED patients, however, far fewer (40%) have image demonstrated DVTs.

2-49. **The answer is C** (Chapter 60). The immobilization of the knee and hip confers the greatest risk to the patient. The risk increases as follows: elbow, shoulder, ankle, knee, and hip. Bed rest also confers an increased risk after 48–72 hours of immobilization.

2-50. **The answer is A** (Chapter 60). The odd ratio (OR) for limb immobility is 2.24 that is the highest amongst a multicenter study of 7940 patients with VTE. Neurologic immobility has an OR of 2.23. Whole body immobilization was 1.76 and traveling >8 hours was not a statistically significant risk factor.

2-51. **The answer is E** (Chapter 60). It is clear that recent surgery is a risk factor for VTE and PE.

What is interesting is that the presentation for PE is usually greater than 10 days after the surgical event. Postop PE risk increases with age, duration of surgery, open surgery, and surgery where venous prophylaxis is not used.

2-52.   **The answer is D** (Chapter 60). The risk peaks in the first week with an incidence of 1 in 500 women. The immobility and increase risk after surgery are likely contributors. Exogenous estrogen, whether for contraception or hormone replacement therapy, increases the risk as well.

2-53.   **The answer is B** (Chapter 60). Dyspnea is the most common chief complaint in patients with a PE. Chest pain is the second most common but is only present in 50% of patients who are diagnosed with a PE. The skilled clinician must not be complacent in the patient with no complaint of chest pain. A PE must still be in the differential.

2-54.   **The answer is D** (Chapter 60). Sinus tachycardia is a common finding on ECG. As the severity of the PE increases, the right heart begins to work harder and the right-sided pressures increase. Once the RV systolic pressures exceed 40 mm Hg, the T-wave inversions, incomplete or complete RBB, and the classic S1 Q3 T3 patterns may emerge.

2-55.   **The answer is A** (Chapter 60). A CT scan gives about 10–20 mSv of radiation and increases the lifetime risk to at least 1 in 500. The risk in young women may be higher given breast radiation. Other life-threatening reactions to CT scans of the chest include anaphylactoid reactions and pulmonary edema, which together occur in about 1 in 1000 patients.

2-56.   **The answer is D** (Chapter 60). The patient met the criteria for the application of the PERC rule. If all criteria are met, the patient has a probability of PE of less than 2%, which is under the commonly accepted threshold for diagnostic testing (see Table 60-7).

2-57.   **The answer is A** (Chapter 60). The Pulmonary Embolism Rule-Out Criteria (PERC) is a well-validated rule to aid the clinician predicts which patients have a very low risk of PE even before any diagnostic testing is done. This allows the clinician, if all criteria are met, to eliminate the diagnosis of PE from the differential diagnosis, thus saving resources and potential complications from unnecessary diagnostic tests.

2-58.   **The answer is A** (Chapter 60). D-dimer test would not be sufficient in this patient as he is a high-risk patient based on the Wells criteria, so a "holding dose" of low-molecular-weight heparin and arrangements for a confirmatory ultrasound on Monday are appropriate. Several reports document the safety of a single dose of low-molecular-weight heparin in patients without contraindications while confirmatory tests are arranged. Admission is not warranted.

2-59.   **The answer is E** (Chapter 60). The condition is phlegmasia cerulea dolens and was first described in the sixteenth century. It is a condition in which the entire venous system is blocked by VTE and limb ischemia is the result. This is limb threatening and should be considered extremely dangerous and a true emergency. The appropriate treatment for this is thrombolysis and possibly surgical thrombectomy. Heparin or a CT will not help this patient, as rapid clot removal or destruction is needed.

2-60.   **The answer is C** (Chapter 61). Patients with acute sympathetic crisis may not have signs of end-organ damage to the brain, heart, or kidneys, but treatment is nevertheless indicated to avoid complications to those organs. The first-line treatment for an acute sympathetic crisis due to cocaine or methamphetamine use is an IV benzodiazepine such as lorazepam or diazepam. Monitor the patient for respiratory depression or sedation. If benzodiazepine therapy is unsuccessful, nitroglycerin, calcium channel blockers, or phentolamine can be used. The text recommends nitroglycerin therapy, followed by nicardipine. Phentolamine is a potent alpha-1 and alpha-2 blocking properties, which beta-blockers are not recommended because of the risk of increased alpha effects in the presence of unopposed beta-blockade. Labetalol has weak alpha-blockage and strong beta-blocking effects, in a ratio of 1 to 7. Esmolol has shorter acting beta-blocking effects but is still not recommended for acute sympathetic crisis.

2-61. **The answer is A** (Chapter 61). ACE inhibitors are contraindicated in pregnant women due to potential teratogenic effects on the fetus. Hydralazine is no longer considered first-line therapy for eclampsia due to an unpredictable therapeutic profile. Nifedipine has been used in preeclamptic women without significant side effects, but should be avoided in other types of nonpregnancy-related hypertensive emergencies. Labetalol and magnesium sulfate are indicated in the treatment of eclampsia.

2-62. **The answer is E** (Chapter 61). Enalaprilat is an intravenous ACE inhibitor that may be indicated in the treatment of patients with heart failure or acute coronary syndrome. Hypotension is the most common side effect with a first dose, so a preliminary test dose of 0.625 mg is recommended. Angioedema, cough, and hyperkalemia are all potential side effects of ACE inhibitors and angiotensin II receptor blockers. Bradycardia is a potential side effect associated with beta-blockers and calcium channel blockers (see Table 61-9).

2-63. **The answer is A** (Chapter 61). See Tables 61-4 and 61-5. Clevidipine is an intravenous, third-generation dihydropyridine calcium channel blocker with ultra-short–acting selective arteriolar vasodilation effects. Clevidipine is titratable and has a half-life of less than a minute. Originally used in cardiac surgery, it is now approved for use in hypertensive emergencies, except for aortic dissection, due to its potential for hypotension and reflex tachycardia. Clevidipine formulation contains 0.2 g of lipid per milliliter.

Patients with serious lipid metabolism disorders may require restrictions of lipid intake if given this drug. Aortic dissection is traditionally first treated with a beta-blocker followed by nitroprusside, since nitroprusside alone causes reflex tachycardia and increased aortic wall stress. Patients with severe COPD or asthma unable to tolerate esmolol may require a switch to a second-generation calcium channel blocker such as nicardipine. In general, however, nicardipine should be avoided in patients receiving beta-blockers.

2-64. **The answer is E** (Chapter 61). Nifedipine is discouraged in the treatment of hypertensive emergencies except preeclampsia. This patient has hypertensive encephalopathy without evidence of ischemic stroke, or hemorrhage, and requires careful BP reduction. The EP must carefully avoid a precipitous drop in BP, which can lead to stroke or MI. Labetalol is the most commonly used parenteral antihypertensive agent in the ED and is indicated in neurologic hypertensive emergencies not complicated by cocaine use. Esmolol is an alternative beta-blocker indicated for use in hypertensive emergencies in patients who also have severe asthma. Fenoldopam is a dopamine receptor agonist used in renal and neurologic hypertensive emergencies. Fenoldopam has an onset of action in 5 minutes, a peak effect in 15 minutes, and a duration of 30–60 minutes. Fenoldopam improves creatinine clearance, urine flow, and sodium excretion and is used in acute renal failure. The drug undergoes non-P450 hepatic metabolism. Concurrent acetaminophen use can increase fenoldopam levels. Nicardipine is a second-generation calcium channel blocker that can be safely used in neurologic hypertensive emergencies but not concomitantly with beta-blockers.

2-65. **The answer is B** (Chapter 61). Fenoldopam undergoes non-P450 hepatic metabolism, and drug levels can increase with concurrent acetaminophen use. See Table 61-5. Enalapril and labetalol undergo first-pass hepatic metabolism. Labetalol and nitroprusside should be avoided in patients with liver failure. Phentolamine undergoes some hepatic metabolism, but some of the drug is also unchanged and excreted renally.

2-66. **The answer is A** (Chapter 61). There is a 60% incidence of pulmonary hypertension in CREST or limited scleroderma. The CREST acronym stands for calcinosis, Raynaud's phenomena, esophageal dysmotility, sclerodactyly, and telangiectasia. The incidence of pulmonary hypertension is 10–30% in patients with hemoglobinopathies, 15–20% in sleep apnea, 2% in portal hypertension, and 0.5% in HIV. Idiopathic pulmonary hypertension is rare. There is indirect evidence that the incidence is high in patients with COPD, but an exact rate is unknown. Pulmonary hypertension denotes elevated pulmonary artery pressure with or without concomitant pulmonary venous elevation and subsequent right ventricular dysfunction. Hemodynamically, the condition defined by a pulmonary artery pressure is >25 mm Hg at rest or >30 mm Hg during exertion. The etiologies are multifactorial, but the final common pathway involves endothelial dysfunction and arterial remodeling. The EP should consider the diagnosis in patients presenting with dyspnea, chest pain, or syncope.

2-67. **The answer is C** (Chapter 61). Patients with hypertensive heart failure and pulmonary edema would be expected to respond well to the decrease in preload and afterload associated with vasodilator therapy. Since patients with aortic stenosis, HCM, and right-ventricular infarction are all preload dependent, standard doses of vasodilator therapy could precipitate profound hypotension. Vasodilators would not be indicated in a patient with volume depletion.

2-68. **The answer is E** (Chapter 61). Transient hypotension is clinically the most important complication of nitroglycerin use, although headache is a very common side effect that usually responds to acetaminophen. Nitroglycerin should be avoided or used with extreme caution in preload-dependent conditions such as aortic stenosis, HCM, and right

ventricular infarct. Nitroglycerin has caused methemoglobinemia in very rare instances. Nitroprusside can cause thiocyanate toxicity, especially when used in patients with renal insufficiency.

2-69. **The answer is A** (Chapter 62). Aortic dissections occur both in patients who have predisposing conditions and in those older than 50 years with chronic hypertension. Patients who are at risk of developing aortic dissection at a young age are those with Marfan's syndrome, Ehlers–Danlos syndrome, and those with a bicuspid aortic valve. Each of these leads to higher intimal wall stress which can, in turn, lead to dissection.

2-70. **The answer is C** (Chapter 62). In a case series of 464 patients with aortic dissections, 60% presented with chest pain, 64% stated the pain was "sharp," and 50% stated it was tearing or ripping. Syncope occurred 10% of the time. In all 90% of the patients stated that the pain associated with their dissection was the worst they had ever felt.

2-71. **The answer is C** (Chapter 62). This patient is likely having an aortic dissection. Aortic dissections are difficult because of the dynamic nature of their presentations. As the dissection travels down the aorta, it can cut off circulation to the brachiocephalic artery, the carotids, the renal vessels, etc. This patient's hypotension was most likely due to his dissection spreading anterograde and causing a pericardial tamponade. Chest x-ray, CT scans, etc., are less helpful than a bedside cardiac echo. The echo can help in the patient with undifferentiated hypotension. It can be done at the bedside, without the need for transporting the critically ill patient to the radiology suite.

2-72. **The answer is A** (Chapter 62). Beta-blockers are favored as the first-line agent in patients with aortic dissection. When antihypertensive therapy is warranted, the main issue is to limit the shear wall forces on the aorta. The importance of the beta-blocker is to prevent rebound tachycardia when nitrates are used. An ideal combination is esmolol followed by nitroprusside since they can be titrated well and have short half-lives. Hydralazine and lisinopril have no role in the antihypertensive therapy of aortic dissection patients.

2-73.   **The answer is B** (Chapter 63). While it is important to recognize all factors that increase cardiovascular disease, a family history of a first-degree relative with an AAA has been shown to be highly predictive. Eighteen percent of patients with an AAA have a first-degree relative who also had an AAA. Diabetes mellitus, hypertension, high cholesterol, and smoking may all be associated with the development of an AAA or cardiovascular disease in general but not as much as a strong family history.

2-74.   **The answer is E** (Chapter 63). The scenario depicted is a classic example of a patient who likely has a leaking or symptomatic AAA. This patient is known to be hypertensive at baseline and is hypotensive in the ED. This is the kind of patient who cannot go to the radiology suite with the limited supervision that is afforded there. This patient is a great candidate for a bedside ultrasound to assess for an AAA. If found, the constellation of abdominal pain, hematuria, and AAA should prompt the ED physician to urgently consult surgery for a possible exploration and repair of his AAA. The other answers all involve leaving the bedside of a potentially critically ill patient.

2-75.   **The answer is A** (Chapter 64). Limb ischemia can be caused by either arterial thrombosis or embolization from the aneurysm. It is the most common serious complication. Rupture can occur, but it is exceedingly rare. Discomfort, pain, or swelling may be present, but they are precursors to the more serious complications.

2-76.   **The answer is C** (Chapter 64). Diabetes and smoking are the two most important risk factors for occlusive arterial disease. In the PARTNERS study, patients older than 50 years with diabetes or a smoking had a prevalence >29%. In other studies, more than 80% of patients with occlusive arterial disease are either former or current smokers. Other risk factors include hyperlipidemia, hypertension, hyperhomocysteinemia, and elevated C-reactive protein. Occlusive arterial disease, defined as an ankle-brachial index <0.9, increases with age, is two to four times more common in men than in women, and more prevalent in non-Caucasians. (See Figure 64-1 for description of ankle-brachial index.)

2-77.   **The answer is E** (Chapter 64). Thrombotic occlusion, of native vessels or bypass grafts, is the most common cause of acute limb ischemia, followed by embolic occlusion. Thrombotic occlusion causes more than 80% of lower limb cases and more than 50% of upper limb cases. Emboli and arteritis, respectively, account for a third and a fourth of the remainder of upper limb cases. Thrombosis can also result from hypercoagulable states or from direct vessel injury, such as catheters, bypass graft sites, or intra-arterial drug injections. The heart is the source of 80–90% of emboli. Atrial fibrillation is associated with at least two-thirds of peripheral embolic, with clot originating from the left atrial appendage. Postinfarction ventricular mural thrombi account for about 20% of limb emboli. Other embolic sources include thrombi from aneurysms and fragmentation of atheromatous plaques. The false lumen of a propagating thoracic aortic dissection can occlude flow into the subclavian or iliofemoral systems.

2-78.   **The answer is E** (Chapter 64). Paralysis and anesthesia are late findings of ischemic injury that portend loss of limb viability. An adequate collateral blood supply may mask signs of ischemia in a severely diseased artery. Pain can be the sole and earliest symptom of ischemia in a patient with underlying peripheral vascular disease. Peripheral nerves and muscles are very sensitive to ischemia, which causes early findings of hypesthesia, hyperesthesia, and muscle weakness. Skin changes associated with complete arterial obstruction include pallor, cyanosis, petechiae or blisters, and decreased temperature. Ultimately, skin and fat necrosis ensue.

2-79. **The answer is C** (Chapter 64). The clinical evaluation is the EP's most important diagnostic tool for assessing potential occlusive arterial disease. Clinically, thrombus has most likely subacutely caused limb-threatening ischemia in a patient with underlying peripheral vascular disease. Pain can be the sole symptom of ischemia in a patient with chronic peripheral vascular disease, but sometimes, total occlusion in a severely diseased artery is silent. An ankle-brachial index <0.25 suggests possibly limb-threatening ischemia. Values between 0.41 and .90 suggest mild-to-moderate peripheral arterial disease. Normal values are 0.91–1.3. See Figure 64-1. Once acute limb ischemia is suspected, the EP should obtain a vascular surgery consultation, before ordering confirmatory imaging. Current practice calls for immediate administration of IV unfractionated heparin: an 80 units/kg followed by an infusion of 18 units/kg/hour. Conservative medical therapy with heparin, without surgery, is generally done in cases such as this one with thrombotic occlusion in the setting of advance atherosclerosis. Aspirin can also be given. Patients with suspected occlusive arterial disease are at risk for reperfusion injury, which is characterized by myoglobinemia, renal failure, and peripheral muscle infarction. About one-third of deaths from occlusive arterial disease are secondary to the metabolic sequelae of revascularization. Baseline electrolytes, myoglobin, and creatine kinase should be ordered, as well as a coagulation panel. If an embolic source, rather than thrombotic source, is suspected, an echocardiogram can rule out a mural thrombus. Bedside studies are usually more available than transthoracic echocardiograms. An ECG can evaluate the presence of atrial fibrillation or ischemia. Serial cardiac biomarkers are indicated to establish acute coronary syndrome. The EP can order a duplex ultrasound to determine complete or incomplete obstruction in the common femoral, superficial femoral, and popliteal vessels, or in bypass grafts. An arteriogram is done to confirm diagnosis and define vascular anatomy and perfusion. Arteriosclerosis is usually evident in patients with a thrombus. An embolus would show an abrupt cutoff of blood flow in a disease-free or minimally diseased vessel. CTA or MRA of the extremity could also be ordered. If an aortic dissection, or aneurysm in the aortoiliac or femoral vessels, is suspected, an aortogram, CT, or MR can be ordered. Definitive treatment of an arterial clot requires a vascular surgeon. Options include percutaneous mechanical thrombectomy and revascularization with percutaneous transluminal angioplasty (PTA) or standard surgery. Timely embolectomy is indicated for acute embolic occlusions.

2-80. **The answer is B** (Chapter 64). Neurogenic claudication, due to spinal stenosis or lumbar radiculopathy, can mimic intermittent vascular claudication. Patients with neurogenic claudication can have bilateral buttock pain, and posterior leg pain triggered by exercise and relieved by rest, but onset of relief is not as immediate as it is in intermittent claudication. Patients with neurogenic claudication have relief of pain with lumbar flexion and worsening pain with upright posture or lumbar extension.

CHAPTER 3

Cutaneous Disorders
Questions

3-1. Which of the following is NOT true of the pictured disease (Figure 3-1)?

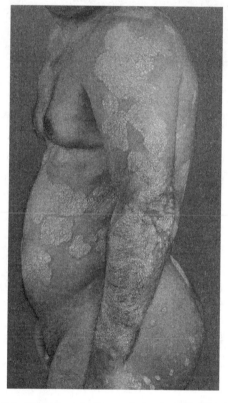

Figure 3-1. Reproduced with permission from Wolff K, Johnson RA, Suurmond R: *Fitzpatrick's Color Atlas & Synopsis of Clinical Dermatology*, 5th Edition. Copyright © 2005 The McGraw-Hill Companies, Inc.

(A) Age of peak incidence occurs in patients in their early 20s.

(B) It has a hereditary predisposition.

(C) Lesions are symmetrical with a predilection for the flexor surfaces.

(D) Stress or alcohol ingestion can be associated with a flare.

(E) The disease is common affecting 1.5–2% of the population.

3-2. The most appropriate treatment for this condition is (Figure 3-2).

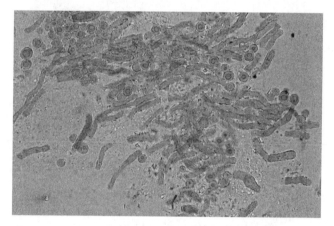

Figure 3-2. Reproduced with permission from Wolff K, Johnson RA: *Fitzpatrick's Color Atlas & Synopsis of Clinical Dermatology*, 6th Edition. Copyright © 2009 The McGraw-Hill Companies, Inc.

(A) Ketoconazole shampoo

(B) Oral antihistamines and topical steroids

(C) Permethrin cream

(D) Selenium sulfide lotion or shampoo

(E) Vaseline

3-3. Which of the following tests can be used to make the definitive diagnosis of this disease (Figure 3-3)?

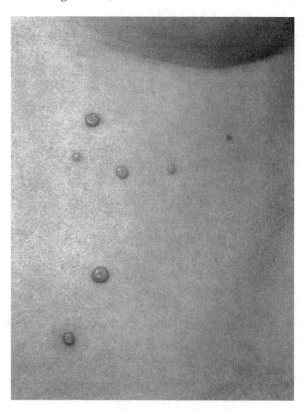

Figure 3-3. Reproduced with permission from Wolff K, Johnson RA, Suurmond R: *Fitzpatrick's Color Atlas & Synopsis of Clinical Dermatology*, 5th Edition. Copyright © 2005 The McGraw-Hill Companies, Inc.

(A) Biopsy showing Donovan bodies

(B) Giemsa stain showing intracytoplasmic inclusion bodies

(C) Potassium hydroxide preparation (KOH prep)

(D) Serology

(E) Tzanck smear

3-4. This picture shows a lesion on the tongue of a HIV-infected individual (Figure 3-4). Which of the following statements about this disease is NOT correct?

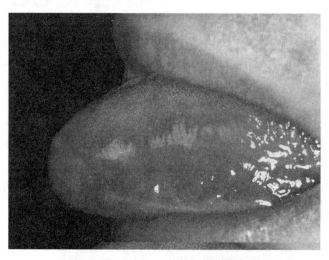

Figure 3-4. Reproduced with permission from Knoop KJ, Stack LB, Storrow AB, Thurman RJ: *The Alas of Emergency Medicine*, 3rd Edition. Copyright © 2010 The McGraw-Hill Companies, Inc.

(A) Diagnosis is confirmed by skin biopsy.

(B) Differential diagnosis includes disseminated fungal infections such as *cryptococcosis, histoplasmosis, coccidioidomycosis,* and *penicilliosis.*

(C) Human herpes virus has been identified in these lesions.

(D) There are several different types of this disease affecting very different populations.

(E) Treatments may include intralesional or systemic chemotherapy.

3-5. This patient presents with a painful, penile lesion with associated tender swelling in the groin (Figure 3-5). What medication would be useful in treating the lesion?

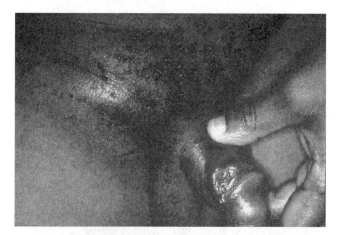

Figure 3-5. Reproduced from Martin DH, Mroczkowski TF: Dermatologic manifestations of STDs other than HIV. *Infect Dis Clin North Am.* 1994:8:550.

(A) Ceftriaxone

(B) Doxycycline

(C) Penicillin

(D) Permethrin cream

(E) Trimethoprim sulfamethoxazole

3-6. The individual pictured here gives a history of working at a local pet store (Figure 3-6). His job is to maintain the fish tanks. Which of the following is NOT true concerning his infection?

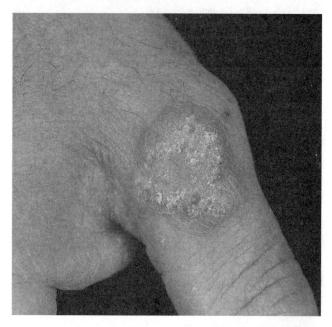

Figure 3-6. Reproduced with permission from Wolff K, Johnson RA, Suurmond R: *Fitzpatrick's Color Atlas & Synopsis of Clinical Dermatology*, 5th Edition. Copyright © 2005 The McGraw-Hill Companies, Inc.

(A) All aquatic environments can support the causative organism of this infection: fresh, salt, and brackish water.

(B) Infection requires exposure to traumatized skin in a contaminated environment.

(C) The infection can be treated with rifampicin or clotrimazole.

(D) There is the development of significant lymphadenopathy with this infection.

(E) Two to three weeks after exposure to this organism, an initial nodule or pustule forms, which then breaks down to form an abscess or ulcer.

3-7. What is the most common organism responsible for this lesion (Figure 3-7)?

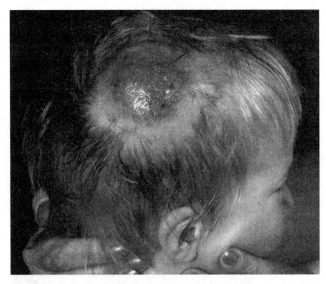

Figure 3-7. Reproduced with permission from Wolff K, Johnson RA: *Fitzpatrick's Color Atlas & Synopsis of Clinical Dermatology*, 6th Edition. Copyright © 2009 The McGraw-Hill Companies, Inc.

(A) *Malassezia furfur*

(B) Microsporum

(C) *Streptococcus pyogenes*

(D) *Staphylococcus aureus*

(E) Trichophyton

3-8. Which of the following statements about this skin disorder is NOT true (Figure 3-8)?

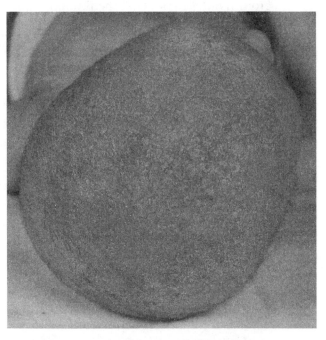

Figure 3-8. Reproduced with permission from Fleischer A Jr, Feldman S, McConnell C, et al: *Emergency Dermatology: A Rapid Treatment Guide.* Copyright © 2002 The McGraw-Hill Companies, Inc.

(A) Adults with AIDS and Parkinson disease are predisposed to severe forms of this.

(B) Fungal culture should be performed in patients up to puberty.

(C) Ketoconazole shampoo and antidandruff shampoo may be used to treat this.

(D) *M. furfur* may play a role in the pathogenesis of this disease.

(E) The rash is intensely pruritic.

3-9. Which of the following is true concerning the condition involving this patient's right ear (Figure 3-9)?

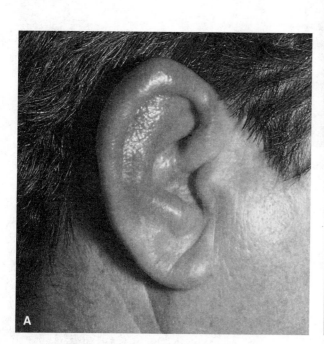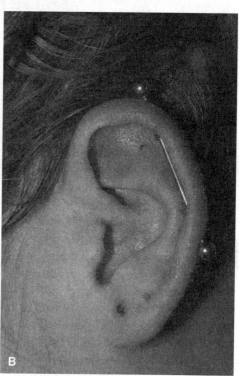

Figure 3-9. Reproduced with permission from Knoop KJ, Stack LB, Storrow AB, Thurman RJ: *The Atlas of Emergency Medicine*, 3rd Edition. Copyright © 2010 The McGraw-Hill Companies, Inc. Photo contributor: Lawrence B. Stack, MD.

(A) Methicillin-resistant *S. aureus* causes this infection.

(B) Oral valacyclovir is the treatment of choice for patients with HIV.

(C) Rapid treatment shortens healing time.

(D) Rash is typically followed by pain.

(E) Treatment is indefinite for patients with this condition.

3-10. Which of the following is true concerning this intensely pruritic rash (Figure 3-10)?

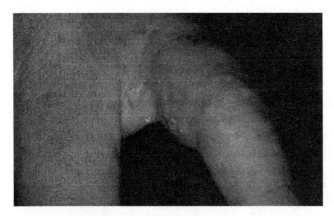

Figure 3-10. Reproduced with permission from Wolff K, Johnson RA: *Fitzpatrick's Color Atlas & Synopsis of Clinical Dermatology*, 6th Edition. Copyright © 2009 The McGraw-Hill Companies, Inc.

(A) Children typically present with a milder rash.

(B) Immunocompromised hosts may develop crusted plaques on the scalp, hands, and feet.

(C) Pruritus is most notable upon awakening.

(D) Rash usually spares the head and neck in children.

(E) Treatment in pregnant women is limited to oral ivermectin.

3-11. Which of the following is NOT correct regarding the prescription of steroids for this eruption (Figure 3-11)?

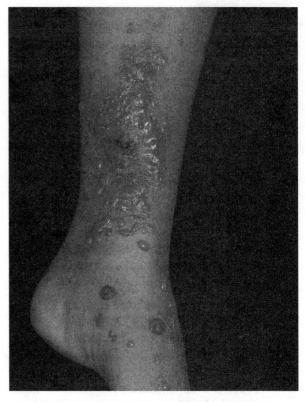

Figure 3-11. Reproduced with permission from Fleischer A Jr, Feldman S, McConnell C, et al: *Emergency Dermatology: A Rapid Treatment Guide*. Copyright © 2002 The McGraw-Hill Companies, Inc.

(A) A short burst of oral prednisone will hasten resolution of this condition.

(B) Fluorinated topical steroids provide increased potency, therefore do not have to be applied as frequently or for as long duration.

(C) If this patient is diabetic or immunocompromised, caution should be used when prescribing oral steroids.

(D) One treatment for an eruption like this on the hand would be intermediate or low potency topical steroids.

(E) The burn rule of 9s can be used to estimate the amount of topical steroid required in a prescription.

3-12. Which of the following is TRUE concerning this condition (Figure 3-12)?

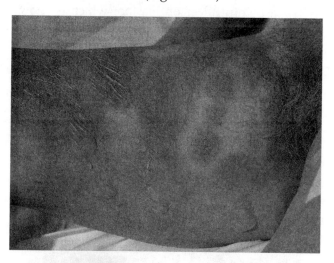

Figure 3-12. Reproduced with permission from Tintinalli JE, Stapczynski JS, Ma OJ, Cline DM, Cydulka RK, Meckler GD: *Tintinalli's Emergency Medicine: A Comprehensive Study Guide,* 7th Edition. Copyright © 2011 The McGraw-Hill Companies, Inc.

(A) Blindness is the most common complication.

(B) Etiology of this condition is unknown.

(C) Scaring is typical.

(D) Fluid and electrolyte imbalances and secondary infections are the most common cause of death.

(E) Symptoms in addition to the rash include diffuse arthralgias.

3-13. Which of the following conditions is associated with the following clinical finding (Figure 3-13)?

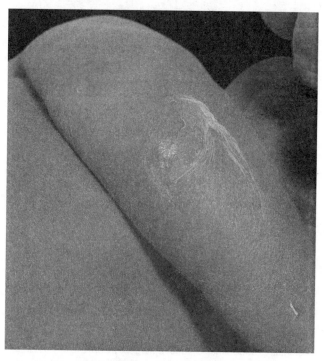

Figure 3-13. Reproduced with permission from Wolff K, Johnson RA: *Fitzpatrick's Color Atlas & Synopsis of Clinical Dermatology,* 6th Edition. Copyright © 2009 The McGraw-Hill Companies, Inc.

(A) Bullous pemphigoid

(B) Eczema herpeticum

(C) Exfoliative erythroderma

(D) Staphylococcus scalded skin

(E) Toxic shock syndrome

3-14. This rash is caused by which of the following (Figure 3-14)?

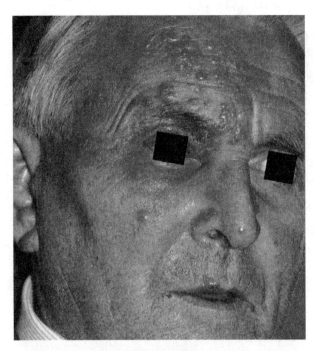

Figure 3-14. Reproduced with permission from Fleischer A Jr, Feldman S, McConnell C, et al: *Emergency Dermatology: A Rapid Treatment Guide.* Copyright © 2002 The McGraw-Hill Companies, Inc.

   (A) Group A streptococcus

   (B) Herpes simplex virus (HSV)

   (C) Human papilloma virus

   (D) *S. aureus*

   (E) Varicella zoster virus

3-15. A 65-year-old male with a history of diabetes and cardiac disease presents complaining of a painful ulcer on his foot which is shown in Figure 3-15. He reports pain in the distal leg when supine and a new appearance of shiny skin with hair loss. What is the MOST important next step in his evaluation and management?

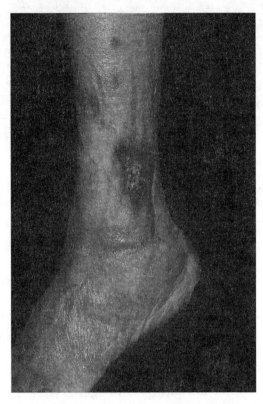

Figure 3-15. Reproduced with permission from Fitzpatrick TB, Johnson RA, Wolff K, Suurmond D: *Color Atlas & Synopsis of Clinical Dermatology*, 4th Edition. Copyright © 2001 The McGraw-Hill Companies, Inc.

   (A) Apply a wet-to-dry dressing with a topical antimicrobial and start oral antibiotics.

   (B) Arrange for outpatient wound management and regular checkups.

   (C) Obtain a wound culture to determine the best antibiotic management.

   (D) Order an arterial duplex and ankle-brachial indices of the leg.

   (E) Order a venous duplex ultrasound.

3-16. Initial ED treatment for a patient with these skin findings includes which of the following (Figure 3-16)?

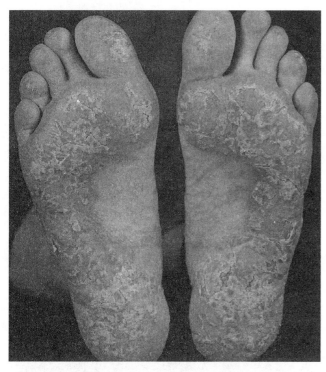

Figure 3-16. Reproduced with permission from Wolff K, Johnson RA, Suurmond R: *Fitzpatrick's Color Atlas & Synopsis of Clinical Dermatology*, 5th Edition. Copyright © 2005 The McGraw-Hill Companies, Inc.

(A) Acitretin

(B) High or ultrahigh potency topical corticosteroids

(C) Methotrexate

(D) Psoralen–ultraviolet light A treatments

(E) Tar-containing solutions

3-17. Which of the following is NOT true about this disease (Figure 3-17)?

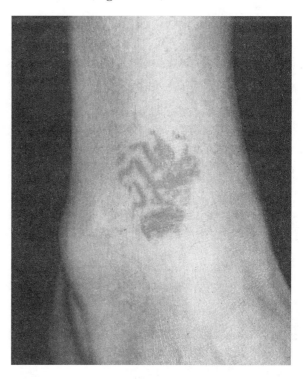

Figure 3-17. Reproduced with permission from Knoop KJ, Stack LB, Storrow AB: *Atlas of Emergency Medicine*, 2nd Edition. Copyright © 2002 The McGraw-Hill Companies, Inc. Photo contributor: Department of Dermatology, National Naval Medical Center, Bethesda, MD.

(A) A complete blood count may demonstrate peripheral eosinophilia.

(B) A single dose of oral albendazole or ivermectin is effective treatment.

(C) Erythematous serpiginous tracts are formed by the causative organism.

(D) It occurs when ringworm larvae migrate into exposed epidermis.

(E) It is commonly found in subtropical or tropical climates.

3-18. Infestation by this organism produces symptoms approximately how long after initial exposure (Figure 3-18)?

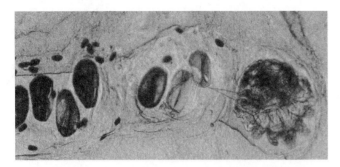

Figure 3-18. Reproduced with permission from Wolff K, Johnson RA: *Fitzpatrick's Color Atlas & Synopsis of Clinical Dermatology*, 6th Edition. Copyright © 2009 The McGraw-Hill Companies, Inc.

(A) Within 1 month
(B) Within 2 weeks
(C) Within 24 hours
(D) Within 3 hours
(E) Within 5 days

3-19. Which of the following medications does NOT typically cause the reaction shown in Figure 3-19?

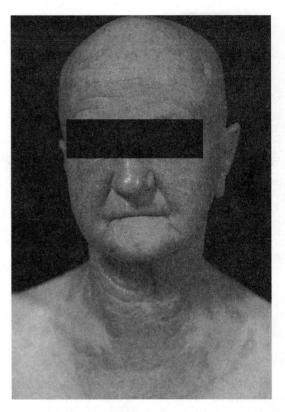

Figure 3-19. Reproduced with permission from Wolff K, Johnson RA: *Fitzpatrick's Color Atlas & Synopsis of Clinical Dermatology*, 6th Edition. Copyright © 2009 The McGraw-Hill Companies, Inc.

(A) Amiodarone
(B) Chlorpromazine
(C) Furosemide
(D) Metoprolol
(E) Tetracycline

3-20. Which of the following is NOT correct regarding the tick-borne illness demonstrated in Figure 3-20?

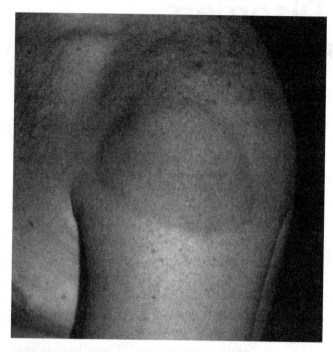

Figure 3-20. Reproduced with permission from Wolff K, Johnson RA, Suurmond R: *Fitzpatrick's Color Atlas & Synopsis of Clinical Dermatology*, 5th Edition. Copyright © 2005 The McGraw-Hill Companies, Inc.

(A) IgG antibodies develop months after infection.

(B) IgM antibodies peak between the third and sixth week of infection.

(C) Most lesions fade within 1 month of presentation.

(D) Pain and/or itching at the site of this lesion are characteristic.

(E) Skin, nervous system, and joints are commonly affected by this infection.

Cutaneous Disorders
Answers and Explanations

3-1. **The answer is C** (Chapter 249). This picture shows a lesion caused by psoriasis. The lesions are typically silver and scaly with erythematous plaques and papules. The areas affected may include scalp, nails, sacrum, gluteal cleft, umbilicus, and typically symmetrical extensor surfaces. The disease is common and has a strong hereditary predisposition. The peak of incidence occurs when people are in their early 20s. It has an insidious onset. Flares can occur with Streptococcal infections, severe sunburns, AIDS, as well as with multiple drugs including beta-blockers, lithium, steroid withdrawal, and antimalarials medications.

3-2. **The answer is D** (Chapter 249). The slide shows a KOH prep obtained from a patient with pityriasis versicolor. This condition is caused by an overgrowth of yeast called *Pityrosporum ovale*, otherwise known as *M. furfur*. It is most common in young adults in the summer months. The lesions are asymptomatic, may be hypo- or hyperpigmented, occurring most commonly on the chest or upper back. Selenium sulfide shampoo may be used daily for a week to treat the lesions. Other treatments may include topical ketoconazole, econazole, miconazole, or clotrimazole. Extensive or refractory pityriasis versicolor can be treated with oral ketoconazole 400 mg single dose, repeated at monthly intervals. Fluconazole 400 mg single dose or itraconazole 200 mg/d/7 days or 400 mg single dose are also effective treatments. Permethrin cream is used to treat scabies lesions. Vaseline may be used to treat psoriatic lesions and may be used in hydrocortisone preparations with *Pityriasis rosea*.

3-3. **The answer is B** (Chapter 249). This picture shows lesions of *Molluscum contagiosum*. These lesions may occur in single or multiple lesions. It is spread skin-to-skin contact and is most common in infants, sexually active adults, and immunocompromised individuals. A Giemsa stain of the keratotic core will show intracytoplasmic inclusion bodies or "molluscum bodies." These lesions usually resolve in 6–24 months without specific treatment. Tape may be applied after showers to prevent friction and spread of the lesions. Other treatments that could be prescribed by a dermatologist include topical cantharidin (blister beetle fluid) applied in the office or imiquimod (Aldara) every day three to five times per week at home to speed the resolution of the lesions. Donovan bodies are seen with granuloma inguinale. KOH prep is used to help visualize the hyphae seen in fungal etiologies of skin lesions. Serology is used for syphilis diagnosis. Tzanck smear is used to help diagnose herpes lesions.

3-4. **The answer is B** (Chapter 249). The picture shows a Kaposi sarcoma (KS) on the face of an HIV-infected individual. There are several types of KS including classic or European, non-HIV-related African endemic, HIV-related, and iatrogenic immunosuppressive-associated KS. The lesion is a vascular neoplasia characterized by multisystem involvement. Herpes human virus-8 has been identified in all variants of the lesions. Differential diagnosis includes other vascular neoplasms such as hemangioma, pyogenic granuloma, and bacillary angiomatosis, as well as ecchymosis, insect bites, stasis dermatitis, and pigmented lesions. Treatment does depend on the extent and type of KS. HIV-related cases have improved with highly active antiretroviral therapy. Intralesional chemotherapy with vinblastine, cryotherapy, radiotherapy, laser surgery, or electrosurgery can be used on individual lesions. More aggressive systemic chemotherapy may be required for extensive mucocutaneous or visceral involvement.

3-5. **The answer is A** (Chapter 248). The picture shows an individual with the painful ulceration of a chancroid, caused by *Haemophilus ducreyi*. Local, painful adenopathy is often present. The diagnosis is made clinically. The disease is sexually transmitted. Treatment may include ceftriaxone, azithromycin, and ciprofloxacin. Other painless ulcerations in the differential diagnosis include HSV that may resemble this disease if the vesicles are already broken.

3-6. **The answer is C** (Chapters 247). The picture shows fish tank granuloma caused by *Mycobacterium marinum*. This infection is distinguished from cat scratch fever and primary tuberculosis by the absence of lymphadenopathy. Treatment may include sulfamethoxazole, trimethoprim, tetracyclines, and rifampicin. It is seen rarely and is associated with frequent exposure to bodies of water or who are fish tank cleaners. The infection requires exposure to abraded or traumatized skin.

3-7. **The answer is E** (Chapter 246). The picture shows tinea capitis with a kerion. The most common cause of kerion development is an inflammatory response with infection of tinea capitis. The most common cause of tinea capitis is Trichophyton. Kerion is an inflamed, boggy plaque with pustules and alopecia. It may cause permanent scarring. Diagnosis is based on positive KOH or fungal culture. Trichophyton invade the hair shaft, so may not have a positive KOH. Wood's light

may also be used to help diagnose, but Trichophyton does not fluoresce. First-line treatment is oral griseofulvin.

3-8. **The answer is E** (Chapter 246). The picture shows infantile seborrheic dermatitis. Adults can have seborrheic dermatitis too. Infantile seborrheic dermatitis occurs most commonly in the first 3 months of life and is also known as "cradle cap." Fungal cultures should be done in children up to puberty to exclude tinea capitis as a cause of the lesions. The rash occurs in areas of active sebaceous glands. Certain medications may exacerbate the lesions. Common ones are buspirone, cimetidine, chlorpromazine, haloperidol, and lithium. The infantile form is nonpruritic, and in adults, it may be mildly pruritic. Seborrheic dermatitis is a chronic disorder and treatment includes 1% ketoconazole shampoo for infants and for adults may include antidandruff shampoo or ketoconazole shampoo for scalp lesions. For the face, 1–2.5% hydrocortisone is mainstay applied twice a day. Higher potency steroids should be avoided.

3-9. **The answer is C** (Chapter 246). The pictures show Ramsey Hunt syndrome in an individual with the characteristic lesions of herpes zoster. Ramsey Hunt syndrome occurs when there is involvement of the facial and auditory nerve from the reactivation of the varicella-zoster virus. Pain or dysesthesia will precede the rash by 3–5 days. Lesions on the auditory canal and tympanic membrane along with a Bell's palsy, deafness, or vertigo may suggest the diagnosis. Treatment includes oral acyclovir or valacyclovir for 1 week. HIV patients should only receive acyclovir due to the risk of hemolytic uremic syndrome with valacyclovir. Treatment should be initiated within 72 hours to shorten healing time, decreases new lesion formation, and prevents postherpetic neuralgia.

3-10. **The answer is B** (Chapter 249). The figure shows the characteristic burrows of a scabies infestation. The rash occurs approximately 30 days after exposure to the mite, *Sarcoptes* *scabei*. The rash will typically be more pruritic at night. The distribution of the lesions is different between adult, children, and immunocompromised hosts. Adults typically have lesions on the feet, ankles, wrist, hands, axilla, groin, and extensor surfaces of the extremities. The lesions spare the head and neck. Children have a more generalized distribution that includes the face, scalp, and neck, as well as the diaper area. Immunocompromised hosts may have crusted, confluent plaques that is termed "crusted" or Norwegian scabies. Treatment includes topical Permethrin 5% cream, Lindane shampoo, as well as oral ivermectin. Lindane and oral ivermectin are not safe to treat pregnant women.

3-11. **The answer is A** (Chapter 247). While oral steroids may be indicated in severe cases of allergic contact dermatitis (poison ivy as displayed in the photo), a short burst will likely precipitate worsening of the patient's symptoms upon withdrawal of the steroid. Therefore, 2–3-week tapered dosing is required to attempt to avoid this rebound effect from systemic steroid therapy. Intermediate or low potency topical steroids can be used for symptomatic management. The rule of 9s, which is typically applied to burn patients, can be used to estimate the amount of topical steroids required, and dosing will be less frequent if fluorinated steroid preparations are prescribed. Caution and close monitoring is advised when prescribing steroids to immunosuppressed or diabetic patients.

3-12. **The answer is D** (Chapter 245). Stevens–Johnson syndrome (SJS) is characterized by dermatologic and mucous membrane involvement. Patients complain of malaise, fever, myalgias, and arthralgias. Skin eruptions typically involve epidermal detachment of less than 30%, no greater than 50% of epidermal surfaces. Ophthalmic involvement can occur in almost 70% of cases. Patients with ophthalmic involvement should be monitored by an ophthalmologist. Precipitants of SJS include infections such as mycoplasma and HSV and medications; however, the cause is unknown in 50% of cases. The most frequent complications of SJS and most common cause of death include fluid and electrolyte imbalances and secondary infections. Patients rarely are left with scars unless they develop a superinfection. Be aware that any patient with ophthalmic involvement should be monitored by an ophthalmologist.

3-13. **The answer is D** (Chapter 245). A positive Nikolsky sign occurs when there is a detachment of the epidermis from the dermis with gentle traction on the skin as demonstrated in the photo. Disease processes that exhibit this finding include staphylococcus scalded skin, toxic epidermal necrolysis, and pemphigus vulgaris. Eczema herpeticum, toxic shock syndrome, HSV, bullous pemphigoid, and exfoliative erythroderma all involve detachment of skin but do not demonstrate a positive Nikolsky sign.

3-14. **The answer is E** (Chapter 246). The photo demonstrates Hutchinson's sign, which is the presence of a vesicular eruption on the tip of the nose in an outbreak of varicella zoster virus known as shingles. Zoster lesions present on the nose indicate involvement of the skin innervated by the anterior ethmoidal branch of the nasociliary nerve. Because the nasociliary nerve also innervates the cornea, such skin lesions may indicate ocular involvement. Although HSV is also from the herpes family of viruses, it does not cause zoster; therefore, it is not associated with Hutchinson's sign. Group A strep on the face typically causes erysipelas, which presents with a well-demarcated erythematous plaque involving the cheeks. *S. aureus* often causes impetigo, both bullous and nonbullous forms, but does not present with the eruption seen in the photo. Human papilloma virus eruptions typically do not involve the face or eyes.

3-15. **The answer is D** (Chapter 247). In a diabetic patient with a history of cardiovascular disease presenting with a leg ulcer, with recent hair loss, increased pain, and shiny skin, vascular insufficiency must be considered.

Measurement of ankle-brachial indices as well as performing an arterial duplex are of utmost importance in this case, as severe vascular insufficiency can require emergent intervention by a vascular surgeon. This takes precedence over determining if there is a coexistent deep vein thrombosis, local wound care, or arranging for outpatient wound management, although all of these interventions may be necessary for this patient eventually. Wound cultures of leg ulcers have been shown to be of questionable value and generally are not helpful unless performed in the operating room during wound debridement.

3-16. **The answer is B** (Chapter 247). The figure demonstrates a silver scaly eruption on a salmon-colored base typical of psoriasis. Initial treatment of psoriasis, especially without the intervention of a dermatologist, is high or ultra-high potency topical corticosteroids, including fluocinonide, clobetasol propionate, or betamethasone dipropionate ointment. Tar-containing soaks followed with application of topical corticosteroids are reserved for areas that are difficult to treat, such as the palms and soles, due to the thickness of the skin. Other treatments employed under the care of a dermatologist, often when initial attempts at topical corticosteroids are insufficient, include systemic biologics, such as methotrexate or cyclosporine, acitretin, and psoralen–ultraviolet light A.

3-17. **The answer is D** (Chapter 247). The photo demonstrates the clinical presentation of cutaneous larva migrans, which is an infection caused by a hookworm. Ringworm is a fungal infection of candidal origin, which is not associated with these clinical findings. Cutaneous larva migrans does occur in tropical and subtropical climates worldwide. It typically presents with a pruritic, erythematous serpiginous tract that marks the migration of the larva in the skin. The main portal of entry is exposed feet, which contact feces infested with the larva. It can cause an otherwise asymptomatic eosinophilia on peripheral blood count. One dose of albendazole or ivermectin is adequate for treatment and eradication of the larva.

3-18. **The answer is A** (Chapters 248 and 249). The image demonstrates scabies. Once exposed, it typically takes the immune system approximately 30 days to respond with the development of the intensely pruritic eruptions, which are an immune response to the scabies mite and its excrement within the skin. All of the other options are too short of a timeline for adequate development of immune response and subsequent symptoms.

3-19. **The answer is D** (Chapter 246). The photo demonstrates a photosensitivity reaction. This occurs most commonly with phototoxic medications, including tetracycline, doxycycline, furosemide, amiodarone, fluoroquinolones, and chlorpromazine. Metoprolol does not exhibit phototoxicity.

3-20. **The answer is D** (Chapter 249). The photo demonstrates a classic presentation of erythema migrans, a stage 1 dermatologic finding associated with Lyme borreliosis. IgM antibodies to this infection are developed prior to IgG, with a peak between 3 and 6 weeks after initial exposure. IgG antibodies can take months to develop and infer previous infection, rather than active acute infection. The erythema migrans rash typically presents as a macule or papule initially, which develops an expanding annular lesion with central clearing. It is not typically pruritic or painful, but a burning sensation is possible. Most of these lesions fade within 1 month of presentation. The spirochete causing this infection can spread to multiple organ systems hematogenously, and has a predilection for the skin, nervous system, and joints, causing the typical clinical findings in stages 2 and 3 of the disease.

Endocrine and Electrolytes Emergencies
Questions

4-1. A 37-year-old male presents to the ED with altered mental status. He was found unconscious in the bathroom at work. On exam, he is arousable to painful stimulus, muttering incoherently. His airway is intact and he has bilateral breath sounds. His initial vital signs are blood pressure (BP) 95/47, P 110, respiratory rate (RR) 14, O_2% 97% on room air, T 99.4. He has dry mucus membranes. Fingerstick glucose is 396. Lab work reveals a normal CBC, 3 + acetone, Na 121, Cl^- 97, HCO_3 9, K 3.0, Mg 2.9, Phos 1.5, AG 29. Which of the following is the first priority in caring for this patient?

(A) IV bicarbonate
(B) IV lactated ringers
(C) IV phosphate
(D) IV potassium
(E) IV saline

4-2. A 75-year-old female is brought to the ED by her family. Her family states that over the last few months, she has been complaining of generalized weakness and fatigue. The family became concerned because she had not wanted to get out of bed the last 2 days despite the fact that she is normally very active. On exam, the patient answers questions slowly, stating that she stopped taking her thyroid medicine and her BP medicine several months ago. Her vital signs are BP 92/61, HR 57, RR 14, 100% RA, T 95.9. Her finger stick glucose is 99. The patient receives warm blankets, IV fluids, and oxygen. She also receives a dose of steroids. Which of the following is the most appropriate next step in the management of this patient?

(A) Atropine
(B) D_5NS
(C) Inotropes
(D) T4
(E) T4 plus T3

4-3. A 37-year-old female presents to the ED complaining of palpitations and dyspnea. Her vital signs reveal tachycardia, hypertension, and a fever of 104.1°F. She is breathing rapidly and her O_2 saturation is 99% on room air. She is thin and anxious. Her ECG shows atrial fibrillation. She denies drug use and has not had any recent illnesses. Her neck is shown below (Figure 4-1). After initiating supportive care, which of the following describes the appropriate treatment priorities for this patient?

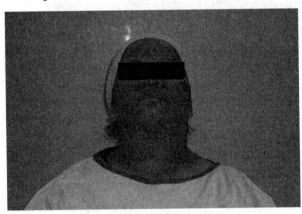

Figure 4-1. Reproduced with permission from Tintinalli JE, Stapczynski JS, Ma OJ, Cline DM, Cydulka RK, Meckler GD: *Tintinalli's Emergency Medicine: A Comprehensive Study Guide*, 7th Edition. Copyright © 2011 The McGraw-Hill Companies, Inc.

(A) Dexamethasone, PTU, iodine, propranolol
(B) Iodine, propranolol, dexamethasone, PTU
(C) Propranolol, dexamethasone, PTU, iodine
(D) PTU, iodine, propranolol, dexamethasone
(E) Propranolol, PTU, iodine, dexamethasone

4-4. What is the most likely cause of the previous patient's symptoms?

(A) Grave's disease
(B) Lithium therapy
(C) Pituitary tumors
(D) Thyroiditis
(E) Toxic nodular goiters

4-5. What is the most common cause of primary adrenal insufficiency (AI) in the United States?

(A) Autoimmune disorders
(B) Adrenal hemorrhage

(C) Drugs
(D) Idiopathic
(E) Infectious

4-6. A 64-year-old female is brought in by her family for right-sided paralysis. The family states the patient was watching TV and had sudden onset of slurred speech 35 minutes ago. When she tried to get up and walk, she was unable to move her right side. The family states that she thinks she has had the flu for a few days but no fever, cough, or abdominal pain. She has a past medical history of diabetes and hypertension. She takes metformin, glyburide, and metoprolol. She has not had any changes in her medications. Her vital signs show a BP of 169/93, heart rate of 56, RR of 12, and her pulse oximetry of 99% on 2 L. She is speaking to you but has a right-sided facial droop and a right-sided motor deficit. Which of the following is the first step in this patient's management?

(A) CT angiogram of head
(B) ECG
(C) Glucose level
(D) Lactate level
(E) MRI of head

4-7. The previous patient's right-sided paralysis resolves after intervention. She is sitting comfortably with her family, eating lunch, and asking when she can go home. Her CBC, chemistry panel, chest x-ray, and urinalysis are all normal. Which of the following is the most appropriate next step in the management of this patient?

(A) Admission for observation
(B) Broad-spectrum antibiotics and admission
(C) Discharge home with oral antibiotics
(D) Discharge home with precautions to return to ED.
(E) Observe for another 2 hours and if normal finger stick, discharge home.

4-8. A 29-year-old male is brought in by EMS after being found by a friend stuporous in his apartment. His friend tells you that the patient is a migrant construction worker from Mexico and had not shown up for work for the past 5 days. As far as the friend knows, the patient has no medical problems and does not use drugs or alcohol. He is unsure about the patient's family medical history. EMS reports that the patient's glucose was "high" (>600). His vital signs reveal hypotension and tachycardia. On exam, the patient is stuporous, has dry mucous membranes, clear lung fields, and poor skin turgor. His abdomen is soft and nontender. The patient receives two large bore IVs and 2 L of normal saline (NS). His vital signs remain normal and the patient is able to answer simple questions. On neurological exam, the patient has profound weakness in his upper and lower extremities. Which of the following electrolyte abnormalities pose the most immediate risk for bad outcome in this patient?

(A) Chloride
(B) Glucose
(C) Magnesium
(D) Potassium
(E) Sodium

4-9. A 52-year-old noninsulin-dependent diabetic male presents to the ED complaining of a 4-cm ulcer to his foot. He states that the pain has gotten much worse. It has become progressively red and warm, and he has had fevers up to 103.1°F today. He states that for the last 2 days his blood sugars have been ranging between 300 and 400. His vital signs are BP 101/69, P 122, RR 16, normal oxygen saturation, and an oral temperature of 102.9°F. On exam, the patient has a 4-cm deep ulcer to the medial calf with significant surrounding erythema and 3–4 cm of streaking up the calf. What is the antibiotic of choice for this patient?

(A) Amoxicillin–clavulanate
(B) Ampicillin–sulbactam
(C) Cephalexin

(D) Imipenem–cilastin
(E) Ticarcillin–clavulanate

4-10. A 34-year-old male with no past medical history presents to the ED complaining of 1 day of nausea, vomiting, and epigastric pain after drinking "a lot" over the weekend. He denies hematemesis, bright red blood per rectum or melena. He states that he has never been much of a drinker but drank excessively this weekend when some college friends were in town. He has vomited more than 15 times and has not been eating much because of the nausea and vomiting. His finger stick glucose is 97 and his vital signs are stable. His exam is significant for dry mucous membranes. He is anicteric. His abdomen is soft with mild discomfort in the epigastric region with no abdominal distention, masses, rebound, or guarding. Which of the following is MOST important in determining the patient's diagnosis?

(A) Electrolytes
(B) Improvement with GI cocktail.
(C) Lipase
(D) Ultrasound of gallbladder
(E) Urine ketones

4-11. Which of the following is a frequent cause of hypokalemia in ED patients?

(A) β-Adrenergic therapy
(B) Diuretic therapy
(C) Lithium therapy
(D) Poor dietary intake
(E) Primary aldosteronism

4-12. A 27-year-old patient with a history of cystic fibrosis presents to the ED complaining of 2 days of gradual onset throbbing headache. She has had no fevers, chills, upper respiratory infection symptoms, and has never gotten headaches before. She is very healthy and has been going to the gym a lot in the last 2 weeks. Her husband states that she has been "grumpy" the last day or two and he has noticed she occasionally has resting "muscle twitches." She does not drink alcohol, smoke, or use illegal drugs. Her last hospitalization was more than 2 years ago. Her vital signs are within normal range and she is afebrile. The patient proceeds to have a grand mal seizure in the ED and while the nurse is giving IV benzodiazepines, the laboratory calls you for a serum sodium level of 109. Which of the following is the most appropriate rate for a 3% sodium chloride infusion?

(A) 5 mL/hour
(B) 50 mL/hour
(C) 150 mL/hour
(D) 250 mL/hour
(E) 400 mL/hour

4-13. A 52-year-old male with no past medical history complains of tremulousness and increased irritability. His primary care provider sent him to the ED because on exam, his sodium was 161 mEq/L, urine osmolality was 226, and his serum osmolality was 283. Which of the following is the most appropriate next step in diagnosis?

(A) Aldosterone level
(B) Cortisol level
(C) Corticotrophin stimulation test
(D) Thyroid-stimulating hormone level
(E) Water deprivation test

4-14. A 16-year-old female with acne complains of blurry vision, anorexia, myalgias, and hair loss. What vitamin is causing these symptoms?

(A) Vitamin A
(B) Vitamin B
(C) Vitamin D

(D) Vitamin E
(E) Vitamin K

4-15. A 46-year-old male with high cholesterol presents with face, neck, and chest burning, itching and redness after taking something from an herb shop to help his cholesterol. Which of the following is the etiology for this patient's symptoms?

(A) Vitamin B_1
(B) Vitamin B_3
(C) Vitamin D
(D) Vitamin E
(E) Vitamin K

4-16. A 49-year-old male with a history of chronic renal insufficiency is referred to the ED for palpitations and fatigue. His potassium level was found to be 6.1 by his primary doctor. Upon arrival, the patient has a heart rate of 56, a widened QRS on ECG, and a BP of 110/76. He is speaking to you, his lungs are clear bilaterally, and his oxygen saturation is 100% on 2 L NC. He has a large bore IV and is placed on the monitor. Which of the following is the most appropriate initial treatment for this patient with severe hyperkalemia?

(A) Albuterol nebulizer
(B) Calcium chloride
(C) Insulin and glucose
(D) Sodium bicarbonate
(E) Sodium polystyrene sulfonate

Use the following case to answer questions 4-17 and 4-18.

A 66-year-old female with no past medical history presents to the emergency department with increasing lethargy. The family states that she is normally healthy, but has been losing weight (unintentionally) over the past few months. The last week, she has been complaining of abdominal pain, frequent urination, and pain in her arms and legs. She has had no cough, headache, fevers, or chills. On exam, the patient is arousable to stimulus but is confused, is afebrile, and has normal vital signs. She is moving all extremities and her exam is unremarkable. Her ECG shows ST segment depressions, widened T waves, and a shortened ST and QT interval. Her glucose on finger stick is 98. Her CBC is within normal limits. The laboratory notifies you because her calcium level is 14.2 mg/dL, magnesium level is 1.1 mEq/L, and phosphate level is 1.9 mEq/L.

4-17. Which of the following is the most appropriate medication for this patient?

(A) Calcitonin

(B) Hydrocortisone

(C) Magnesium

(D) Normal saline

(E) Phosphate

4-18. Which of the following is the most likely explanation for this patient's hypercalcemia?

(A) Hyperparathyroidism

(B) Lithium toxicity

(C) Malignancy

(D) Paget's disease

(E) Sarcoidosis

4-19. You are called to see a 35-year-old liver transplant patient on immunosuppressant therapy who has been admitted for vomiting and diarrhea but is boarding in the ED. The nurse is concerned because the hospitalist ordered a blood gas and she cannot get a hold of them to address the abnormal values. The patient is hemodynamically stable and has received 2 L of NS. The blood gas shows pH 7.44, pCO_2 48, HCO_3 32.6, base excess 7.3, pO_2 100. What is the patient's acid–base status?

(A) Metabolic acidosis

(B) Metabolic acidosis with respiratory alkalosis

(C) Metabolic alkalosis

(D) Metabolic alkalosis with respiratory acidosis

(E) Normal acid–base status

4-20. A 24-year-old female vegetarian (no dairy/animal by-products) training for a marathon for 1 month presents with persistent cracked lips, a reddened tongue, and eczema of the face and genitalia. What vitamin deficiency is causing her symptoms?

(A) Vitamin A

(B) Vitamin B_1

(C) Vitamin B_2

(D) Vitamin B_{12}

(E) Vitamin K

4-21. A 39-year-old alcoholic presents with ataxia, confusion, and confabulations. What vitamin deficiency is causing these symptoms?

(A) Vitamin A

(B) Vitamin B_1

(C) Vitamin B_6

(D) Vitamin B_{12}

(E) Vitamin C

4-22. A 67-year-old female presents with bilateral hand and feet paresthesias, decreased proprioception, anemia, and an elevated lactate dehydrogenase level. What vitamin deficiency is causing her symptoms?

(A) Vitamin A

(B) Vitamin B_1

(C) Vitamin B_2

(D) Vitamin B_{12}

(E) Vitamin K

4-23. A 20-year-old male presents to the ED complaining of several weeks of fatigue. He has not had any fevers, chills, cold symptoms, or cough. He has never traveled out of the country. His vital signs are all within normal range. On review of systems, he does state that he has frequent urination and has been drinking more fluids than normal because he feels that he is always thirsty. He ate lunch an hour ago and his finger stick is 279. His serum acetone is negative and his anion gap, potassium, bicarbonate, and sodium levels are all within normal limits. His serum glucose is 283. He receives 2 L of NS in the ED and 6 units of subcutaneous insulin. His repeat glucose is 119. Which of the following is the most appropriate step in this patient's care?

(A) Admit to the hospital for new onset diabetes rehydration and insulin.

(B) Admit to the hospital for fasting glucose and oral glucose tolerance test (OGTT).

(C) Discharge home with diabetic instructions and follow-up in 24–48 hours.

(D) Discharge home with metformin and follow-up with 24–48 hours.

(E) Schedule for outpatient fasting glucose and oral glucose tolerance test (OGTT).

4-24. Which of the following causes an anion gap acidosis solely by the production of lactate?

(A) Ethylene glycol

(B) Iron

(C) Ketoacidosis

(D) Methanol

(E) Uremia

Endocrine and Electrolytes Emergencies
Answers and Explanations

4-1. **The answer is E** (Chapter 220). In patients with diabetes mellitus, it is very important to prioritize therapeutic interventions. The order of therapeutic priorities is volume resuscitation first and foremost. Patients often have a fluid deficit of 5–10 L. Potassium deficits should be addressed next. Diabetic ketoacidosis (DKA) patients often have profound total-body potassium deficits. For an initial potassium level between 3.3 and 5.3 mEq/L, with established urine output, potassium should be replaced at a rate of 10 mEq KCL per hour for 4 hours. Insulin may be given, but only after volume resuscitation and potassium deficits have been addressed. It may be administered at a bolus of 0.1 units/kg and followed by a drip of 0.1 units/kg per hour. In general, IV phosphate therapy should only be initiated if the serum level is <1.0 mg/dL. Routine use of IV bicarbonate is not recommended in the treatment of DKA.

4-2. **The answer is E** (Chapter 223). After supportive care has been initiated, the next steps involve replacing thyroid hormones and identifying and treating the precipitating factors. In this case, the patient was noncompliant with medications. It is important not to wait for lab results before initiating treatment. IV T4 should be given in combination with T3 because conversion of T4 to T3 in myxedema coma is often reduced. T4 alone has a slow and steady onset of action. T3 alone has a more rapid onset but levels fluc-

tuate rapidly. Causes of hypothyroidism include autoimmune (Hashimoto's), ablation, thyroiditis, infiltrative disease, congenital, panhypopituitarism, neoplasms, drugs such as amiodarone, lithium, or iodine, and idiopathic.

4-3. **The answer is D** (Chapter 224) The treatment of thyroid storm is complicated because the physician must take into account the neogenesis of thyroid hormone. Stopping the thyroid gland from synthesizing new thyroid hormone needs to occur prior to starting iodine therapy as this will prevent the stimulation of new thyroid hormone. After supportive care, thionamides (PTU or methimazole) should be given to decrease the new hormone production. PTU is preferred over methimazole because it also can inhibit the conversion of T4 to T3. At least 1 hour later, iodine therapy may be started. This will block the release of thyroid hormone. If there is concern for either amiodarone-induced or iodine overload-induced hyperthyroidism, lithium should be used instead of iodine. Propranolol is given to help block the direct effects of the thyroid hormone. It is contraindicated in reactive airway disease, CHF, pregnancy, and diabetes. Glucocorticoid therapy, either dexamethasone or hydrocortisone, block peripheral conversion of T4 to T3 and improve survival rates from thyroid storm.

4-4. **The answer is A** (Chapter 224). The most common cause of hyperthyroidism is Grave's disease. In general, hypothyroidism is 10 times more common in women than in men. Grave disease is most common in the third and fourth decades of life. It is caused by an autoimmune thyroid-stimulating antibody. Toxic multinodular and toxic nodular goiters are the next most frequent etiologies; however, these usually present in older patients, often with a history of an uncomplicated goiter. Other less common causes are thyroiditis, pituitary adenomas, metastatic thyroid cancer, and dermoid tumors. Lithium, iodine, and thyroid medications can also cause hyperthyroidism.

4-5. **The answer is A** (Chapter 225). Approximately 70% of primary AI is caused by autoimmune disorders. Adrenal hemorrhage and thrombosis are usually caused by meningococcal sepsis, coagulation disorders (including anticoagulation therapy), Waterhouse-Frederickson syndrome, trauma, and antiphospholipids syndrome. Drugs such as ketoconazole and adrenolytic agents such as metyrapone, aminoglutethimide, and mitotane can also cause primary AI. Worldwide, the most common infectious agent causing primary AI is tuberculosis. In the United States, the most common infectious agent is HIV/AIDS.

4-6. **The answer is C** (Chapter 218). Although neurological causes such as cerebrovascular events and transient ischemic attacks are high on the differential diagnosis, it is important to recognize that hypoglycemia may manifest in a stroke-like syndrome. In any patient where stroke is suspected, a bedside glucose level should be attained prior to the patient receiving further evaluation.

4-7. **The answer is A** (Chapters 161 and 219). Hypoglycemia is a known complication in the treatment of diabetes. In patients who are taking sulfonylureas, a search for underlying causes should be sought. This patient has no evidence of an infection, so treatment with antibiotics is not indicated. Patients on sulfonylureas, medium- to long-acting

insulins, or meglitinides should be admitted for serial glucose monitoring and treatment.

4-8. **The answer is D** (Chapter 222). This patient is likely suffering from a hyperosmolar hyperglycemic state (HHS). His glucose is greater than 600 mg/dL. While all of the labs are helpful, the most important electrolyte abnormality is hypokalemia and should be anticipated. As treatment of HHS with fluids and insulin often alter the serum potassium levels, the importance of monitoring of serum potassium levels and repletion cannot be overemphasized. Serum sodium is often abnormal in patients with HHS. They often have low sodium levels. In severe hyperglycemia, the sodium must be corrected for with the formula: corrected [Na] = measured [Na] + [1.6 × (glucose − 100)]/100.

4-9. **The correct answer is D** (Chapter 219). Lower extremity infections in diabetic patients are classified as non–limb-threatening, limb threatening, or life threatening. Non–limb-threatening infections do not involve deep structures or bone and are often from a recent injury. The patient will have no signs of systemic toxicity or leukocytosis and may be treated with cephalexin, clindamycin, dicloxacillin, or amoxicillin–clavulanate. Patients with limb-threatening infections will have a wound with greater than 2 cm of surrounding cellulitis, ascending lymphangitis, an area of large necrotic tissue, involvement of bone or deep structures, full-thickness ulceration or abscess, and gangrene surrounding the ulcer or lower extremity ischemia. Limb-threatening patients may be treated with ampicillin–sulbactam, ticarcillin–clavulanate, second-generation cephalosporin, clindamycin plus ciprofloxacin or ceftriaxone, or an oral fluoroquinolone plus oral clindamycin. Patients with a life-threatening infection will exhibit signs of sepsis such as fever, leukocytosis, hypotension, tachycardia, tachypnea, altered mental status, and metabolic abnormalities. They should be treated with imipenem–cilastatin, ampicillin–sulbactam plus tobramycin, or vancomycin plus metronidazole plus aztreonam.

4-10. **The answer is A** (Chapter 221). Although alcoholic ketoacidosis (AKA) is most common in chronic alcoholics, it also occurs in first time binge drinkers. Patients usually present with nonspecific complaints of abdominal pain, nausea, and vomiting. The anion gap in AKA is positive and ranges between 16 and 33 and is caused by ketonemia, primarily from β-hydroxybutyrate. The blood glucose ranges from low to mildly elevated. Urine ketones may be often low or negative initially as the nitroprusside reagent used to measure urine and serum ketones only measure acetoacetate. Acetone and β-hydroxybutyrate are not reactive and are more common early in the process of AKA. Gastritis can accompany AKA; however, improvement of symptoms with a "GI cocktail" does not rule out AKA, and without a high suspicion, AKA might be missed. Pancreatitis may also accompany AKA, but this patient does not have a history and physical consistent with pancreatitis. The patient's exam and history are also not consistent with gallbladder disease, so an ultrasound would not aid in making the diagnosis of AKA.

4-11. **The answer is B** (Chapter 21). Frequent causes of hypokalemia in ED patients are alkalosis, gastrointestinal loss (vomiting, diarrhea, nasogastric suctioning, etc.), and diuretic therapy. Other less common causes are from sweat loss, other causes of renal loss (primary or secondary aldosteronism, renal tubular acidosis, postobstructive diuresis, licorice ingestion, and osmotic diuresis), extracellular to intracellular potassium shifts such as hypokalemic periodic paralysis, and increased plasma insulin. Symptoms of hypokalemia such as hypertension, orthostatic hypotension, dysrhythmias, weakness, cramps, paralysis, and hyporeflexia usually present when potassium levels are below 2.5 mEq/L. Potassium should be replaced either orally with 20 mEq of K^+ every 60 minutes until anticipated results are achieved, or through a peripheral IV. No more than 40 mEq should be added to each liter of IV fluid and infusion rates should be no greater than 20 mEq/hour.

4-12. **The answer is B** (Chapter 21). It is important to know how to treat seizures caused by hyponatremia as too rapid of a correction may lead to central pontine myelinolysis. Administration of 3% saline should be considered when hyponatremia is severe (<120 mEq/L), develops rapidly (>0.5 mEq/L, decrease in serum Na per hour), or when patients are in extremis (i.e., seizure or coma). The dosage is 25–100 mL/hour and requires close observation of serum sodium levels. To reduce the risk of complications from rapid correction of sodium deficits, sodium levels should not rise more than 0.5–1.0 mEq/L per hour. If seizures are present, the rise in sodium can be increased to 1.0–2.0 mEq/L per hour. In patients with hyponatremia, it is important to assess volume status. This patient presents with a euvolemic hyponatremia, most likely caused by her cystic fibrosis. In patients who present with hyponatremia and volume overload (pulmonary edema, ascites, pitting edema), syndrome of inappropriate antidiuretic hormone should be considered.

4-13. **The answer is E** (Chapter 21). The patient has diabetes insipidus (DI), which can be central or nephrogenic. In DI, patients have increased sodium levels, abnormally low urine osmolality, and an increased serum osmolality. His irritability and tremulousness is a result of his elevated serum osmolality. To determine if the DI is central or peripheral, the patient must undergo a water deprivation test. In DI, the urine will fail to show increasing urine osmolality. Once this occurs, aqueous vasopressin is administered subcutaneously. Central DI will respond to the vasopressin causing an increase in urine osmolality. Patients with nephrogenic diabetes will fail to show increases in their urine osmolality. Patients with hypoaldosteronism, for which an aldosterone level might be useful, often present with postural hypotension, anorexia, weight loss, asthenia, hyperpigmentation, and/or elevated potassium levels. Serum cortisol levels can be utilized to detect Addison disease, hypopituitarism, and Cushing syndrome. A corticotrophin stimulation test is used to differentiate between primary or secondary adrenal insufficiency. A thyroid-stimulating hormone level would help differentiate thyroid abnormalities, which do not usually present with elevations of sodium.

4-14. **The answer is A** (Chapter 199). Vitamin A comes in two primary forms: retinol, which is commonly used to treat acne, and 3-dehydroretinol. Symptoms of overdose include blurred vision, appetite loss, abnormal skin pigmentation, loss of hair, and occasionally pseudotumor cerebri. Treatment is withdrawal of vitamin A.

4-15. **The answer is B** (Chapter 199). Vitamin B_3, niacin, is both a prescribed and over-the-counter therapy for high cholesterol. In doses greater than 100 mg, niacin ingestion triggers a histamine release with resultant vasodilation causing uncomfortable face, neck, and chest flushing and itching. Antihistamines can be used to ameliorate the symptoms. Vitamin B_1, thiamine, is not generally stored in the body in significant quantities and thus does not generally cause problems with large dose ingestions. Vitamin D toxicity generally requires massive doses (1000–3000 IU/kg) with symptoms manifesting in 2–8 days. Patients can present with anorexia, nausea, abdominal pain, lethargy, weight loss, polyuria, constipation, confusion, and coma. Treatment involves discontinuing vitamin D supplements and the reduction in calcium intake. Vitamin E is composed of eight different fat-soluble compounds. At high doses, vitamin E increases vitamin K requirements and inhibits platelet aggregation. Fatigue, nausea, and blurry vision may also be encountered in adults who ingest toxic doses of vitamin E. Vitamin K is important in several steps of the coagulation pathway. Toxic doses can cause hemolytic anemia, kernicterus, and hemoglobinuria in premature

infants. In adults, it may cause renal and liver damage.

4-16. **The answer is B** (Chapter 21). While all the answers are therapeutic interventions, it is important to recognize which drug should be given first in a patient with elevated potassium and a wide QRS. Calcium chloride is a cardiac membrane stabilizer and has an onset of action within 1–3 minutes and lasts between 30 and 50 minutes. Calcium carbonate may also be used, but calcium chloride has three times the amount of calcium as calcium carbonate. Albuterol may be given to help shift potassium intracellularly, but its onset of action is approximately 15–30 minutes. It lasts between 2 and 4 hours. Insulin and glucose also work to shift potassium into the cell and has an onset of action of approximately 30 minutes and lasts between 4 and 6 hours. Sodium bicarbonate also shifts potassium intracellularly and works within 5–10 minutes and lasts between 1 and 2 hours. Sodium polystyrene sulfonate acts to increase GI potassium excretion. Its time of onset is 1–2 hours and its effects last 4–6 hours.

4-17. **The answer is D** (Chapter 21). Treatment of hypercalcemia should begin in the ED if patients are symptomatic or if the calcium level is greater than 14 mg/dL. The first component of treatment is for volume repletion with NS. Once volume repletion has been accomplished, furosemide may be added to increase the renal calcium excretion. To decrease absorption of calcium from the bones, calcitonin may be given. Hydrocortisone has been shown to be useful in patients with hypercalcemia caused by sarcoidosis, vitamin D toxicity, multiple myeloma, leukemia, or breast cancer. IV phosphates are no longer used in patients with elevated calcium levels.

4-18. **The answer is C** (Chapter 21). The most common causes of hypercalcemia in the ED are malignancy, particularly lung, breast, kidney, myeloma, and leukemia. Primary hyperparathyroidism is also a frequent cause of elevated calcium levels, but is not as common in the ED. Drugs such as lithium and thiazides can also raise calcium levels. Granulomatous diseases are also known to increase serum calcium levels.

4-19. **The answer is D** (Chapter 19). It is important to recognize that the pH is the least important component of an ABG in assessing a patient's acid–base status. Acidosis is any process that increases the H^+ concentration. Any condition that decreases it is called an alkalosis. Acid–base disorders are further separated into respiratory or metabolic. Respiratory disorders represent changes in the pCO_2, whereas metabolic disorders represent changes in the HCO_3. This patient has an elevated HCO_3 and a mildly elevated pCO_2, which represents the poorly understood relationship between pCO_2 in the alveoli and H^+. Metabolic alkalosis is classified as either chloride sensitive or chloride insensitive.

4-20. **The answer is C** (Chapter 199). Vitamin B_2, riboflavin, is found in meats, dairy, and leafy green vegetables. It is not stored in the body and must be replaced daily. It is important in the metabolism of fats, proteins, and carbohydrates. Vigorous exercise will significantly increase the body's need for riboflavin.

4-21. **The answer is B** (Chapter 199). Wernicke–Korsakoff syndrome is a complication seen most often in malnourished chronic alcoholics who are suffering from a vitamin B_1 deficiency. Wernicke encephalopathy is believed to be the result of an acute deficiency thiamine. Korsakoff syndrome is believed to be a chronic long-term sequela of Wernicke encephalopathy. The administration of thiamine prior to administering D_{50} to avoid precipitation of Wernicke encephalopathy is unfounded. Thiamine is excreted in the urine and therefore toxic levels are relatively unheard of.

4-22. **The answer is D** (Chapter 199). Vitamin B_{12} deficiency causes pernicious anemia. Vitamin B_{12} takes several forms: cyanocobalamin, hydroxocobalamin, aquocobalamin, nitrito-cobalamin, coenzyme B_{12}, and methylcobalamin. Deficiencies are usually a result of absorption problems rather than dietary deficiencies. It is a potent molecule and thus small doses are needed to correct the deficiency.

4-23. **The answer is C** (Chapter 219). Diabetes mellitus may be diagnosed in three ways: symptoms of diabetes plus a random glucose ≥ 200 mg/dL, a fasting plasma glucose ≥ 126 mg/dL, or a 2-hour plasma glucose level ≥ 200 mg/dL during an oral glucose tolerance test. Patients who are nonpregnant adults, stable, do not have life-threatening metabolic decompensation, and with no comorbid illnesses are safe to be discharged with appropriate diabetes instructions with follow-up within 1–2 days. Although metformin is a relatively safe drug to start, it is not recommended to start in the ED.

4-24. **The answer is B** (Chapter 19). Elevated anion gaps are usually associated with metabolic acidosis. While the differential for elevated anion gap acidosis is broad, it is important to separate out processes that cause the elevation directly and those that cause it indirectly by producing lactate. Without this separation, important components in the differential for lactic acidosis will be missed. Biguanides, cyanide, iron, and theophylline are not unmeasured ions causing an elevated anion gap. These substances actually raise the anion gap by producing a lactic acidosis.

Environmental Disorders
Questions

5-1. A 40-year-old homeless alcoholic man presents to the ED complaining of foot numbness. He has been sleeping in a drainage culvert to stay out of the wind. Nighttime temperatures have been well above freezing, but it has rained steadily for the past 5 days. His feet are pale and numb. They develop severe burning pain on rewarming. What is the most likely diagnosis?

(A) Chilblains
(B) Cold urticaria
(C) Frostbite
(D) Trench foot
(E) Panniculitis

5-2. Which of the following describes the most appropriate treatment for frostbite?

(A) Debridement of blisters and early amputation to prevent spread of tissue damage
(B) Immediate rewarming by any means possible in the field
(C) Heparin and prophylactic antibiotics in all cases
(D) Rapid rewarming in warm water bath and aloe vera cream for blisters
(E) Early mobilization for lower extremity injuries and CT scan to assess degree of injury

5-3. Which of the following conditions is most likely to be observed in an alcoholic man found in an alley in January with a core temperature of 31°C?

(A) Delta wave on the ECG
(B) Coma

(C) Hypercoagulability
(D) Respiratory distress
(E) Volume overload

5-4. An 82-year-old man is brought in by ambulance during a summer heat wave unresponsive with a rectal temperature of 41°C and dry skin. He lives alone in a trailer without air conditioning. No medications were found by emergency medical services (EMS) on the scene. Which of the following is the most appropriate initial management?

(A) Cooling to body temperature of 37°C by immersion bath
(B) CT scan of brain, serum and urine toxicological screens, and cooling blanket
(C) Evaporative cooling and fluid resuscitation
(D) Rectal acetaminophen, blood cultures, and broad-spectrum antibiotics
(E) Thyroid function tests and administration of dantrolene sodium

5-5. A 47-year-old man was moving wooden logs at a construction site when he was bit on the hand by "some bug." The bite was immediately painful and is now red and swollen. His arm began to ache and he now presents hypertensive with severe back pain. Which of the following is the most likely culprit?

(A) Bark scorpion (*Centruroides exilicauda*)
(B) Black widow spider (*Latrodectus mactans*)
(C) Brown recluse spider (*Loxosceles reclusa*)
(D) Hobo spider (*Tegenaria agrestis*)
(E) Yellow jacket (Hymenoptera)

5-6. Which is the best immediate treatment for anaphylaxis due to a Hymenoptera sting?

(A) Corticosteroids and H2-receptor antagonists

(B) Epinephrine intramuscularly and antihistamines

(C) Epinephrine intravenously and antivenom

(D) Removal of stinger and nonsteroidal anti-inflammatory agent

(E) Venom immunotherapy and discharge with a prescription for an epinephrine autoinjector (e.g., Epi-pen™).

5-7. Which of the following is an indication for polyvalent Crotalidae Immune Fab (CroFab™) administration after a rattlesnake bite?

(A) Elevated platelets

(B) Hypertension

(C) Localized pain and redness

(D) Progressive pain and swelling

(E) Normal prothrombin time (PT)

5-8. A 35-year-old woman presents with a red, swollen, hot foot that is draining pus out of a wound she sustained while snorkeling in the ocean last week. Which of the following organisms is the LEAST likely to be implicated?

(A) *Aeromonas* spp.

(B) *Mycobacterium marinum*

(C) Beta-hemolytic streptococci

(D) *Staphylococcus aureus*

(E) *Vibrio* spp.

5-9. Which of the following diving injuries is correctly paired with its appropriate treatment?

(A) Arterial gas embolism—heparin and thrombolytics

(B) Decompression sickness—recompression with hyperbaric oxygen

(C) Nitrogen narcosis—recompression with hyperbaric oxygen

(D) Pulmonary barotrauma—recompression with hyperbaric oxygen

(E) Sinus barotrauma—immediate otolaryngology consult

5-10. Which of the following submersion injury patients has the best prognosis?

(A) 8-year-old child pulled from an icy lake after a brief submersion; no cardiopulmonary resuscitation (CPR) was required on scene

(B) 75-year-old man with Alzheimer's who was recovered from his neighbor's swimming pool after a witnessed fall and submersion; CPR was performed by bystanders and the patient remained unconscious on arrival to the ED

(C) 16-year-old boy found floating in a swimming pool after drinking at a party; bystanders performed CPR and CPR was ongoing in ED

(D) 30-year-old man with history of epilepsy who had a seizure in a hot spring and was asystolic on arrival of the paramedics

(E) 2-year-old child who fell into a warm fresh water lake; bystanders performed CPR and patient was resuscitated by the paramedics

5-11. A 48-year-old alcoholic woman is brought in by EMS from a house fire. The patient is awake and on oxygen. Which of the following is true in evaluating and managing her respiratory status?

(A) Absence of stridor or wheezing excludes lower airway edema

(B) Carboxyhemoglobin (COHb) measurement is not helpful

(C) Inhalation injury is excluded if the initial chest radiograph is normal

(D) Intubation should be avoided if she has circumferential neck burns

(E) Singed nasal hair, soot in mouth, and carbonaceous sputum are useful indicators of smoke inhalation

5-12. Which of the following is NOT correct treatment for the burn patient?

(A) Fluids to maintain urine output at 1 mL/kg/hr for a child with 50% body surface area (BSA) partial thickness burns

(B) High doses of intravenous morphine for a 20% BSA partial thickness burn in a 30-year-old healthy man

(C) Referral to a burn center for an 18% BSA partial thickness burn in a 69-year-old diabetic man

(D) Prophylactic systemic antibiotics and tetanus toxoid for a 3% BSA full-thickness burn to the arm in a 45-year-old woman with no known medical problems

(E) Topical bacitracin ointment and 24-hour recheck for a 5% BSA partial-thickness burn to leg of a 16-year-old boy

5-13. Which of the following statements is TRUE regarding chemical burns?

(A) Acids generally require longer irrigation times than alkalis.

(B) Acetic acid burns may be associated with serious systemic toxicity.

(C) Earlier irrigation is associated with improved prognosis.

(D) The is no benefit to use of calcium gluconate over irrigation with water in hydrofluoric acid burns.

(E) Most chemical burns to the eye can be treated with delayed outpatient ophthalmology referral.

5-14. Which of the following is NOT a complication of high-voltage electric injury?

(A) Blunt trauma from being hurled from the source

(B) Cardiac or respiratory arrest

(C) Compartment syndrome

(D) Fern pattern burn

(E) Tetanic contractions

5-15. A 37-year-old man is brought in by EMS from a golf course after a lightening strike. He was rapidly resuscitated on the scene. Which of the following is LEAST likely to be observed in this patient?

(A) Cataracts

(B) Compartment syndrome ✓

(C) ECG abnormalities

(D) Lower extremity paralysis

(E) Tympanic membrane rupture

5-16. A 30-year-old man presents with hallucinations, tachycardia, and ataxia after eating some mushrooms his roommate brought home from a camping trip. What is the most appropriate therapy?

(A) Activated charcoal and monitoring of liver enzymes

(B) Atropine and intravenous fluids

(C) Immediate evaluation for liver transplant

(D) Intravenous hydration and antiemetics

(E) Supportive care and observation with benzodiazepines if need for sedation

5-17. Ingestion of which of the following plants is NOT associated with life-threatening toxicity?

(A) Castor bean

(B) Foxglove

(C) Jimsonweed

(D) Oleander

(E) Water hemlock

5-18. Which of the following medications is the best choice for treating mild to moderate acute mountain sickness?

(A) Acetazolamide

(B) Dexamethasone

(C) Ginkgo biloba

(D) Nifedipine

(E) Sildenafil

5-19. In which of the following patients is hyperbaric oxygen treatment indicated after a carbon monoxide (CO) exposure?

(A) Asymptomatic 85-year-old woman with history of dementia whose mental status is at baseline according to family

(B) Asymptomatic 30-year-old man with COHb of 17%

(C) Asymptomatic woman who is 36 weeks pregnant with COHb of 5%

(D) 5-year-old girl with a headache and vomiting

(E) 60-year-old man with chest pain and ST segment elevations on ECG

5-20. A 5-year-old child is brought in by parents for headache, vomiting, and dyspnea but no fever. The parents have similar but milder symptoms. They have been staying in their mountain cabin that is heated by a propane heater. Which of the following tests is most likely to be abnormal?

(A) COHb level

(B) Chest radiograph

(C) CT of the brain

(D) Influenza swab

(E) Pulse oximetry

Environmental Disorders
Answers and Explanations

5-1. **The answer is D** (Chapter 202). Trench foot occurs when feet are exposed to cold and wet conditions, but not freezing. It is most often seen in military situations. Frostbite is an injury due to freezing that could superficially resemble trench foot. Chilblains are inflammatory lesions that typically occur on the hands of women after cold exposure. Cold urticaria is a hypersensitivity reaction to cold temperatures. Panniculitis involves necrosis of subcutaneous fat due to prolonged cold, but not freezing temperatures, and occurs mainly in children and the thighs and buttocks of women horseback riders.

5-2. **The answer is D** (Chapter 202). Frostbite should never be rewarmed in the field if there is a chance of refreezing. Rapid rewarming should be done with a water bath at 40–42°C after there is no chance for refreezing. Dry heat should not be used. Elevation, immobilization, and meticulous wound care will aid in healing. Debridement of blisters is controversial, but application of aloe vera cream is considered beneficial. Amputation and soft tissue debridement should be deferred, as full demarcation of devitalized tissue may take weeks. MRI and radionuclide angiography with bone scan (but not CT) have been used for early assessment of tissue viability. Heparin is not beneficial, but tissue plasminogen activator (TPA) has been used successfully to prevent amputation. Prophylactic antibiotics are controversial in all but deep or clearly infected cases. Tetanus prophylaxis is indicated.

5-3. **The answer is B** (Chapter 203). Hypothermia causes multiple metabolic changes. As temperature decreases, the victim becomes initially uncoordinated, progressively confused, and finally comatose. Respiratory depression (not distress) occurs, and cough and gag reflexes are also diminished. Hypothermic patients are prone to bleeding due to inhibition of platelet function, alterations in coagulation cascade enzyme function, and may be associated with disseminated intravascular coagulation. Patients with hypothermia are usually volume depleted for a variety of reasons, and may have renal dysfunction secondary to rhabdomyolysis. Patients are at risk for cardiac arrhythmias. The ECG may show the classic Osborne or J-wave, a terminal deflection at the end of the QRS complex. A delta wave is a slurring of the QRS complex seen in patients with Wolff–Parkinson–White syndrome.

5-4. **The answer is C** (Chapter 204). The likely diagnosis is heat stroke. CT scan of the brain, toxicological screens, endocrine evaluation, and search for infection may be important in this patient to rule out other causes of hyperthermia. However, the initial goal is rapid cooling and fluid resuscitation with normal saline. The goal temperature should be 39°C to avoid overshoot hypothermia, and is best accomplished by evaporative cooling. Immersion cooling makes patient airway management and cardiac monitoring difficult and is not advised. Cooling blankets work too slowly for a patient with heat stroke. Ice packs to groin, neck, and axilla may be useful adjunctive cooling measures. Acetaminophen and dantrolene have no role in treatment of heat stroke.

5-5. **The answer is B** (Chapter 205). Black widow spider bites are typically felt by the victim and can rapidly progress from local pain to severe cramps in large muscle groups. Patients may have associated hypertension. Treatment consists of adequate analgesia and Latrodectus antivenom. In contrast, Brown recluse spider bites are often initially painless. The wound may progress from erythematous lesion to blistering and necrosis and leave a poorly healing ulcer. Associated systemic symptoms, including hemolysis and disseminated intravascular coagulation are rare. Hobo spider bites may present similarly to Brown recluse bites. Headache, nausea, and fatigue are the most commonly associated systemic symptoms. Bark scorpion venom contains a neurotoxin that causes local pain and paresthesias. Severe cases may demonstrate cranial nerve dysfunction, excessive motor activity, nausea, vomiting, tachycardia, and agitation. Yellow jacket stings are typically painful and cause a local erythematous reaction with swelling which can mimic cellulitis. In sensitized individuals, they can cause anaphylaxis.

5-6. **The answer is B** (Chapter 205). Anaphylaxis from a Hymenoptera sting should be treated like any other cause of anaphylaxis. Intramuscular epinephrine is the mainstay of treatment. Antihistamines, both H1- and H2-blockers, may be helpful adjuncts but should not delay or precede administration of epinephrine. Corticosteroids may prevent delayed reactions but do not treat acute anaphylaxis. Beta-agonists such as albuterol are helpful adjuncts for patients who are wheezing. Intravenous epinephrine is reserved for patients with hypotension refractory to initial treatment or those in cardiac arrest. No antivenom is currently commercially available. Discharge with epinephrine autoinjector (e.g., Epi-pen™) is appropriate for all patients who recover from acute anaphylaxis. Outpatient referral for desensitization with venom immunotherapy is recommended for those patients with anaphylaxis due to Hymenoptera stings.

5-7. **The answer is D** (Chapter 206). CroFab™ is indicated in any rattlesnake victim with progressive signs and symptoms, evidence of systemic toxicity such as hypotension or altered mental status (AMS), serious neurological toxicity (e.g., limb paralysis), or serious hematologic toxicity such as elevated PT or falling (not elevated) platelet count.

5-8. **The answer is A** (Chapter 207). The most common cause of infection in seawater-associated wounds is bacteria found as part of normal skin flora including staph and strep species. Vibrio species are the most commonly implicated marine-specific organisms. *Mycobacterium marinum* is an atypical mycobacterium that causes cutaneous granulomatous disease associated with both fresh- and salt-water exposure. Aeromonas organisms are seen in fresh water-associated infections.

5-9. **The answer is B** (Chapter 208). Decompression sickness and arterial gas embolism are treated with recompression using hyperbaric oxygen (HBO) in a specially designed chamber. Nitrogen narcosis occurs at depths of 100 feet seawater or greater and improves upon ascent. Pulmonary barotrauma (e.g., pneumothorax) should be treated with tube thoracostomy drainage but does not require recompression with HBO unless there is an associated arterial gas embolism. Sinus barotraumas is best treated symptomatically with decongestants, whereas inner ear barotrauma may require otologic intervention.

5-10. **The answer is A** (Chapter 209). Submersion victims requiring CPR on the scene or in the ED have a generally poor prognosis. Initial presentation and extent of required resuscitation are associated with the degree of anoxic insult. Asystole associated with warm water drowning is a particularly poor prognostic indicator. Rare reports describe recovery in both children and adults following icy water submersion; therefore prolonged resuscitative measures may be indicated in these patients. Victims who do not require CPR on the scene or in the ED usually have complete re-covery. Patients who present asymptomatic with normal oxygenation and normal pul-monary exam after submersion injury may be observed for 4–6 hours and safely discharged home if there is no evidence of deterioration.

5-11. **The answer is E** (Chapter 210). Inhalation in-jury is suspected based on history and pres-ence of physical signs of airway involvement including facial burns, singed nasal hair, soot in mouth, carbonaceous sputum, hoarseness, and wheezing. Upper airway edema can oc-cur rapidly and presents early. Stridor may be present. In contrast, lower airway edema may not be evident for up to 24 hours and respiratory signs may be absent initially. Ac-cordingly, the initial chest radiograph may be normal. Up to 50% of intubated burn pa-tients will go on to develop acute respiratory distress syndrome (ARDS). COHb should be measured in all patients suspected of inhala-tion injury and may help confirm prolonged smoke exposure. Circumferential neck burns are an indication for early intubation due to the potential for airway edema. Other in-dications for early intubation include full-thickness burns of the face or perioral region, respiratory distress, progressive hoarseness, stridor or air hunger, respiratory depression or AMS, supraglottic edema, and inflamma-tion on laryngoscopy.

5-12. **The answer is D** (Chapter 210). Prophylactic systemic antibiotics are not indicated for any burns. Tetanus prophylaxis is indicated when the patient's tetanus status is not up to date or is unknown. Topical antibiotics such as baci-tracin, 1% silver sulfadiazine cream and triple antibiotic ointment are appropriate dressings for minor burns. The Parkland formula and others may be used to calculate fluid re-quirements in adults and children with major burns, but these are only guides. Maintain-ing urine output at 1 mL/kg/hr is a reason-able goal for fluid administration in children. Burn patients may require high doses of opi-ates to achieve adequate analgesia. Patients with full-thickness burns, those with associ-

ated inhalation injury, children, elderly, and those with underlying medical problems that could complicate management are all criteria for referral to a burn center.

5-13. **The answer is C** (Chapter 211). Immediate co-pious irrigation with water is the mainstay of treatment for most chemical burns. Prognosis is related to the amount of chemical involved and the duration of exposure. Thus, earlier irrigation is associated with improved out-comes. Many chemical agents causing burns are also associated with systemic toxicity, particularly acids such as hydrofluoric acid, chromic acid, and phenol. However, acetic acid, which is found in hair products and can cause extensive scalp burns, is not gen-erally associated with systemic symptoms. Some chemical burns require treatment with specific antidotes, for example, calcium glu-conate is required to detoxify the damag-ing fluoride ion in hydrofluoric acid burns. Chemical burns to the eye are a serious emer-gency and require immediate, copious irriga-tion and ophthalmology consult.

5-14. **The answer is D** (Chapters 212 and 213). High-voltage DC electricity can throw the victim from the electrical source causing blunt traumatic injuries. High-voltage AC in-jury can result in tetanic contractions where the victim cannot let go of the source of injury. High-voltage injury is associated with deep tissue destruction and may cause compart-ment syndrome. Any type of electrical injury may cause cardiac or respiratory arrest. Fern pattern burns, also known as Lichtenberg fig-ures, are seen with lightning injuries. These are not true burns and resolve quickly.

5-15. **The answer is B** (Chapter 213). Patients struck by lightning may sustain cardiac and/or respiratory arrest but have a good prognosis with resuscitation. Prolonged CPR may be indicated. Lightning injury is as-sociated with cardiac arrhythmias, ST seg-ment abnormalities, and other ECG changes. Lower extremity paralysis following light-ning injury is termed keraunoparalysis and is usually temporary. Cataracts are a common ocular complication of lightning injury, even in patients without evidence of direct injury to head or eyes. Development of cataracts may be delayed for weeks to years. Tympanic membrane perforation can be seen due to blast injury. Unlike high-voltage electrical injuries, electrical injury from lightning tends to be superficial and skeletal muscle injury is rare in the absence of associated blunt trauma. Hence, compartment syndrome is not associated with lightning injuries.

5-16. **The answer is E** (Chapter 214). Psilocybe and Gymnopilus mushrooms can cause euphoria, hallucinations, tachycardia, and other neurological symptoms but are not associated with GI toxicity. Treatment is supportive with benzodiazepines as needed. Inocybe and Clitocybe mushrooms can cause the SLUDGE syndrome due to their cholinergic properties and toxicity may be treated with atropine. Many different types of mushrooms are associated with GI symptoms and can be treated with supportive care including antiemetics. Decontamination with activated charcoal is also indicated in most cases of mushroom poisoning presenting with GI symptoms as empiric treatment for *Amanita phalloides* and *Amanita bisporigera* poisoning. These two mushrooms are associated with delayed liver toxicity and liver failure.

5-17. **The answer is C** (Chapter 215). Jimsonweed is commonly ingested for its hallucinogenic properties. It can cause an anticholinergic toxidrome that is not usually life threatening. Castor beans contain ricin toxin, one of the most potent naturally occurring toxins. Oleander and foxglove both contain cardiac glycosides resembling digitalis and can cause fatal cardiac dysrhythmias. Water hemlock contains cicutoxin that may be rapidly fatal.

5-18. **The answer is A** (Chapter 216). Acetazolamide is the drug of choice for treating acute mountain sickness. Corticosteroids are effective, but are generally reserved for severe cases of acute mountain sickness or high-altitude cerebral edema. Sildenafil and nifedipine can be used for prophylaxis of high-altitude pulmonary edema due to their ability to lower pulmonary artery pressure. There is conflicting evidence on the use of Ginkgo biloba for prevention of acute mountain sickness and no studies have evaluated its used for treatment.

5-19. **The answer is E** (Chapter 217). Although the benefits of hyperbaric oxygen for carbon monoxide poisoning remain controversial, AMS or coma, focal neurological deficits, pregnancy with COHb >15%, COHb level >25%, and evidence of acute myocardial ischemia are all accepted indications for HBO. Children and elderly may be more susceptible to the toxic effects of CO poisoning, but the indications for HBO are the same as in adults.

5-20. **The answer is A** (Chapter 217). Exposure to propane-fueled heaters is a common source of CO. Frequently whole families may fall ill. COHb level is likely to be abnormal and would explain this child's symptoms. Positive influenza swab is less likely given the exposure history. CT of the brain can show hypoattenuation in the globus pallidus after significant CO exposure, but these lesions may take up to 24 hours to develop. Chest radiograph is typically normal. Pulse oximetry does not reflect the systemic hypoxia of CO poisoning because the device cannot distinguish between oxyhemoglobin and COHb.

CHAPTER 6

Eye, Ear, Nose, Throat, and Oral Emergencies
Questions

6-1. Which of the following is the one opthalmologic emergency in which measurement of visual acuity and eye exam should not precede treatment?

(A) Acute monocular visual loss

(B) Acute red eye with photophobia

(C) Blunt trauma to the eye

(D) Chemical burn to the eye

(E) Foreign body to the eye using high-powered tool

6-2. You pick up a patient's chart that states "acute blindness for 1 hour with pain." Which of the following diagnoses is likely the cause of this patient's symptoms?

(A) Acute optic neuritis if you notice that there is a Marcus Gunn pupil and the posterior chamber is clear

(B) Acute retinal artery occlusion secondary to carotid cholesteatoma if visual loss is bilateral

(C) Hysterical blindness if the patient exhibits no lateral nystagmus when vertical lines are passed before the eyes

(D) Occipital stroke

(E) Uveitis

6-3. A 66-year-old woman with a history of hypertension and allergy to "sulfa" complains of acute onset of left eye pain, headache, and vomiting. She has photophobia. Her eye is pictured below (Figure 6-1). Her intraocular pressure (IOP) is 60 mm Hg. What medication is contraindicated?

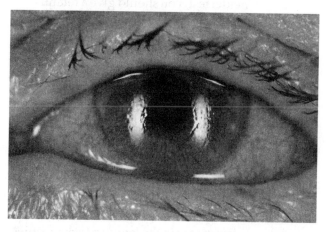

Figure 6-1. Reproduced with permission from Knoop KJ, Stack LB, Storrow AB, Thurman RJ: *The Atlas of Emergency Medicine*, 3rd Edition. Copyright © 2010 The McGraw-Hill Companies, Inc. Photo contributor: Kevin J. Knoop, MD, MS.

(A) Acetazolamide

(B) Ciprofloxacin

(C) Morphine sulfate

(D) Pilocarpine

(E) Timolol

6-4. A 45-year-old man comes in with acute eye pain that occurred suddenly while grinding a metal sculpture without safety goggles. His vital signs and visual acuity are normal. Eyes are grossly normal except for redness in the affected eye and mild photophobia after topical anesthesia. What is the most appropriate diagnostic test and treatment for the following slit-lamp exam findings?

(A) If you see injected conjunctiva, quiet anterior chamber, a positive Seidel test on fluorescein stain, you should get a computed tomography (CT) to rule out intraocular foreign body, give intravenous antibiotics, a tetanus booster, and request an ophthalmology consultation.

(B) If you see injected conjunctiva, quiet anterior chamber and a punctate corneal abrasion in the temporal inferior quadrant on fluorescein stain with a negative Seidel test, you should give a tetanus booster, treat with topical antibiotics, and obtain an ophthalmology consult in 24 hours.

(C) If you see injected conjunctiva, quiet anterior chamber, a superficial piece of metal at the visual axis with a rust ring, you should remove the piece with an eye spud, remove the rust ring with a burr, give topical antibiotics, a tetanus booster, and obtain ophthalmology follow-up in 24 hours.

(D) If you see injected conjunctiva with a black tissue in the temporal sclera, quiet anterior chamber, negative fluorescein stain uptake, you should give topical antibiotics, a tetanus booster, and ophthalmology follow-up in 24 hours.

(E) If you see injected conjunctiva with normal sclera, clear cornea, small amount of blood in the anterior chamber, check the IOP, give pain meds, cycloplegics, and referral for recheck by ophthalmology within 24 hours.

6-5. A 75-year-old woman with new onset atrial fibrillation presents with acute visual loss in the right eye for 20 minutes. She has a pale retina with a cherry red macula. What is the appropriate diagnosis and corresponding treatment?

(A) She has acute central retinal artery occlusion and she should be treated with acetazolamide, topical beta-blockers, and ocular massage. Emergent ophthalmologic consultation is recommended and tPA infusion considered.

(B) She has acute central retinal vein thrombosis and she should be treated with aspirin and emergent ophthalmologic consultation.

(C) She has an acute occipital stroke and should receive tPA infusion.

(D) She has acute optic neuritis and should be treated with intravenous steroids and immediate ophthalmologic consultation is recommended.

(E) She has a vitreal hemorrhage and needs to be upright, and should avoid aspirin and nonsteroidal anti-inflammatory drugs and follow up with the ophthalmologist in 24 hours.

6-6. An otherwise healthy 45-year-old woman with no significant past medical history comes in complaining of 12 hours of diplopia. On exam she has a dilated right pupil and can only abduct and look up with her right eye when range of motion is tested. What is her likely diagnosis?

(A) Aneurysm
(B) Diabetes mellitus
(C) Carotid dissection
(D) Werneike encephalopathy
(E) Vertebral artery dissection

6-7. A 12-year-old boy with sickle cell disease was hit in the eye with a fist. His visual acuity is normal. On physical exam he has mild periorbital edema, mild enophthalmos, and upward gaze diplopia, fundus is normal. Slit-lamp exam is shown (Figure 6-2). His IOP measures 30 mm Hg. What is the most appropriate treatment for this patient?

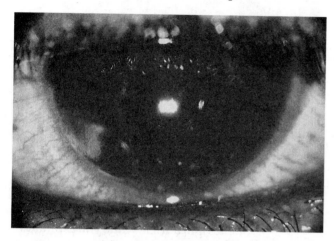

Figure 6-2. Reproduced with permission from Knoop KJ, Stack LB, Storrow AB, Thurman RJ: *The Atlas of Emergency Medicine*, 3rd Edition. Copyright © 2010 The McGraw-Hill Companies, Inc. Photo contributor: Dallas E. Peak, MD.

(A) He is best treated with topical beta-blockers, steroids, cycloplegics, and intravenous acetazolamide to reduce IOP; get an orbital CT and immediate ophthalmic consultation.

(B) He is best treated with topical beta-blockers, steroids, and cycloplegics, and intravenous acetazolamide to reduce IOP; get an orbital CT and ophthalmic follow-up within 24 hours.

(C) He is best treated with topical beta-blockers, steroids, and cycloplegics to reduce IOP; get a CT of the orbits and immediate ophthalmology consultation.

(D) He is best treated with topical beta-blockers, steroids, and cycloplegics to reduce IOP; get a CT of the orbits and follow up with ophthalmology in 24 hours.

(E) He is best treated with topical cycloplegics and acetazolamide to reduce IOP and urgent ophthalmology consult.

6-8. A 39-year-old woman comes in complaining of red eyes and watery discharge. On exam, there is conjunctival injection, chemosis, watery discharge, as well as auricular adenopathy. No uptake was noted with fluorescein staining and anterior chamber was clear on slit-lamp exam. Which of the following is recommended?

(A) Antibiotic drops

(B) Cycloplegic drops

(C) Needle biopsy of the lymph node

(D) Ocular decongestant drops

(E) Urgent ophthalmology consult

6-9. A 7-year-old girl scraped her cornea with an apple stem. Her visual acuity is 20/20. She has moderate photophobia and is rubbing her eye and crying. On slit-lamp exam, she has a 6-mm superficial linear abrasion of her cornea in the temporal inferior quadrant. Seidel test is negative. Anterior chamber is quiet. What is the most appropriate treatment?

(A) Erythromycin ointment, an eye patch, pain medication, and ophthalmology follow-up in 24 hours

(B) Homoatropine drops, tobramycin drops, an eye patch, pain medication, and ophthalmology follow-up in 24 hours

(C) Homoatropine drops, erythromycin ointment, pain medication, and ophthalmology follow-up in 24 hours

(D) Tobramycin eye drops, topical steroids, pain medication, and ophthalmology follow-up in 24 hours

(E) Tobramycin drops, atropine drops, pain meds, and ophthalmology follow-up in 24 hours

6-10. Which of the following statements about acute hearing loss and tinnitus is most accurate?

(A) Antidepressants are the most commonly implicated drugs in tinnitus.

(B) Metoprolol is the most commonly implicated drug causing tinnitus.

(C) Sudden hearing loss (SHL) by definition is hearing loss occurring within 10 days.

(D) Side effects of medications cause the majority of cases of tinnitus.

(E) Tinnitus may be heard by the examiner.

6-11. Which of the following statements is most accurate about outer ear infections?

(A) *Candida* and *Aspergillus* are the most common cause of otomycosis and best treated with topical antifungals.

(B) Cortisporin solution eardrops are safe with perforated tympanic membranes (TMs).

(C) Otitis externa (OE) is best treated with gently irrigation with hydrogen peroxide and suctioning, alkalinizing agents, topical antimicrobials, and steroids.

(D) Patients with a history of diabetes and HIV, or elderly presented with OE and trismus, cranial nerve palsies, or any systemic signs should get CT of the brain.

(E) Topical ofloxacin is contraindicated in OE with perforated TM in a 6-year-old child.

6-12. Which of the following statements about otitis media (OM) is most accurate?

(A) Approximately 70% of all OM is viral.

(B) 70% of all OM is secondary to *Streptococcus* and *Moraxella*.

(C) Initial treatment of choice for OM in patients older than 2 years is pain management and for patients younger than 2 years is second-generation cephalosporins.

(D) OM with fever, posterior auricular erythema and tenderness, headache, papilledema, and sixth nerve palsy

should get CT and be treated with broad-spectrum antibiotics.

(E) OM with fever and posterior auricular erythema and tenderness should get mastoid radiographs or a CT and be treated with broad-spectrum antibiotics and close follow-up with otolaryngology

6-13. A 22-year-old man is brought in after being caught in an avalanche while back country skiing. Among his injuries, he has white non-tender right auricle and a swollen ecchymotic left auricle and perforated left TM without hemotympanum. You should:

(A) Place lukewarm (35–38°C) gauze soaks on the right auricle while you give IV antibiotics. Do not violate the skin of the left auricle.

(B) Place lukewarm (35–38°C) gauze soaks on the right auricle while you aspirated the subcutaneous blood from the left auricle and give IV antibiotics.

(C) Place warm (38–40°C) gauze soaks on the right auricle, debride the vesicles that form, incise and debride the subcutaneous blood from the left auricle, and place a sutured bolster dressing.

(D) Place warm (38–40°C) gauze soaks on the right auricle, do not debride vesicles that form, incise and debride the subcutaneous blood, and place a sutured bolstered dressing on the left auricle.

(E) Place warm (38–40°C) gauze soaks on the right auricle while you aspirated the subcutaneous blood from the left auricle and place a sutured bolster covered with silver sulfadiazine and gentle dressing.

6-14. A 40-year-old homeless man returns to the ED for the third visit in 5 days having been diagnoses with pharyngitis and given penicillin that was then switched to clindamycin on the last visit 2 days ago complaining of persistent and worsening sore throat and having run out of his pain medications. On exam, he has fever and mild tachycardia; there is no facial swelling. He can open his mouth only 2 finger breaths and oropharynx reveals dry erythematous mucous membranes without lesion, normal soft palate, and tonsils except for marked erythema bilaterally; he is handling his secretions but wincing and speaking with a soft voice secondary to "pain." What is the most appropriate course of action?

(A) Change his antibiotics to a macrolide noting concerns for "drug seeking behavior" and discharge home.

(B) Emergently intubate the patient, give intravenous antibiotics, and order a CT scan.

(C) Give intravenous narcotics, cephalexin, and order a CT scan.

(D) Give intravenous narcotics, clindamycin, and order a CT scan.

(E) Perform a 3-point needle aspiration.

6-15. A 54-year-old woman, with a history of alcohol abuse, presents with a well-demarcated 4 cm raised, puffy, warm, erythematous patch without fluctuance on her right cheek that started as a bug bite 6 hours ago. What is the most likely diagnosis?

(A) Cellulitis

(B) Erysipelas

(C) Facial abscess

(D) Impetigo

(E) Panniculitis

6-16. Which of the following is most accurate about salivary gland enlargement?

(A) 80% of sialoliths occur in the parotid gland (Stenson's duct) because of its more viscous secretions.

(B) Mumps is most commonly caused by paramyxovirus, follows a viremic prodrome, can be associated with orchitis, and is more severe in children than in adults.

(C) Submandibular gland stones are best treated with massage and lemon drops.

(D) Suppurative parotitis is not affected by the use of antihistamines and tricyclic antidepressants.

(E) Suppurative parotitis should be treated by minimal stimulus to the gland.

6-17. A 50-year-old man with a history of hypertension comes in complaining of spontaneous copious bleeding from his nose over the past 2 hours despite applying pressure. On physical exam, his blood pressure is 190/100, other vital signs are normal. He has bright red blood oozing from the septum in the right nares. What is the most appropriate next step?

(A) Administer an antihypertensive medication, then spray the nares with a vasoconstrictor, apply steady pressure for 15 minutes; if the bleeding continues, place a 5-cm nasal sponge and discharge with cephalexin and follow up in 2 days.

(B) Administer an antihypertensive medication, then spray the nares with a vasoconstrictor, apply the tip of a silver nitrate stick with gently pressure for 3 minutes.

(C) Spray the nares with vasoconstrictor, apply steady pressure for 15 minutes; if the bleeding continues, place a 5-cm nasal sponge and discharge with cephalexin, ibuprofen, and follow up in 2 days.

(D) Spray the nares with vasoconstrictor, apply steady pressure for 15 minutes; if the bleeding continues, place a 5-cm nasal sponge and discharge with cephalexin, and follow up in 2 days.

(E) Spray the nares with a vasoconstrictor, apply steady pressure for 15 minutes; if the bleeding continues, then place thrombogenic foam to the bleeding surface prior to trying nasal tamponade.

6-18. A 20-year-old man comes in after receiving a blow to the face during a basketball game. He complains of pain in her nose. His exam is shown in Figure 6-3.

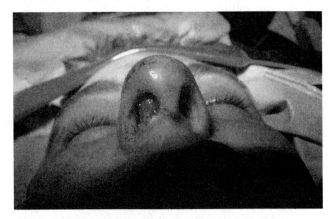

Figure 6-3. Reproduced with permission from Knoop KJ, Stack LB, Storrow AB, Thurman RJ: *The Atlas of Emergency Medicine*, 3rd Edition. Copyright © 2010 The McGraw-Hill Companies, Inc. Photo contributor: Lawrence B. Stack, MD.

What is the appropriate management?

(A) If clinical exam suggests an isolated nasal fracture, incise the lesion and pack the nares.

(B) If clinical exam suggests an isolated nasal fracture, perform closed reduction of the above lesion with a blunt elevator, then send for CT to assess extent of fracture and alignment.

(C) Order CT and if no fracture appreciated, send home with vasoconstrictors and analgesics to follow up with otolaryngology in 2–48 hours.

(D) Order a CT of the facial bones to assess extent of nasal fracture.

(E) Order plain films of the face including waters view to assess for nasal fracture.

6-19. Which of the following statements are most accurate about sinus disease?

(A) Acute sinusitis is best treated with saline irrigation, topical decongestants, and antibiotics

(B) Ethmoid sinusitis is the leading cause of orbital cellulites.

(C) Macrolides and trimethoprim–sulfamethoxazole are recommended as first-line treatment.

(D) Meningitis, cavernous sinus thrombosis, and intracranial abscesses occur in up to 15% of sinusitis.

(E) Most acute rhinosinusitis is bacterial in origin.

6-20. A 25-year-old Japanese tourist presents to the ED complaining of inability to close her jaw after yawning widely this morning. She was in her normal state of health prior. No history of trauma. On physical exam, she has a gaping jaw with the mandibular teeth protruding anterior to the alveolar teeth. What is the most appropriate management?

(A) Administer 2 cc of 2% lidocaine to the preauricular space bilaterally, grab the posterior mandibular molars with padded thumbs, and exert steady pressure downward and posteriorly.

(B) Administer IV anesthesia, grab the anterior inferior molar with padded thumbs, and exert anterior rotational torque.

(C) Obtain a panorex radiograph, administer intravenous antibiotics, and call an oral surgery consult.

(D) Obtain a panorex radiograph, administer intravenous narcotics and muscle relaxants, and exert steady pressure on the mentus posteriorly.

(E) Obtain a panorex radiograph, administer intravenous narcotics and muscle relaxants, grab the posterior mandibular molars with padded thumbs, and exert steady pressure downward and posteriorly.

6-21. Which of the following is TRUE?

(A) Episodes of cold sensitivity lasting seconds at a time and recurring several times a day over greater than 1 week is a sign of *irreversible pulpitis* and should be referred for root canal within 48 hours.

(B) Pain over an erupting wisdom tooth is *pericoronitis* and is treated with saline irrigation.

(C) Pain at a percussed tooth with mild gingival edema with scant expressible pus and a panorex showing slight widening of the periodontal ligament space is best treated with oral antibiotics and referral for root canal or extraction.

(D) Episodes of paroxysmal tooth pain and a normal exam should be considered drug seeking behavior and discharge only with nonnarcotic pain medication.

(E) Pain and cold sensitivity after biting a hard kernel showing chip fracture with exposed dentin is best treated with pain medication, antibiotics and 24 hour dental follow-up.

6-22. A 37-year-old smoker presents with severe pain at the site of his third mandibular molar extraction 2 days ago. He is afebrile and has no trismus, facial, or gingival swelling. The space at the site of his third molar is without bleeding or exudate but is exquisitely tender. Which of the following is TRUE?

(A) This man presents with common postextraction pain and should be given an inferior alveolar nerve block and analgesics and be seen by his dentist in 24 hours.

(B) This man presents with early postextraction infectious complication and should have a CT scan to rule out masticator space infection and then should be treated with IV antibiotics and analgesics and be seen by his dentist in 24 hours.

(C) This man presents with *postextraction alveolar osteitis* due to fibrin clot loss at the site of extraction and is at risk for bleeding. He should be given an in-

ferior alveolar nerve block, irrigation and packing with thrombin impregnated gauze, and be seen by his dentist in 24 hours.

(D) This man presents with *postextraction alveolar osteitis* and should have a panorex radiograph to rule out retained root tip or foreign body and then be given an inferior alveolar nerve block, irrigation and packing with oil of clove-soaked gauze, and be seen by his dentist in 24 hours.

(E) This man presents with *postextraction mandibular osteomyelitis* and is at risk for developing *Ludwig's Angina*. He should undergo CT and treated with IV antibiotics and analgesics and urgent dental referral.

6-23. A 32-year-old HIV-positive man presents with painful teeth, bleeding gums, and foul metallic taste in his mouth (Figure 6-4). On exam he has a low-grade fever, fetid breath, and the following dental exam. What is this patient's diagnosis?

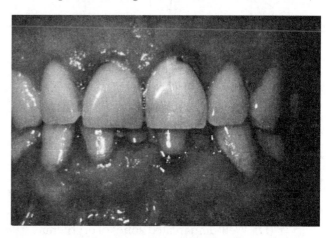

Figure 6-4. Reproduced with permission from Knoop KJ, Stack LB, Storrow AB, Thurman RJ: *The Atlas of Emergency Medicine*, 3rd Edition. Copyright © 2010 The McGraw-Hill Companies, Inc. Photo contributor: Department of Dermatology, National Naval Medical Center, Bethesda, MD.

(A) Acute necrotizing ulcerative gingivitis

(B) Hand, foot, and mouth disease

(C) Herpes gingivostomatitis

(D) Phenytoin-induced gum disease

(E) Vitamin deficiency

6-24. Which of the following statements is TRUE with respect to oral ulcerative disease?

(A) Aphthous ulcers involve the nonkeratinized surfaces of the mouth especially the labial and buccal mucosa and is best treated with topical steroids.

(B) Hand, foot, and mouth disease is commonly associated with Coxsackie-type A16 virus and is characterized by petechiae on the posterior pharynx and the lips and is best treated with pain medication.

(C) Herpangina is caused commonly by Coxsackie's group viruses, which causes painful ulcers on keratinized tongue, gingival, hard palate, and is best treated with pain medication.

(D) Herpetic gingivostomatitis involves primarily nonkeratinized surfaces of the mouth especially the buccal mucosa and soft palate and is best treated with oral antivirals.

(E) Traumatic ulcers are best treated with pain medication and topical steroids.

6-25. Which of the following statements regarding oral lesions is most accurate?

(A) *Erythroplakia*, red patches, that persist and cannot be attributed to other diseases are more common than *leukoplakia* but less likely to be associated with malignancy.

(B) Lymphoma is the most common form of oral cancer.

(C) Most common site for oral cancer is the posterior aspect of the tongue.

(D) Well-demarcated zones of erythema on the tongue with atrophy of filiform papillae is known as *erythroplakia* and is a precancerous lesion.

(E) White plaques that cannot be scraped off the buccal mucosa known as *leukoplakia* requires biopsy as 20% of the time they show dysplastic changes.

6-26. A 22-year-old man complains of having tripped and hit his front tooth against the edge of the table. He has no complaints except for a chipped tooth with sensitivity to air passing over it. Physical exam shows his right incisor with a chip from the bottom third of the tooth (see Figure 6-5). It is exquisitely tender to palpation, no bleeding, no laxity, with normal overlying gingiva. What is the most appropriate management?

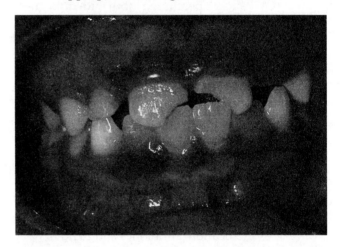

Figure 6-5. Reproduced with permission from Knoop KJ, Stack LB, Storrow AB, Thurman RJ: *The Atlas of Emergency Medicine*, 3rd Edition. Copyright © 2010 The McGraw-Hill Companies, Inc. Photo contributor: James F. Steiner, DDS.

(A) Give the patient oil of clove for topical anesthesia, prescribe oral analgesics, and follow up with dentist in 24 hours.

(B) Give the patient oral analgesics and antibiotics and follow up with dentist in 24 hours.

(C) Cover the dried exposed tooth with calcium hydroxide base, prescribe oral analgesics and antibiotics, and then follow up with dentist in 24 hours.

(D) Cover the dried exposed tooth with glass ionomer dental cement base and prescribe oral analgesics and antibiotics then follow up with a dentist in 24 hours.

(E) Cover the dried exposed tooth with glass ionomer dental cement base and prescribe oral analgesics then follow up with a dentist in 24 hours.

6-27. A 16-year-old comes to the ED after having been punched in the mouth 30 minutes ago. He is holding his two front teeth in his hand, which are complete from crown to root. His physical exam is normal except for two avulsed front teeth, minimal gingival ecchymosis, and a stable alveolar ridge. What is the best course of action?

(A) Rinse the dry teeth under sterile saline, rinse the socket thoroughly cleaning out any debris, and then immediately reimplant the teeth and splint.

(B) Soak the teeth in Hank's balanced salt solution for 30 minutes, then push the teeth firmly into the tooth sockets, securing them to the surrounding teeth with periodontal dressing and follow up with a dentist within 24 hours.

(C) Suspend the teeth in Hank's balanced salt solution, sterile normal saline or milk, get a CT scan to rule out alveolar ridge fracture, give pain medications, and have the patient follow up with a dentist within 24 hours.

(D) Suspend the teeth in Hank's balanced salt solution, sterile normal saline or milk, give pain medications, and have the patient follow up with a dentist within 24 hours.

(E) Washing the teeth with sterile normal saline, gently place the teeth and the sockets and secure the teeth to the surrounding teeth with periodontal dressing, and follow up with a dentist within 24 hours.

6-28. A 5-year-old boy comes in 20 minutes after having tripped into a table edge; his mother brings in one front tooth suspended in milk. His physical exam is normal except for ecchymotic gingiva over his anterior alveolar ridge, which is stable. His one incisor is completely avulsed and suspended in milk. His other incisor is extremely loose but still in the socket. You should:

(A) Extract the loose tooth and follow up with a dentist within 24 hours.

(B) Extract the loose tooth, soak both teeth in Hank's balanced salt solution for 30 minutes, then push the teeth firmly into the tooth sockets, securing them to the surrounding teeth with periodontal dressing, and follow up with a dentist within 24 hours.

(C) Leave the avulsed tooth out, secure the loose incisor to surrounding teeth with periodontal dressing, and follow up with a dentist within 24 hours.

(D) Leave the loose tooth and follow up with a dentist within 24 hours.

(E) Push the avulsed tooth firmly into the tooth socket, securing them to the surrounding teeth with periodontal dressing, and follow up with a dentist within 24 hours.

6-29. A 24-year-old student presents with 5 days of low-grade fever, cough, and worsening sore throat. On physical exam, she has a petechial pattern on her soft palate, grade II tonsils with erythema, and no exudates and nontender cervical adenopathy. What is the most appropriate plan of action?

(A) Ask her about a history of exposures to HIV, mononucleosis, and influenza and treat with salt gargling, oral hydration, and analgesics.

(B) Ask her about recent antibiotics and immune status and treat with fluconazole, oral hydration, and analgesics.

(C) Give her single-dose oral dexamethasone and discharge with salt gargling, oral hydration, and analgesics.

(D) Test her for Group A Beta-Hemolytic Streptococci (GABHS) using the rapid antigen test and, if negative, treat with salt gargling, oral hydration, and analgesics.

(E) Test her for heterophile antibody and treat with acyclovir, oral hydration, and analgesics.

6-30. Which of the following statements is most accurate about peritonsillar abscesses?

(A) A physical exam suggestive of peritonsillar abscess with negative needle aspiration requires imaging to rule out abscess.

(B) Acute tonsillectomy is contraindicated especially in children.

(C) Adjuvant steroids have not been found to be helpful.

(D) Needle aspiration effectively treats 65% of patients and often incision and drainage will be required.

(E) The proper technique of needle aspiration is application of topical anesthesia followed by introduction of an 18-gauge needle halfway between the base of the uvula and the maxillary alveolar ridge penetrating no more than 2 cm.

6-31. A 55-year-old diabetic woman complains of 1 week of lower anterior molar pain and now with 24 hours of sore throat, difficulty swallowing, and sweats. On physical exam (see Figure 6-6), she is anxious and having difficulty breathing. She has significant trismus and so the pharynx is not visualized. Her tongue appears elevated and she is unable to protrude it beyond her teeth, and the sublingual space is indurated and elevated. What is the next best course of action?

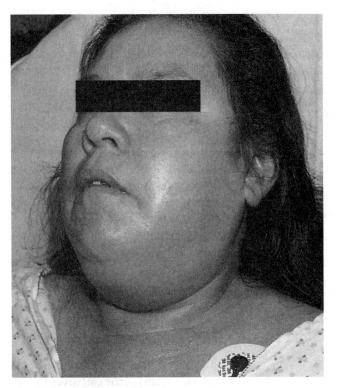

Figure 6-6. Reproduced with permission from Knoop KJ, Stack LB, Storrow AB, Thurman RJ: *The Atlas of Emergency Medicine*, 3rd Edition. Copyright © 2010 The McGraw-Hill Companies, Inc. Photo contributor: Jeffrey Finkelstein, MD.

(A) Administer broad-spectrum antibiotics and drain the submandibular abscess.

(B) Perform a cricothyroidotomy, administer intravenous fluoroquinolone, order a CT scan, and emergent head and neck surgery consultation.

(C) Perform rapid sequence endotracheal intubation, administer intravenous ampicillin–sulbactam, order a CT scan, and emergent head and neck surgery consultation.

(D) Perform rapid sequence endotracheal intubation, administer intravenous fluoroquinolone, order a CT scan, and emergent head and neck surgery consultation.

(E) Perform awake fiberoptic endotracheal intubation, administer intravenous ampicillin–sulbactam, order a CT scan, and emergent head and neck surgery consultation.

6-32. Which of the following statements about neck masses is most accurate?

(A) In adults older than 40 years, the most common cause of unilateral neck masses is Hodgkin lymphoma.

(B) In adults older than 40 years, up to 75% of neck masses persisting more than 6 weeks are malignant.

(C) Midline masses suggest branchial cleft cysts.

(D) Neck masses in adolescents and young adults are usually due to congenital cyst inflammation.

(E) Single tender solitary thyroid nodules are usually malignant or premalignant.

6-33. One week prior to presentation, an 18-month-old girl was being fed a half orange by squeezing it into her mouth and she began coughing and gasping. She was admitted to the intensive care unit overnight for trace vocal cord edema that resolved. She returns now with 3 days of cough and fever (101°F) and a focal right-sided wheeze. She has no stridor, her voice and cry are normal. Chest x-ray shows a right lower lobe infiltrate. What is the most appropriate next step?

(A) Albuterol nebulizer and antibiotics to cover aspiration pneumonia and 24 hours follow-up

(B) Albuterol nebulizer, antibiotics, and immediately referral for bronchoscopy

(C) Albuterol nebulizer and a chest CT to rule out pulmonary embolism

(D) Albuterol nebulizer, chest percussion, antibiotics to cover aspiration pneumonia, and admission for observation

(E) Albuterol nebulizer, oral steroids, and antibiotics to cover aspiration pneumonia and 24 hours follow-up

6-34. A 36-year-old man brought in by ambulance after his falling off his horse when he was struck in the neck with a tree limb. He comes in complaining of neck pain and dysphagia. On physical exam, he is speaking with hoarse voice, has edema and crepitus over his anterior midline neck. What is the best course of action?

(A) Administer intravenous dexamethasone and racemic epinephrine nebulizer and obtain a CT of the neck

(B) Perform an immediate cricothyroidotomy then consult ENT for a definitive airway placement

(C) Perform an immediate fiberoptic endotracheal intubation

(D) Perform an immediate fiberoptic endotracheal intubation, if the laryngeal lumen cannot be visualized then perform a cricothyroidotomy

(E) Placed a cervical collar and obtain a CT scan of the neck

6-35. A 65-year-old woman recently started on lisinopril presents with 2 hours of swelling of her lips and tongue. She has no stridor or wheezing and her sublingual space is normal. What is the best course of action?

(A) Give diphenhydramine 50 mg and methylprednisolone 125 mg intravenously. Admit to the intensive care unit.

(B) Give epinephrine 0.3 mg subcutaneously, diphenhydramine 50 mg, and methylprednisolone 125 mg intravenously. Avoid nasopharyngoscopy; the patient can be discharged after several hours of observation if clinically improved.

(C) Give epinephrine 0.3 mg subcutaneously, diphenhydramine 50 mg, and methylprednisolone 125 mg intravenously. Perform nasopharyngoscopy; if there is laryngeal edema, perform a cricothyroidotomy and admit to the intensive care unit.

(D) Give epinephrine 0.3 mg subcutaneously, diphenhydramine 50 mg, and methylprednisolone 125 mg intravenously. Perform nasopharyngoscopy; if there is no laryngeal edema, the patient can be discharged after observing for several hours if clinically improved.

(E) Give racemic epinephrine nebulizer, diphenhydramine 50 mg, and methylprednisolone 125 mg intravenously. Admit to the intensive care unit.

6-36. Which of the following statements about the management of tracheostomy tubes is most accurate?

(A) Patients with tracheostomies and respiratory distress should first be suctioned through the inner cannula with sterile saline and preoxygenation.

(B) Patients with tracheostomies and respiratory distress should first have the inner cannula removed and cleaned and be suctioned through the tracheotomy tube.

(C) Patients with tracheostomies and respiratory distress should first have the tracheostomy tube removed and be suctioned through the stoma.

(D) Patients with tracheostomies less than 7 days old can be manipulated by an ED physician if the proper technique is used.

(E) When pediatric tracheostomy tubes are crusted or clogged, only the inner cannula should be removed for cleaning.

Eye, Ear, Nose, Throat, and Oral Emergencies
Answers and Explanations

6-1. The answer is D (Chapter 236). Full vital signs, including visual acuity, the vital sign of the eye, and a full eye exam should be done before initiating treatment except for chemical exposure to eye, in which high volume irrigation must be initiated as soon as possible. A few drop of topical anesthetic are often indicated prior to the full exam in cases of acute eye pain, but a full exam including visual acuity, field of vision testing, pupillary exam, slit lamp, and fundoscopic exam should be done. Blunt trauma may require eye speculum for examination if the lids are swollen shut.

6-2. The answer is A (Chapter 236). A normal exam with a Marcus Gunn pupil suggests optic neuritis or other causes of afferent papillary defect. Initial findings of optic neuritis may include problems with color vision and visual field defects. Acute retinal artery occlusion is monocular. Hysterical blindness is suggested when nystagmus *does* occur when confronted by moving vertical lines. Occipital stroke causes hemianopsia. Uveitis is almost universally painful and associated with photophobia. It may cause blurry vision but not usually visual loss.

6-3. The answer is A (Chapter 236). The proper management of acute angle glaucoma is intravenous analgesics, antiemetics, mannitol and acetazolamide, topical beta-blockers, and steroids to lower IOP, followed by a miotic. However, in this patient, acetazolamide is contraindicated with her allergy to sulfonamides. Miotics (pupillary constrictors) not mydriatics (pupillary dilators) are effective when the IOP has been brought under control by the other measures and pull the iris away from the cornea to avoid recurrence. There is no role of antibiotics. Emergent ophthalmic consultation is needed for definitive treatment.

6-4. The answer is A (Chapter 236). The Seidel test is performed by brushing a moistened fluorescein strip across the anesthetized cornea then under blue light checking for streaming indicative of corneal violation from a foreign object. Black tissue imbedded in the sclera is suggestive of uveal tissue herniation through a rent in the sclera caused by a foreign body. Any suspicion of FB violation of the eye, even with no obvious evidence of injury, should be worked up with a CT or ultrasound. If the mechanism of injury is highly suspicious treat with intravenous antibiotics, a tetanus booster, and get a ophthalmic consultation. A negative Seidel's test with a superficial corneal abrasion does not require CT or intravenous antibiotics. Rust rings or foreign bodies located in the *visual axis* should not be removed by an emergency physician but be deferred to the ophthalmologist. Do not attempt to measure IOP if globe rupture from penetrating or blunt trauma is suspected.

6-5. The answer is A (Chapter 236). Central retinal artery occlusion is commonly caused by an embolus originating from a thrombus in the heart as occurs in atrial fibrillation or a cholesterol plaque from an arterial source. There is no good evidence-based treatment for acute retinal artery occlusion, but tPA can be considered if administered within 20 hours of symptoms. Central vein thrombosis presents with a "blood and thunder" retina. A vitreal hemorrhage would usually obscure visualization of the retina or appear as a pre-retinal bleed, not a cherry red macula. Optic neuritis presents with decreased color perception before visual loss, and a normal fundus with normal or edematous optic disk. Occipital strokes manifest as hemianopsia not monocular visual loss.

6-6.   The answer is A (Chapter 236). This patient is presenting with a third nerve palsy and pupil dilation. Acute CN III palsy with ipsilateral pupillary dilatation is a posterior circulation aneurysm until proven otherwise. The expanding aneurysm causes compression on the pupillomotor fibers that ride on the outside of the third verve. Emergent blood pressure management, neuroimaging, and neurosurgical consultation are indicated. Although diabetes and hypertension are the most frequent causes of third nerve palsy, they are usually papillary sparing as the mechanism is secondary to insufficiency of the vasa vasorum (penetrating feeding vessels into the nerve), thus causing ischemia to the central fibers first. Carotid dissection would cause a Horner syndrome, which presents as miosis not dilation along with ptosis and anhydrosis and does not affect the third nerve. Werneike encephalopathy affects the abductors or CN VI rather than CN III and is associated with altered mental status. CN palsy of IV is most common after acceleration/deceleration injury and presents with subtle diplopia.

6-7.   The answer is D (Chapter 236). This patient presents with two complications from blunt injury to the eye: a traumatic hyphema and a blowout fracture of the orbit with entrapment. Traumatic hyphema occurs because of bleeding from a ruptured iris vessel. Treatment involves keeping the head elevated, paralyzing the iris with cycloplegics, topical prednisone, and lowering the IOP with

topical beta-blockers. If IOP is elevated, carbonic anhydrase inhibitors (CAIs) are indicated EXCEPT in sickle cell anemia in which the CAI can lower the pH of the aqueous humor and cause sickling of the cells thereby clogging the outflow tract of the trabecular matrix. Intravenous mannitol may be used as an alternative. Hyphemas occupying greater than one-third of the anterior chamber should be seen by an ophthalmologist emergently. Re-bleeding occurs in 3–5 days in up to 30%. In general, patient with hyphemas occupying less than one-third of the anterior chamber can be referred to an ophthalmologist for close outpatient follow-up. Blowout fractures should be evaluated with CT to rule out sinus fracture and oral antibiotics are often recommended. All blowout fractures should be referred to ophthalmologist for a full dilated exam in the next 3 to 10 days to rule out retinal tears or detachment (CT or ultrasound may help). Immediate bedside consultation is not indicated unless the consult ophthalmologist prefers to admit hyphemas.

6-8.   The answer is D (Chapter 236). This patient has a classic case of viral conjunctivitis. Supportive care is in order. Ocular decongestants and artificial tears can provide some relief. Symptoms may take weeks to resolve. Antibiotics are not warranted when there is no sign of purulent discharge. Flare, cell and photophobia are signs of iritis, which should trigger a workup for systemic disease and is treated with steroids and cycloplegics. This patient has a clear anterior chamber.

6-9.   The answer is C (Chapter 236). Cycloplegics help considerably decrease the pain from corneal abrasion, though adjunct oral pain medications are often needed. Homatropine is recommended rather than atropine, as the effects of atropine can last up to 2 weeks. Both tobramycin and erythromycin are adequate topical antimicrobial agents, but abrasions from organic sources have potential for fungal infections and should not be patched. There is no role for steroids in the treatment of corneal abrasion.

6-10. The answer is E (Chapter 237). Tinnitus can be divided into objective, heard by the examiner (i.e., secondary to AV malformations, arterial bruits, mechanical abnormalities), and subjective tinnitus (i.e., secondary to cochlear/neuro sensory insult from toxins or vascular insufficiency). Pharmacological side effects are the cause of tinnitus in 10% of cases. Aspirin, followed by nonsteroidal anti-inflammatory drugs, and antibiotics such as amniogycosides are the most commonly implicated pharmacological causes of tinnitus. Antidepressants are not implicated in tinnitus; in fact, they are the only class of drug found to be useful in alleviating idiopathic tinnitus. SHL is defined as hearing loss occurring within 3 days or less, and "idiopathic" is the most common cause of SHL, though infectious causes such as mumps, genetic degenerative diseases, vascular insufficiency from a variety of causes, and toxic affects of drugs need to be considered in the differential.

6-11. The answer is D (Chapter 237). Any patients with a history of being immunocompromised presenting with OE, or patients with persistent OE despite 2 weeks of treatment, or any patients with associated cranial nerve palsy or fever, should get a CT to rule out malignant OE, which requires parenteral antibiotics, admission, and ENT consultation. *Staphylococcus aureus* and *Pseudomonas aeruginosa* along with *Enterobacteriaceae* and *Proteus* are the most common organism implicated in OE. Otomycosis is seen in tropical climates and in the immunocompromised. *Aspergillus*, and *Candida*, accounts for most of the cases and are best treated with systemic antifungals, and *Aspergillus* may require itraconazole. OE is best treated with gently irrigation with hydrogen peroxide and suctioning, *acidifying agents*, topical antimicrobial, and sometimes steroids. Cortisporin Otic preparations have not been approved by the Food and Drug Administration (FDA) for OE with perforations due to the theoretical concern of the neomycin (aminoglycoside) toxicity on the inner ear. However, the ENT literature recommends the *suspension* but not the *solution*, which is more easily absorbed across the round window. Ofloxacin is the only antibiotic drop approved by the FDA for OE with perforated TM. Topical ofloxacin would be the treatment of choice for OE with perforated TM in a 6-year-old boy and is the only FDA-approved medication in kids.

6-12. The answer is A (Chapter 237). In one study, viruses were found to be the causal agent in 70% of all OM when an organism could be cultured. When bacteria were causal, *Streptococcus*, *Haemophilus*, and *Moraxella* were most common. Treatment of choice for OM in patients older than 2 years is pain management with 48 hours recheck. Amoxicillin, high dose for 7–10 days, is still the initial treatment of choice with change to alternative agents if no improvement after 72 hours. Acute mastoiditis, a complication of OM, requires admission and IV antibiotics with urgent myringotomy. OM with systemic symptoms, signs of mastoiditis, and elevated intracranial pressure are best imaged with magnetic resonance imaging, which is more sensitive than CT to rule out lateral sinus thrombosis, an ominous complication of OM.

6-13. The answer is D (Chapter 237). This patient has both frostbite of his right ear and traumatic injury of his left ear. Frostbite injuries should be quickly rewarmed with aseptic warm (38–40°C) saline-soaked gauze with good adjuvant analgesia. Vesicles that form should not be debrided but allowed to reabsorb naturally. The left ear with a hematoma needs to be debrided to prevent necrosis of the cartilage and formation of the cauliflower ear. Incision and drainage with sutured bolster dressing has found to have best outcome. Antibiotics should be reserved for immunocompromised patients. Silver sulfadiazine should not be used for burn care from the clavicle upward for cosmetic reasons as it can cause skin pigmentation changes. Sterile pledget bolster may be coated with nonsulfa antibiotic ointment.

6-14. The answer is D (Chapter 241). Trismus without swelling suggests pterygomandibular space abscess which can be diagnosed by CT. Constitutional symptoms of masticator space infections include fever, malaise, pain, dehydration, and no visible edema. Airway compromise is rare but should be considered if the trismus does not abate with pain medication; the patient is vomiting; there is a large phlegmon on CT; or other signs of impending airway compromise. Clindamycin or ampicillin–sulbactam would be the antibiotics of choice as the offending organism is usually anaerobic.

6-15. **The answer is B** (Chapter 238). This patient presents with the classic appearance of erysipelas, rapidly spreading raised red puffy appearance sharply defined borders. Cellulitis, chemical or infectious, is more diffuse in appearance. Impetigo presents with amber crusting, as it is more of a superficial epidermal infection. Whether this patient had erysipelas or cellulitis, intravenous ampicillin–sulbactam would be the treatment of choice. The most common pathogen in erysipelas is *Streptococcus pyogenes* and in cellulitis is *S. aureus* and *S. pyogenes*. Facial abscess can be diagnosed with clinical exam or bedside ultrasound and is best treated with incision and drainage.

6-16. **The answer is C** (Chapter 238). Submandibular gland stones are best treated with analgesics, massage, sialogogues, and antibiotics if superinfection is suspected. Eighty percent of sialoliths occur in the *submandibular gland* (Wharton's duct) because of its more viscous secretions and uphill course. Suppurative parotitis occurs in states of dehydration, and can be brought on by medications that dehydrate of decrease salivary flow such as antihistamines or tricyclic antidepressants. It occurs in patients with compromised salivary flow and retrograde migration of bacteria into the duct; the treatment should involve antibiotics that cover staphylococcus and anaerobic bacteria, but also maneuvers that stimulate salivary flow, such as hydration, massage, applied heat, and stimulatory sialogogues such as lemon drops. In contrast to viral infection, the onset is rapid and

without prodrome and shows erythema and warmth usually absent in viral parotitis. Viral parotitis is usually benign in children but can be severe in adults. Treatment is supportive.

6-17. **The answer is E** (Chapter 239). High blood pressure usually resolves as the epistaxis and patient's anxiety are controlled. Persistent, extremely high blood pressure should be addressed once the epistaxis is brought under control. Current treatment algorithm recommendations for acute anterior epistaxis are have the patient blow out all clots, spray the nares with vasoconstrictor, apply steady pressure for 15 minutes, and if direct pressure fails, chemical cautery is the next appropriate step with a silver nitrate stick. Thrombogenic foams and gels are becoming an increasing good option to be considered when chemical cautery fails. If the above measures fail, nasal tamponade with sponge or balloon is indicated. Nasal sponge and antistaphylococcal antibiotics are appropriate treatments for epistaxis that does not subside with direct pressure. Aspirin and nonsteroidal anti-inflammatory drugs should be avoided for 3–4 days.

6-18. **The answer is A** (Chapter 239). This picture shows a septal hematoma for which urgent incision and drainage, followed by nasal packing, is indicated. Imaging studies are usually not indicated for isolated nasal fractures since the fracture is best assessed by clinical exam. Closed reduction of an acute nasal fracture without significant edema can be attempted if there is fracture with obvious displacement or misalignment, followed by packing and external splinting and close follow-up.

6-19. **The answer is B** (Chapter 239). Acute sinusitis, like OM, is usually viral. Thus, acute sinusitis is best treated supportively with saline irrigation and decongestants. Postseptal/orbital cellulitis occurs most frequently from spread of paranasal sinusitis; the ethmoid sinus is most frequently implicated, probably due to perforation of the thin lamina papyracea of the medial wall.

Meningitis, cavernous sinus thrombosis, and intracranial abscesses are rare, but important, complications of sinusitis. Amoxicillin is the recommended first-line therapy for most adults.

6-20. **The answer is A** (Chapter 238). This patient presents with a spontaneous atraumatic anterior dislocation. A radiograph is not required as the diagnosis is clinical unless the reduction is unsuccessful or difficult. This procedure does not require a consult service unless there are other issues or time constraints. The proper method would be anesthesia either locally or with IV narcotics and muscle relaxants, and then grab the posterior mandibular molars with padded thumbs and exert steady pressure downward and posteriorly.

6-21. **The answer is C** (Chapter 240). *Acute periradicular periodontitis* infection extends to the apex of the tooth and is best treated with oral antibiotics, analgesics, and prompt root canal or tooth extraction. Episodes of cold sensitivity lasting seconds at a time recurring several times a day over greater than 1 week is a sign of *reversible pulpitis* and should be treated with antibiotics and pain meds and referred to a dentist. If the duration of symptoms last longer than minutes or hours at a time, the likelihood for *irreversible pulpitis* is high and usually best treated with root canal or extraction. Pain over an eruption wisdom tooth known as *pericoronitis* is usually secondary to severe inflammation from impacted food under the gingival flap and can progressed to masticator space tissue infections and should be treated with saline irrigation, oral antibiotics, and pain medications. Patient with complaint of dental pain and a normal exam should be worked up for sources of referred pain. Exposed dentin is best treated with emergent cover with glass ionomer to prevent pulpitis, pain medications, and urgent dental referral.

6-22. **The answer is D** (Chapter 240). Although third molar extraction can be complicated by deep masticator space infection, this is unlikely in the afebrile patient without trismus or gingival edema and thus a CT and intravenous antibiotics are not indicated. Third molar infection is not usually associated with the sublingual/submandibular space infections. *Ludwig angina* typically arises from more anterior periodontal infections. This patient does have postoperative pain and could probably be managed with local anesthesia and oral analgesics, but this patient's presentation is most consistent with *postextraction alveolar osteitis* or "dry socket" and is most properly managed with a panorex radiograph to rule out retained root tip or foreign body and then be given an inferior alveolar nerve block, irrigation and packing with oil of clove-soaked gauze, and be seen by his dentist in 24 hours. Thrombin-impregnated gauze is not indicated in the absence of bleeding.

6-23. **The answer is A** (Chapter 240). This patient has acute necrotizing ulcerative gingivitis also known as *Vincent's disease* or *trench mouth* considered an opportunistic infection with lowered host immunity—anaerobic bacteria such a *Treponema* invade otherwise healthy tissue. HIV is the most important predisposing factor. Treatment consists mainly of bacterial control with chlorhexidine washes, professional debridement, analgesics, and oral antibiotics that cover anaerobes nutritional support and follow-up with an oral surgeon within 24 hours. However, it can be difficult to differentiate from herpes gingivostomatitis. Herpes gingivostomatitis usually has more systemic symptoms and a *lack of interdental papilla involvement*. Hand, foot, and mouth disease involves other surfaces of the mouth as well, not just the gingival. Phenytoin causes gingival hyperplasia and bleeding.

6-24. **The answer is A** (Chapter 240). The location of mouth ulcerations can help differentiate the pathological entities. Aphthous ulcers involve the nonkeratinized surfaces of the mouth (buccal and labial mucosa and soft palate) and are best treated with topical steroids. Herpes simplex ulcer or herpetic gingivostomatitis involves primarily keratinized surfaces of the mouth (gingival hard palate, outer lip) and is treated with pain medications, oral hydration, and oral antivirals. Herpangina caused commonly by Coxsackievirus causes shallow painful ulcerations primarily on nonkeratinized mucosa (soft plate, tonsillar pillars, sparing the buccal mucosa, and keratinized surfaces) and is best treated with pain medication. Hand, foot, and mouth disease is commonly associated with Coxsackie type A16 virus and is characterized by vesicles and ulcers of all surfaces of the oral cavity surfaces and is best treated with pain medication. Traumatic ulcers are best treated supportively with removal of the offending source (i.e., sharp tooth or ill-fitting dentures) and pain medication.

6-25.   **The answer is C** (Chapter 240). The most common site for oral cancer is the posterior aspect of the tongue and is usually nontender. Well-demarcated zone of erythema on the tongue with atrophy of filiform papillae is known as erythema migrans or geographic tongue and is a common benign finding. *Leukoplakia* requires biopsy especially if found on the floor of the mouth, tongue, or vermillion border but only as 2–4% of the time they show dysplastic changes. *Erythroplakia*, red patches that persist and cannot be attributed to other diseases, is less common than *leukoplakia* but more likely to be associated with malignancy. Squamous cell carcinoma of the tongue is the common form of oral malignancy.

6-26.   **The answer is E** (Chapter 240). This patient presents with a Ellis class II fracture, which accounts for 70% of tooth fractures. The treatment of Ellis class II (dentin exposed) is dry the fractured surface of the tooth and seal with glass ionomer dental cement to decrease dental contamination by oral bacteria and give 24 hours dental follow-up. In Ellis class III fracture with pulp exposed, the surface should be covered with calcium hydroxide base and then covered with glass ionomer dental cement as is Ellis II fractures. Oral analgesics are indicated. Topical analgesics

should be avoided. No antibiotic treatment is necessary.

6-27.   **The answer is B** (Chapter 240). Total avulsion of the tooth requires reimplantation as soon as possible and can be successful if done within 3 hours of avulsion. Teeth should be kept moist with the mouth, or suspended in Hank's balanced salt solution, sterile normal saline, or milk in transport. If the teeth have been dry for 20–60 minutes, they should be soaked in Hank's balanced salt solution for 30 minutes. The socket can be gently rinsed with saline for clot removal but as little manipulation of the socket as possible should occur. Radiography is not necessary if physical exam does not suggest alveolar fracture. The teeth should be placed in the sockets with gentle firm pressure and securing them to the surrounding teeth with periodontal dressing and follow-up with a dentist within 24 hours.

6-28.   **The answer is A** (Chapter 240). Avulsed primary teeth are never reimplanted. Severe luxations generally require extraction, as they are a risk for aspiration and risk damage to the underlying teeth. Posttraumatic sequelae are variable and require close dental follow-up.

6-29.   **The answer is A** (Chapter 241). This patient presents with classic viral pharyngitis and should be queried about risk factors for the three viral causal organism that require diagnostic testing—mononucleosis, influenza, and HIV. However, acute diagnostic testing is usually not warranted. More than 90% of primary infections with HIV are associated with acute pharyngitis developing 2–4 weeks postexposure, but antibody titer may not be positive for up to 4–6 months. If suspicion for HIV is high, an HIV RNA viral load may be drawn. Up to 25% of patients with mononucleosis in the first week of symptoms have a false-negative test. She does not meet three of the four CDC criteria for GABHS, which are tonsillar exudates, tender anterior cervical adenopathy, absence of cough, and history of fever, so testing is not recommended. She has no signs of significant soft-tissue edema threatening airway compromise and so there is no role for dexamethasone. Fungal pharyngitis presents with hyperemia and exudates and usually has buccal mucosal involvement. There is no role for acyclovir in this scenario.

6-30. **The answer is A** (Chapter 241). A physical exam suggestive of peritonsillar abscess with negative needle aspiration requires CT or intraoral ultrasound to rule out abscess despite the fact that the most common mimic is peritonsillar cellulitis. Needle aspiration will effectively treat 90%. The proper technique is described in answer C except the needle should penetrate no more than 1 cm because the internal carotid artery lies just lateral and posterior to the tonsil. Adjuvant single-dose steroids improves severity and duration of symptoms, given in conjunction with 10 days of broad-spectrum antibiotics. Acute tonsillectomy may be considered if general anesthesia is required for incision and drainage.

6-31. **The answer is E** (Chapter 241). This patient presents with classic sublingual, submandibular space infection known as *Ludwig's angina*. The tongue can be rapidly displaced posteriorly occluding the airway. The airway of choice is awake fiberoptic endotracheal intubation or awake tracheotomy. A CT of neck and intravenous antibiotics (penicillin, ampicillin–sulbactam and clindamycin) are the preferred choice, and incision and drainage by head and neck surgeon is the appropriate treatment.

6-32. **The answer is B** (Chapter 241). In patients older than 40 years, 75% of persistent neck masses are neoplastic. The most common cause of unilateral neck masses is squamous cell carcinoma of the upper gastrointestinal tract. They can be initially mobile and then fixed as the cancer invades surrounding tissue. Other tumors are neoplasms of the salivary gland and thyroid and lymphomas.

They can become superinfected and present as abscesses. Neck masses in adolescents and young adults are usually due to infection. Midline masses suggest thyroglossal duct cysts. Single tender solitary thyroid nodules are usually benign.

6-33. **The answer is B** (Chapter 241). This patient shows classic history of foreign body aspiration. There is choking episode followed by asymptomatic period then recurrent unilateral obstructive pneumonia and/or wheezing. The patient's choking and coughing believed to be secondary to laryngeal exposure to the acidic orange juice was actually from aspiration of a seed. Children usually present with a history of choking or dysphagia, but 60% exhibit mild or absent signs and symptoms at initial presentation. Food is the most common aspired foreign body in children. All suspected foreign body aspirations require bronchoscopy.

6-34. **The answer is C** (Chapter 241). The primary goal in the management of acute laryngeal fracture is maintenance of the airway. The best approach is endotracheal intubation over a flexible bronchoscope. If the laryngeal lumen cannot be visualized because of edema or bleeding, then emergent tracheotomy at a level lower than usual should be perform. Cricothyroidotomy is contraindicated. Dexamethasone and racemic epinephrine are helpful in reducing edema after an airway has been placed.

6-35. **The answer is D** (Chapter 241). Angioedema can occur as an adverse effect to angiotensin-converting enzyme inhibitor therapy, usually within the first week of beginning therapy. Other etiologies are IgE-mediated allergic reaction, congenital loss of C1 esterase inhibitor (presents at an earlier age), and idiopathic. Subcutaneous epinephrine and racemic epinephrine nebulizer are both appropriate. Nasopharyngoscopy is indicated and admission is indicated if there is any laryngeal edema or the patient does not improve clinically.

6-36. **The answer is A** (Chapter 242). Tracheostomy tube obstruction with mucous plugging is common. It is best treated with preoxygenation (as suctioning may cause transient hypoxia) and then placing of sterile saline into the trachea and suctioning through large flexible catheters through the inner cannula. If this does not succeed, remove the inner cannula and clean with hydrogen peroxide and rinse with water. Sometimes, the entire tracheostomy tube needs to be removed and cleaned. Tracheostomy tubes less than 7 days in maturation should be manipulated only by otolaryngology surgeons. Pediatric tracheostomies do not have inner cannulas.

Gastrointestinal Emergencies
Questions

7-1. When evaluating a patient for suspected acute bowel perforation, what is the MOST appropriate initial imaging modality?

(A) Cholescintigraphy

(B) Computed tomography (CT) of the abdomen with contrast

(C) Magnetic resonance imaging (MRI) of the abdomen

(D) Plain abdominal films

(E) Ultrasonography of the abdomen

7-2. Which of the following statements is TRUE in patients with abdominal pain?

(A) Early administration of opioid analgesia should be avoided as it will obscure physical findings, delay diagnosis, or lead to increased morbidity/mortality.

(B) Elevated serum lipase is highly sensitive and specific for the diagnosis of acute pancreatitis.

(C) Normal serum lactate rules out mesenteric ischemia.

(D) Normal WBC reliably excludes surgical disease.

(E) The therapeutic value of placing a nasogastric tube in patients who are actively vomiting is well established.

7-3. Which of the following statements is TRUE in elderly patients with abdominal pain?

(A) Symptoms tend to manifest sooner.

(B) Cholecystitis is the most common surgical disease in these patients.

(C) Fever is a reliable marker for serious abdominal infection.

(D) It is not crucial to determine the etiology in the emergency department (ED) prior to admission.

(E) The presence of diarrhea reliably excludes mesenteric ischemia.

7-4. In the United States, what is the MOST common cause of acute nausea and vomiting?

(A) Central nervous system tumor

(B) Diabetic ketoacidosis

(C) Nonsteroidal anti-inflammatory drugs (NSAIDs)

(D) Pregnancy

(E) Viral gastroenteritis

7-5. A 60-year-old male presents to your ED complaining of nausea and vomiting. Two hours ago he had the onset of epigastric abdominal pain. About 1 hour ago he started having intense nausea and multiple episodes of bilious emesis. He denies any history of coronary artery disease or NSAID use. His ECG done at the time of presentation is normal. What is the most likely cause of his emesis?

(A) Achalasia

(B) Gastric outlet obstruction

(C) Large bowel obstruction

(D) Myocardial infarction

(E) Small bowel obstruction

7-6. What is the MOST common cause of traveler's diarrhea in patients returning from Latin America?

(A) *Clostridium difficile*

(B) *Escherichia coli*

(C) Invasive bacteria (*Campylobacter jejuni, shigella, salmonella*)

(D) Norovirus

(E) Protozoa

7-7. Which of the following statements is TRUE regarding infectious diarrhea?

(A) A Wright stain is a good screening test for the presence of invasive organisms.

(B) Antibiotics should be avoided in the treatment of infectious diarrhea because they can lead to a prolonged *Salmonella* carrier state.

(C) *Entamoeba histolytica, Giardia intestinalis,* and *Cryptosporidium parvum* cause short-lived, self-limited episodes of infectious diarrhea.

(D) Patients with severe abdominal pain, fever, and bloody stools should have stool studies sent for invasive bacterial organisms and *E. histolytica.*

(E) Trimethoprim/sulfamethoxazole is the treatment of choice in patients with infectious diarrhea.

7-8. Which of the following statements is TRUE regarding this patient's diagnosis? (See Figure 7-1)

(A) Antidiarrheal medications are good preventative agents.

(B) Colonic perforation is not a complication.

(C) It is associated with advanced cases of ulcerative colitis and Crohn disease.

(D) It is not associated with *C. difficile* colitis.

(E) The disease process is limited to the mucosa and submucosa.

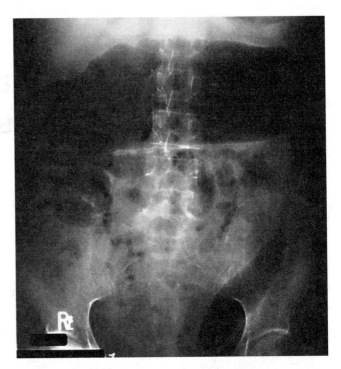

Figure 7-1. Reproduced from Kaiser AM, Beart RW: Images in clinical medicine: chronic ulcerative colitis with megacolon. *N Engl J Med.* 2003;349:358.

7-9. An 82-year-old man with dementia is transported from his nursing home secondary to abdominal distention for the past 24 hours. His vital signs are unremarkable except for a low-grade temperature of 99.5. On abdominal exam, he has hypoactive bowel sounds. His abdomen is distended and diffusely tender. He has soft, brown stool in his rectal vault. Plain abdominal films show a dilated colon from the cecum to the splenic flexure. A subsequent CT scan of the abdomen does not reveal a mechanical cause for the condition. What is the MOST likely diagnosis?

(A) Hirschsprung disease

(B) Intestinal pseudoobstruction (Ogilvie syndrome)

(C) Mechanical colonic obstruction

(D) Mesenteric ischemia

(E) Toxic megacolon

7-10. Which of the following conditions is a cause of ACUTE constipation?

(A) Amyloidosis

(B) Hyperparathyroidism

(C) Hypomagnesemia

(D) Parkinson disease

(E) Volvulus

7-11. Which of the following statements is TRUE regarding upper gastrointestinal (UGI) bleeding?

(A) A patient with an aortoenteric fistula will classically present with a self-limited "herald" bleed that precedes massive intestinal hemorrhage.

(B) Bright red blood or maroon rectal bleeding rules out an UGI bleed.

(C) Erosive gastritis and esophagitis are the most common causes of UGI bleeding.

(D) Mallory–Weiss syndrome is an UGI bleed secondary to a full-thickness esophageal tear from repeated episodes of vomiting.

(E) The passage of a nasogastric tube in patients with varices may provoke further bleeding.

7-12. A 23-year-old male presents to the ED complaining of black stools. He states he has been having an upset stomach and diarrhea for the past 2 days. He started taking an over-the-counter, bismuth-containing medication, with relief of his symptoms. However, today he noticed the onset of black stools and became alarmed. He has a normal exam except for black stool in his rectal vault that is guaiac negative. Lab results show hemoglobin of 15 gm/dL and BUN:creatinine ratio of <20. Which of the following is MOST appropriate?

(A) Discharge without any further testing and with reassurance

(B) Initiation of oral proton pump inhibitor and close follow-up

(C) Insertion of a nasogastric tube to evaluate for an UGI bleed

(D) Intravenous proton pump inhibitor and admission

(E) Type and screen for possible transfusion of packed red blood cells

7-13. Which of the following features predicts adverse outcomes in patients with upper GI hemorrhage?

(A) A history of cirrhosis or ascites on examination

(B) A history of melena

(C) Coffee-ground emesis in the nasogastric lavage

(D) Initial hematocrit less than 40%

(E) Initial systolic blood pressure less than 110 mm Hg

7-14. What is the MOST common cause of LOWER GI bleeding?

(A) Adenomatous polyps

(B) Diverticular disease

(C) Infectious colitis

(D) Inflammatory colitis

(E) Malignancy

7-15. A 74-year-old woman with a history of congestive heart failure presents with diffuse abdominal pain that started 2 hours ago. She describes the pain as severe and she is in significant distress secondary to pain. She has a temperature of 100.5, a heart rate of 110, and a blood pressure of 95/60 mm Hg. Her cardiovascular exam is remarkable for an irregular heart beat. She has a distended abdomen with hypoactive bowel sounds and diffuse tenderness to palpation on abdominal exam. There is no focal tenderness, rebound, or guarding. On rectal examination, there is profuse soft, dark brown stool that is guaiac positive. Lab results are remarkable for WBC of 16 and a lactic acid of 4.0. After fluid resuscitation and antibiotics, what is the MOST appropriate next step in the management of this patient?

(A) CT scan of the abdomen

(B) GI consult for endoscopy

(C) Medical admission for observation

(D) Right upper quadrant ultrasound

(E) Surgical consult

7-16. Which of the following statements is TRUE?

(A) Angiography requires a slow rate, lower GI bleed to detect the site of bleeding.

(B) Endoscopy is less accurate than arteriography or scintigraphy in localizing lower GI bleeding.

(C) Gastrointestinal bleeding leads to a drop in BUN levels.

(D) Hematochezia originates from an upper GI source 10% of the time.

(E) Technetium-labeled red cell scans (scintigraphy) require a relatively brisk, lower GI bleed to detect the site of bleeding.

7-17. A 55-year-old man presents to the ED complaining of new difficulty with initiation of swallowing. His symptoms are associated with halitosis and a sensation of fullness in his neck. He denies pain with swallowing or a sensation of food "getting stuck." He denies a prior history of heartburn or constitutional symptoms. He does not smoke or drink alcohol. His exam and basic labs, including a CBC, are normal. What is the MOST likely diagnosis?

(A) Esophageal stricture

(B) Neoplasm

(C) Plummer–Vinson syndrome

(D) Schatzki ring

(E) Zenker diverticulum

7-18. Which of the following is TRUE regarding esophageal perforation?

(A) Boerhaave syndrome is responsible for more than 30% of esophageal perforations.

(B) Iatrogenic perforation is the most frequent etiology.

(C) Most iatrogenic perforations occur through the left posterolateral wall of the distal esophagus.

(D) Proximal perforations tend to be more severe than distal perforations.

(E) The absence of mediastinal emphysema rules out esophageal perforation.

7-19. The x-ray is MOST consistent with which diagnosis (Figure 7-2)?

(A) Aortic knob dilation

(B) Artifact

(C) Esophageal coin impaction

(D) Subcutaneous coin impaction

(E) Tracheal coin impaction

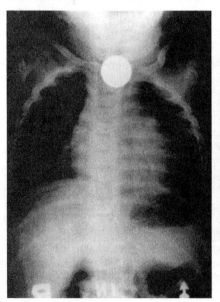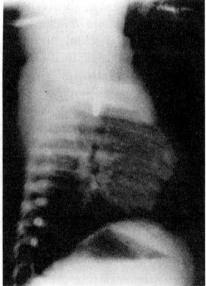

Figure 7-2. Reproduced from Effron D (ed.): *Pediatric Photo and X-Ray Stimuli for Emergency Medicine*, vol. 11. Columbus, OH: Ohio Chapter of the American College of Emergency Physicians, 1997, case 27.

7-20. Which of the following statements is TRUE regarding esophageal foreign bodies?

(A) Button batteries lodged in the esophagus can be managed expectantly.

(B) Button batteries do not need further follow-up once they have passed the esophagus.

(C) Endoscopic retrieval is the preferred method to remove small drug packets in body packers.

(D) Intestinal perforation from ingested sharp objects is rare once they have passed distal to the stomach.

(E) Objects that are irregular, sharp, particularly wide, or long are at risk for becoming lodged distal to the pylorus.

7-21. Which of the following statements is TRUE regarding peptic ulcer disease?

(A) All patients with dyspepsia require endoscopy.

(B) Diet and alcohol use are predisposing factors to the development of peptic ulcer disease, but emotional stress is not.

(C) GI barium studies are the test of choice for diagnosing peptic ulcers.

(D) The majority of peptic ulcers are caused by infection with *Helicobacter pylori* or by the use of NSAIDs.

(E) The incidence of peptic ulcer disease is increasing in the United States.

7-22. Which of the following statements is TRUE regarding *H. pylori* infection?

(A) Eradication of infection dramatically reduces 1-year recurrence rates for duodenal and peptic ulcers.

(B) Infection is not a risk factor for adenocarcinoma of the stomach.

(C) Infection is present in <50% of patients with duodenal and gastric ulcers.

(D) Most infected people will develop peptic ulcer disease.

(E) Serologic studies are superior over stool antigens for diagnosing infection.

7-23. Match the CORRECT drug used to treat peptic ulcer disease and its associated mechanism of action.

(A) Antacids—block secretion of acid at the proton pump.

(B) H2 receptor antagonists—inhibit histamine receptor of parietal cells.

(C) Misoprostol—protects ulcer from acid exposure by forming a sticky gel.

(D) Proton pump inhibitor—buffer gastric acid.

(E) Sucralfate—prostaglandin analog that increases bicarbonate production.

7-24. What is the MOST frequent cause of acute pancreatitis?

(A) Alcohol

(B) Drug induced

(C) Gallstones

(D) Hypercalcemia

(E) Hypertriglyceridemia

7-25. What is the imaging modality of choice in the ED for diagnosing acute cholecystitis?

(A) CT of the abdomen

(B) Endoscopic retrograde cholangiography (ERCP)

(C) Magnetic resonance cholangiopancreatography (MRCP)

(D) Plain radiographs

(E) Ultrasound

7-26. Which of the following causes prehepatic jaundice?

(A) Alcohol

(B) Drugs

(C) Hemolysis

(D) Toxins

(E) Viral infection

7-27.   How is hepatitis A most commonly transmitted?

   (A) Asymptomatic children to adults
   (B) Contaminated food
   (C) Improper food handling
   (D) Lack of hand washing
   (E) Oyster consumption

7-28.   In the setting of liver failure secondary to *Amanita phalloides*, what has been shown to be the most sensitive clinical marker for fatality?

   (A) Diarrhea in less than 8 hours of symptom onset
   (B) Electrolyte imbalance
   (C) Fever of 104°F
   (D) Hypotension
   (E) Tachycardia

7-29.   Which of the following test results MOST accurately predicts spontaneous bacterial peritonitis?

   (A) Low serum glucose
   (B) High protein in peritoneal fluid
   (C) High protein in serum
   (D) Neutrophil count greater than 250/μL in the peritoneal fluid
   (E) Total white count greater than 500/μL

7-30.   A 22-year-old nonpregnant female presents with acute nausea, vomiting, abdominal pain, and jaundice. Her diagnostic tests reveal an AST of 1500 and ALT of 2000. Which factor will determine if the patient should be admitted?

   (A) ALT >1000
   (B) AST >2000
   (C) Bilirubin >20
   (D) Glucose >200
   (E) INR greater than 25% normal

7-31.   What is the MOST common location of pain in a pregnant woman with appendicitis?

   (A) Right upper quadrant
   (B) Right lower quadrant
   (C) Left upper quadrant
   (D) Left lower quadrant
   (E) Umbilicus

7-32.   An 18-year-old male presents with abdominal pain that began approximately 8 hours ago. Initially, he experienced nausea with periumbilical pain that is now primarily in the right lower quadrant. He has never been hospitalized or had any surgeries. On exam, his temperature is 100.6°F, and his abdominal exam reveals tenderness at McBurney's point. What should be the next step?

   (A) CBC and urinalysis
   (B) CT scan of the abdomen/pelvis
   (C) Plain films of the abdomen
   (D) Surgical consultation
   (E) Ultrasound of the abdomen

7-33.   A 64-year-old Caucasian male presents with new left-sided abdominal pain for 1 day. He has no prior episodes of this pain. He also complains of constipation in addition to his pain. On exam, he has reproducible tenderness in the left lower quadrant. His urinalysis is negative. A CBC reveals a mild leukocytosis with a white cell count of 12,000 no bands or left shift. After receiving pain medication, the symptoms improve. What is the most appropriate next step?

   (A) Admit to the hospital for observation
   (B) CT scan
   (C) Discharge home with antibiotics
   (D) Surgery consultation
   (E) Ultrasound

7-34. A 58-year-old obese female presents with abdominal pain localized to the left lower quadrant. A CT scan of the abdomen and pelvis reveals sigmoid diverticulitis with mesenteric abscess measuring 5 cm. Appropriate disposition of this patient is:

(A) Discharge home with PO antibiotics for 2 weeks

(B) Discharge home with PO antibiotics for 2 weeks with a 48-hour recheck

(C) Discharge home after surgery consultation with PO antibiotics

(D) Admit for 24-hour observation

(E) Admit for IV antibiotics and surgery consultation.

7-35. What is the most common cause of large bowel obstruction in a 65-year-old patient?

(A) Adhesions

(B) Hernia

(C) Mesenteric ischemia

(D) Neoplasm

(E) Volvulus

7-36. If you suspect a patient has a small or large bowel obstruction, the diagnostic study of choice is:

(A) Abdominal series (plain films)

(B) Barium enema

(C) Barium swallow

(D) CT scan

(E) MRI

7-37. Which type of hernia is the most common in women?

(A) Epigastric

(B) Femoral

(C) Inguinal

(D) Spigelian

(E) Umbilical

7-38. A 38-year-old male presents with scrotal pain after lifting heavy boxes while at work. On exam, you detect an indirect inguinal hernia. He is nontoxic appearing, has normal vitals and a soft abdomen. He is in mild pain and has some tenderness when you examine him. What should be your next step?

(A) Call surgery for admission

(B) Call surgery to take patient to the OR

(C) Order a CT scan

(D) Place ice packs on groin, give analgesia, and attempt reduction

(E) Send a CBC, lipase, and chemistry panel and observe

7-39. A hernia that is firm, painful, and nonreducible in a stable patient without signs of toxicity is which type of hernia?

(A) Femoral

(B) Incarcerated

(C) Indirect

(D) Reducible

(E) Strangulated

7-40. A 15-year-old female who works after school at a day care presents with an inguinal mass. Her sister was recently diagnosed with cervical cancer, and she is worried she may have cancer. She noticed the mass after lifting an infant at school. It is soft and reducible. On exam, you palpate a mass in the inguinal region on the right. What should occur NEXT to solidify a diagnosis and reassure the patient?

(A) CBC

(B) CT scan

(C) Rectal exam

(D) Ultrasound

(E) Urinalysis

7-41. What is the most common cause of rectal bleeding?

(A) Anal fissures

(B) Colon cancer

(C) Diverticulosis

(D) Hemorrhoids

(E) Ulcerative colitis

7-42.   Which anorectal abscess can be appropriately treated in the ED?

(A) Intersphincteric

(B) Ischiorectal

(C) Perianal

(D) Submucosal

(E) Supralevator

7-43.   A 28-year-old pregnant female (32 weeks of gestation) presents to the ED complaining of painful bowel movements. The pain has been present for 24 hours, and is extremely painful. She is unable to sit during the exam and must lay on her side. On rectal exam, two thrombosed external hemorrhoids are visualized. What is the MOST appropriate next step?

(A) Clot excision

(B) Laxatives

(C) Sitz baths

(D) Surgery consultation

(E) Topical hydrocortisone

7-44.   Which of the following confirms appropriate placement of a nasogastric tube?

(A) Air bubbles when proximal end of tube is placed in water

(B) Epigastric auscultation of air insufflated through the tube

(C) Patient choking or coughing

(D) Patient's inability to speak

(E) pH testing of aspirates (pH >6 indicates gastric placement)

7-45.   A 54-year-old male with cirrhosis presents with a distended abdomen and shortness of breath. An ultrasound reveals significant peritoneal fluid consistent with ascites. A paracentesis was performed. More than 4 L of fluid was removed from the patient. Once the paracentesis is complete, the patient's nurse notifies you that the paracentesis site is leaking. What is the most appropriate next step in management?

(A) Consult a surgeon

(B) Perform another paracentesis to remove more peritoneal fluid

(C) Place a dry dressing and recheck in 1 hour

(D) Place a purse string suture, apply a dry dressing, and recheck in 30 minutes

(E) Send a chemistry panel

7-46.   What is the most common complication after colonoscopy?

(A) Hemorrhage

(B) Infection

(C) Perforation

(D) Splenic rupture

(E) Volvulus

7-47.   A patient presents complaining of nausea, diarrhea, dizziness, and epigastric discomfort immediately after eating a meal. The symptoms recur after each meal with a near syncopal episode today. She had a gastric bypass procedure 3 months ago. What is the most likely cause of her symptoms?

(A) Anastomotic leak

(B) Cholecystitis

(C) Dumping syndrome

(D) Gastroesophageal reflux disease (GERD)

(E) Enterocutaneous fistula

7-48.   A nurse notifies you that an inpatient who had a cholecystectomy 14 hours ago has developed a fever of 101. He is not complaining of shortness of breath, chest pain, or abdominal pain. The rest of his vitals are BP 120/80, RR 18, P 74, and oxygen saturation of 98% on room air. His lungs are clear, heart is regular, abdomen is nontender, and surgical scar appears intact. What is the most likely cause of his fever?

(A) Atelectasis

(B) Deep vein thrombosis

(C) Intra-abdominal infection

(D) Pneumonia

(E) Urinary tract infection

Gastrointestinal Emergencies
Answers and Explanations

7-1. **The answer is D** (Chapter 74). It is important to recognize that surgical consultation should not be delayed awaiting the results of imaging in the acute abdomen. If imaging is obtained in cases of suspected acute bowel perforation, then the most appropriate initial imaging modality is plain abdominal films as they are relatively easy to obtain, and free air visible on a plain abdominal film mandates immediate surgical evaluation without the need for additional imaging. However, abdominal plain films cannot rule out perforation. Up to 20% of patients with perforation will not demonstrate free air. Ultrasonography is the preferred modality for the evaluation of the biliary tract. It may be a more sensitive test than abdominal plain films for the detection of free air, but it is highly operator dependent, requires specialized equipment, and is limited by obesity and overlying gas. While CT scan of the abdomen is superior in identifying free air when compared with plain abdominal films, it is associated with significant delays due to the administration of contrast and radiologist interpretation. Cholescintigraphy and MRI of the abdomen do not have a role in the initial evaluation of suspected acute bowel perforation.

7-2. **The answer is B** (Chapter 74). An elevated serum lipase has a sensitivity of 90% and a specificity of 93% for the diagnosis of acute pancreatitis. It is important to be aware of the limitations of laboratory testing in patients with acute abdominal pain. Laboratory information alone should not be relied upon for the diagnosis. Up to 25% of patients

with mesenteric ischemia will have a normal serum lactate on presentation. A significant number of patients with acute appendicitis and/or perforation have normal WBC. Opioid analgesics do not obscure physical findings, delay diagnosis, or lead to increased morbidity/mortality in patients with undifferentiated abdominal pain and should not be withheld. The therapeutic value of nasogastric tube placement in patients with abdominal pain has not been demonstrated. Instead, the clinician should liberally administer antiemetics in patients who are actively vomiting.

7-3. **The answer is B** (Chapter 74). Cholecystitis is the most common surgical disease in elderly patients with abdominal pain, followed by small bowel obstruction, perforated viscus, appendicitis, and large bowel obstruction. Fever is not a reliable marker for surgical disease. Instead the elderly patient with a serious abdominal infection may be hypothermic. Elderly patients who present to the ED with abdominal pain have a high mortality that doubles if the diagnosis is not made correctly at the time of admission. Diarrhea occurs in 31–40% of patients with mesenteric ischemia. When compared with younger patients, elderly patients present later, with more mild and vague symptom. However, despite this atypical presentation, they have more serious illness.

7-4. **The answer is E** (Chapter 75). Acute nausea and vomiting can be a symptom of many disorders. It is important to consider a broad differential when evaluating a patient with acute nausea and vomiting. While all of the answers are known to cause acute nausea and vomiting, viral gastroenteritis is the most common cause in the United States.

7-5. **The answer is E** (Chapter 75). Pain preceding nausea and vomiting is associated with an obstructive process. The content of the emesis is helpful in determining if an obstruction is present. Bilious emesis is associated with small bowel obstruction. Esophageal disorders such as Achalasia result in regurgitation of swallowed food particles. Gastric outlet obstruction results in emesis composed of food particles, but devoid of bile. Large bowel obstruction is associated with emesis of feculent material. While it is important to consider acute coronary syndrome in elderly patients with epigastric abdominal pain, a normal ECG and the presence of bile in the emesis point to small bowel obstruction as the most likely cause.

7-6. **The answer is B** (Chapter 76). Diarrhea is a common occurrence in travelers returning from developing countries. Toxin and nontoxin-producing strains of *E. coli* account for most identifiable cases in Mexico and South America. The invasive bacteria are more commonly seen in travelers to southern Asia. In the United States, the most common cause of infectious diarrhea is the norovirus, accounting for 50–80% of cases. *C. difficile* and protozoa are known to cause infectious diarrhea, but they are not the most common cause of traveler's diarrhea in patients returning from Central and South America.

7-7. **The answer is D** (Chapter 76). Patients with severe pain, fever, and bloody stool are at increased risk for infection with *C. jejuni, shigella, salmonella, E. coli O157:H7*, and *E. histolytica*. The Wright stain allows for the detection of fecal leucocytes. Traditionally, the Wright stain was used to differentiate between invasive and noninvasive infectious diarrhea. However, the Wright stain has a sensitivity of 52–82% and does not adequately screen for invasive diarrhea. Recent literature does not show

that treating infectious diarrhea with antibiotics leads to a prolonged *Salmonella* carrier state. *E. histolytica, G. intestinalis*, and *C. parvum* lead to episodes of prolonged diarrhea (>7 days). Ciprofloxacin is the antibiotic of choice in all patients with infectious diarrhea who do not have a contraindication to antimicrobial treatment (pediatric age group, allergy, pregnancy, drug interaction). Trimethoprim/sulfamethoxazole is a second-line antibiotic due to resistant organisms.

7-8. **The answer is C** (Chapter 76). Toxic megacolon develops in advanced cases of inflammatory and *C. difficile* colitis when the disease process begins to extend through all layers of the colon. The loss of muscular tone within the colon leads to dilation, localized peritonitis, and, if left untreated, eventual perforation. Most authors recommend avoiding antidiarrheal medications in patients with suspected inflammatory or *C. difficile* colitis because they may precipitate toxic megacolon.

7-9. **The answer is B** (Chapter 77). Intestinal pseudoobstruction is a clinical disorder with the signs and symptoms, and radiographic appearance of acute, large bowel obstruction with no evidence of distal colonic obstruction. The colon may become massively dilated. If not decompressed, the patient risks perforation, peritonitis, and death. The exact mechanism is unknown, but thought to be secondary to an imbalance in the colonic autonomic innervation. Predisposing factors include advanced age, recent surgery, underlying neurologic disorders, and critical illness. Mechanical colonic obstruction is unlikely given the results of the CT scan. Plain radiographs in mesenteric ischemia are generally normal or nonspecific. Toxic megacolon is a complication of inflammatory or infectious colitis. Patients with toxic megacolon are acutely ill with signs of systemic toxicity.

7-10. **The answer is E** (Chapter 77). Acute constipation is secondary to intestinal obstruction until proven otherwise. Common causes of intestinal obstruction include rapidly growing tumors, strictures, hernia, adhesions, inflammatory conditions, and volvulus. Hyperparathyroidism, hypomagnesemia, and Parkinson disease cause chronic constipation.

7-11. **The answer is A** (Chapter 78). An aortoenteric fistula secondary to a preexisting aortic graft is an unusual, but important, cause of intestinal bleeding. Classically, these patients will have a self-limited "herald" bleed that precedes massive hemorrhage. Peptic ulcer disease, not erosive gastritis and esophagitis, is the most common cause of UGI bleeding. Bright red or maroon rectal bleeding originates from an UGI bleed 14% of the time. Concerns that nasogastric tube passage may provoke bleeding in patients with varices are unwarranted.

7-12. **The answer is A** (Chapter 78). When bismuth combines with sulfur in the GI tract, bismuth sulfate is formed which is black. However, unlike with melena, stool guaiac testing will be negative. Given that the patient has a normal exam, a normal hemoglobin, and he gives the history of taking a bismuth-containing medication that accounts for his guaiac-negative black stools, he can be safely discharged home without further testing. The other interventions would be appropriate in a patient with a high clinical suspicion for a GI bleed.

7-13. **The answer is A** (Chapter 78). Clinical features predicting adverse outcomes include initial hematocrit less than 30%, initial systolic blood pressure lower than 100 mm Hg, red blood in the NG lavage, a history of cirrhosis or ascites on examination, and a history of vomiting red blood.

7-14. **The answer is B** (Chapter 79). The most common source for GI bleeding is from a site proximal to the ligament of Treitz (UGI bleed). Most UGI bleeds are secondary to peptic ulcer disease. However, in patients with an established lower GI source of bleeding, the most common etiology is diverticular disease, followed by colitis, adenomatous polyps, and malignancy.

7-15. **The answer is E** (Chapter 79). The most likely diagnosis is mesenteric ischemia secondary to low arterial flow or thromboembolism given the history of congestive heart failure, clinical findings consistent with atrial fibrillation, and pain out of proportion to exam. Mesenteric ischemia is a surgical emergency that will often lead to bowel necrosis and overwhelming sepsis if left untreated. Despite aggressive treatment, prognosis is poor with a survival of 50% if diagnosed within 24 hours. Immediate surgical consultation is required as soon as the diagnosis is suspected to increase the patient's chance of survival. CT scan of the abdomen should be obtained after surgical consultation, but should not delay taking the patient to the operating room. Mesenteric ischemia is a more likely diagnosis than a GI bleed. Therefore, GI consultation for endoscopy is not appropriate prior to surgical consultation. Every attempt should be made to make the diagnosis in the ED prior to admission. A delay in diagnosis by admitting the patient to a nonsurgical service will lead an adverse outcome. Right upper quadrant ultrasound looking for cholecystitis may be appropriate, but should not delay surgical consultation for possible mesenteric ischemia.

7-16. **The answer is D** (Chapter 79). Hematochezia is associated with lower GI bleeding. However 10–14% of the time hematochezia is associated with an upper GI source. Endoscopy is more accurate than arteriography or scintigraphy in localizing lower GI bleeding. Angiography requires a relatively brisk bleeding rate (at least 0.5 mL/min) to detect the site of lower GI bleeding. Technetium-labeled red cell scans are more sensitive than angiography in localizing the site of lower GI bleeding. They can localize the site of bleeding at a rate as low at 0.1 mL/min.

7-17. **The answer is E** (Chapter 80). This patient has symptoms of transfer dysphagia (difficulty in initiating a swallow) associated with halitosis and a sensation of fullness in the neck, most consistent with Zenker diverticula. Zenker diverticula typically develop in middle-aged men and result from a progressive out-pouching of the pharyngeal mucosa just above the upper esophageal sphincter. Esophageal strictures occur in the distal esophagus and interfere with lower sphincter function. Patients typically complain of solid food dysphagia a few seconds after swallowing is initiated (transport dysphagia). Esophageal strictures develop over time as a consequence of GERD or other chronic inflammatory conditions. Esophageal neoplasm must be considered in any patient older than 40 years who develops new onset dysphagia. However, given the constellation of symptoms, neoplasm is not the most likely diagnosis. This patient should be referred to a gastroenterologist to rule out a neoplastic process. Plummer–Vinson syndrome is a disorder associated with intermittent solid food dysphagia, esophageal webs, and iron-deficiency anemia. A Schatzki ring is a fibrous, diaphragm-like structure near the gastroesophageal junction that is present in up to 15% of the population. It is the most common cause of intermittent dysphagia with solids. A frequent presenting sign is the esophageal impaction of poorly chewed meat.

7-18.   **The answer is B** (Chapter 80). It is important to distinguish between iatrogenic and spontaneous causes of esophageal perforation. Iatrogenic perforation from esophageal instrumentation accounts for the majority of cases. Spontaneous perforations can be due to Boerhaave syndrome, caustic ingestions, and pill esophagitis among others. Boerhaave syndrome is a full-thickness perforation of the esophagus due to a sudden rise in intraesophageal pressure such as in forceful emesis or coughing. It accounts for 10–15% of perforations. Most spontaneous perforations occur through the left posterolateral wall of the distal esophagus. Distal perforations tend to be more severe as they can leak esophageal contents into the mediastinum, pleural, or peritoneal spaces. This can result in fulminant necrotizing mediastinitis, pneumonitis,

or peritonitis. The absence of mediastinal emphysema does not rule out esophageal perforation.

7-19.   **The answer is C** (Chapter 80). Esophageal coin impactions appear as a radio-opaque, circular object on AP films. Conversely, tracheal coin impactions appear as a radio-opaque, circular object on lateral films.

7-20.   **The answer is E** (Chapter 80). Most objects continue through the GI tract uneventfully once they have passed through the pylorus. However, irregular, sharp, wide (>2.5 cm) or long (>6 cm) objects are at risk for becoming lodged distal to the pylorus. A button battery lodged in the esophagus is a true emergency as perforation can occur within 6 hours of ingestion. These patients should undergo immediate endoscopic removal. Button batteries that have passed the esophagus can be managed expectantly with 24 hours follow-up. Repeat films should be obtained in 48 hours to ensure that the battery has passed the pylorus. Endoscopic retrieval is contraindicated in body packers because of the risk of iatrogenic packet rupture. So long as there is no evidence of rupture, these packets should be allowed to traverse naturally through the GI tract with the use of whole bowel irrigation to aid the process if necessary. Intestinal perforation from ingested sharp objects that have passed distal to the stomach is common (35%). Therefore, the recommendation is to remove sharp objects by endoscopy while they are still in the stomach or duodenum. If the object passes distal to the duodenum, then daily films will be necessary to document the object's passage. If the object does not pass within 3 days, then surgical retrieval may be necessary.

7-21.   **The answer is D** (Chapter 81). The majority of peptic ulcers are caused by infection with *H. pylori* or by the use of NSAIDs. Not all patients with dyspepsia require endoscopy. Patients with "alarm features" are at increased risk for gastric or esophageal cancer as well as other potentially serious conditions and should be referred for endoscopy. Alarm features include age >55, unexplained weight loss, early satiety, persistent vomiting, dysphagia, anemia or GI bleeding, abdominal mass, persistent anorexia, or jaundice. Emotional stress is a predisposing factor for the development of peptic ulcer disease, while diet and alcohol are not. UGI endoscopy has a sensitivity and specificity of greater than 95% for the visualization of an ulcer and is more sensitive and specific than GI barium studies. The incidence of peptic ulcer disease is decreasing in the United States. The decrease is thought to be secondary to improved standard of living, lack of *H. pylori* infection, and increased use of proton pump inhibitors.

7-22. **The answer is A** (Chapter 81). Eradication of infection reduces 1-year recurrence rates from 35% to 2% for duodenal ulcers and from 39% to 3% for gastric ulcers. Eradication is typically done with "triple therapy" that includes a proton pump inhibitor, clarithromycin, and either amoxicillin or metronidazole. Infection is a definite risk factor for adenocarcinoma of the stomach. In addition, *H. pylori* is a causative agent of mucosa associated lymphoid tissue (MALT) lymphoma. Ninety-five percent of patients with duodenal ulcer and 70% of patients with gastric ulcers are infected. Only 10–20% of infected people develop peptic ulcer disease. *H. pylori* antigens can be detected in the stool with a sensitivity and specificity of greater than 90%. Serologic studies that detect immunoglobulin G antibodies to *H. pylori* have sensitivity and specificity of 76–84% and 79–90%, respectively.

7-23. **The answer is B** (Chapter 81). Histamine receptor antagonists inhibit the H2 receptors of the gastric parietal cells, thereby suppressing acid secretion. Antacids buffer gastric acid, and are mainly used as needed for breakthrough ulcer pain in patients taking concurrent proton pump inhibitor or H2 blockers until healing occurs. Misoprostol is a prostaglandin analog that increases mucous bicarbonate production by increasing mucosal blood flow. Misoprostol may pre-

vent ulcer formation in patients on concurrent NSAID therapy. Proton pump inhibitors decrease acid by blocking its secretion at the proton pump on gastric parietal cells. When compared with H2 blockers, proton pump inhibitors heal ulcers faster. Sucralfate protects ulcer from acid exposure by forming a sticky gel to allow healing.

7-24. **The answer is C** (Chapter 82). Gallstones are the leading cause of acute pancreatitis, accounting for at least 35–40% of cases. Alcohol is the second most frequent cause. Hypertriglyceridemia accounts for 1–4% of cases. Drugs account for <2% of cases.

7-25. **The answer is E** (Chapter 82). Right upper quadrant ultrasound is the imaging modality of choice for diagnosing acute cholecystitis in the ED. It has a sensitivity of 94% and a specificity of 78% for detecting acute cholecystitis. A sonographic Murphy sign has a high PPV for acute cholecystitis. Ultrasonography is readily available in the ED. CT scan of the abdomen is useful in diagnosing acute cholecystitis when ultrasound results are equivocal. ERCP and MRCP are useful for the evaluation of the biliary tree to delineate the cause of obstruction, but are not readily available from the ED. ERCP has the advantage of being both diagnostic and therapeutic. MRI of the abdomen is useful when ultrasonography and CT findings are inconclusive. While it has the highest sensitivity for signs of cholecystitis, it is not as readily available.

7-26. **The answer is D** (Chapter 83). Prehepatic jaundice is caused by any form of hemolysis, or an inborn error of bilirubin metabolism that overwhelms the liver's ability to conjugate bilirubin. The most common causes of hepatic jaundice are viral infection, toxins, drugs, and alcohol. As hepatocytes necrose, the liver's ability to conjugate bilirubin is impaired, and the levels of both unconjugated and conjugated bilirubin rise in the blood. Posthepatic jaundice is caused by a physical obstruction of conjugated bilirubin excretion, typically a pancreatic tumor or a gallstone in the common bile duct, or more uncommonly parasitic infestation or biliary atresia.

7-27. **The answer is A.** Hepatitis A is transmitted by the fecal-oral route. Although it is popularly associated with improper food handling or oyster consumption, the most common transmission occurs from asymptomatic children to adults. Hepatitis A infection has an incubation period of 15–50 days, followed by a prodrome of nausea, vomiting, and malaise. About a week into the illness, patients may note dark urine (bilirubinuria). A few days later, they develop clay-colored stools and jaundice. Hepatitis A does not have a chronic component, and death from hepatic failure is rare.

7-28. **The answer is A** (Chapter 83). There are three stages in the presentation of mushroom poisoning. In the first stage, 6–24 hours after ingestion, patients experience abdominal pain, fever, nausea, vomiting, pronounced diarrhea, tachycardia, hyperglycemia, hypotension, and electrolyte imbalance. From 24 to 48 hours after ingestion, the second stage of poisoning brings reduction in symptoms, even as the liver deteriorates precipitously. Fulminant liver failure marks the third stage, and the patient will experience coagulopathy, hepatic coma, shock, renal failure, extreme electrolyte imbalance, and seizures. The onset of diarrhea at less than 8 hours after ingestion has been demonstrated to be a sensitive marker for fatality (i.e., death or liver transplantation). In addition, all patients with international normalized ratio (INR) ≥6 at 4 days from ingestion have required liver transplantation. Overall, various case series have demonstrated that 10–30% of patients who ingest *A. phalloides* will develop hepatic failure and need transplantation. The rapid progression of initial symptoms to full hepatic failure makes transplantation difficult.

7-29. **The answer is D** (Chapter 83). Ascitic fluid is tested for cell count, glucose and protein, Gram stain, and culture to identify bacterial peritonitis. A total white blood cell count greater than 1000/μL or a neutrophil count greater than 250/μL is diagnostic for spontaneous bacterial peritonitis. Low glucose or high protein values suggest infection. Gram stains and culture results can be falsely negative 30–40% of the time, and empiric antibiotics should be started in the ED based on clinical suspicion. Culture sensitivity is increased by using 10 mL of ascitic fluid per blood culture bottle. Additional studies of ascites that can help with inpatient evaluation are cytology, albumin, LDH, and tumor markers.

7-30. **The answer is C** (Chapter 83). Patients with acute hepatitis require supportive treatment with pain management and fluid resuscitation. Consider admission for high-risk patients including the elderly and pregnant women. Admit those who have a bilirubin ≥20 mg/dL, prothrombin time 50% above normal, hypoglycemia, low albumin, or any signs of GI bleeding.

7-31. **The answer is B** (Chapter 84). It is important to remember that appendectomy is the most common nonobstetrical surgical procedure in pregnant women. The right lower quadrant is the most common location of pain in patients with an acute appendicitis. Pregnant women are no exception. However, one must consider appendicitis in other areas of the abdomen especially right upper quadrant because the uterus can displace the intestines into the abdominal cavity as the uterus grows.

7-32. **The answer is D** (Chapter 84). Surgical consultation is recommended for any patient with a classic history for appendicitis. However, surgeons may request imaging before they will take the patient to the operating room.

7-33. **The answer is B** (Chapter 85). In stable patients with a history of confirmed diverticulitis and a similar acute presentation, no further diagnostic evaluation is necessary unless the patient fails to improve with conservative medical treatment. If a prior diagnosis has not been confirmed or the current episode differs from the past episode, diagnostic imaging is required to rule out other intra-abdominal pathology and evaluate for complications. CT is the preferred imaging modality given its ability to evaluate the severity of disease and the presence of complications.

7-34. The answer is E (Chapter 85). The majority of uncomplicated diverticulitis improves with bowel rest (liquid diet) and antibiotics (Table 7-1). It is estimated that conservative treatment in this group of patients has a 70–100% success rate. In cases where uncomplicated diverticulitis is confirmed with CT, the success rate is 97%. Most patients should be able to follow this regimen as an outpatient. Complicated diverticulitis generally requires admission. In addition to the standard regimen of bowel rest and IV antibiotics, patients will need specific treatments directed at the complications. Complicated diverticulitis is often referred to by the Hinchey Classification scheme: Stage 1 refers to small, confined pericolic or mesenteric abscesses; Stage 2 refers to larger abscesses, often confined to the pelvis; Stage 3 refers to perforated diverticulitis where a ruptured abscess causes purulent diverticulitis; and Stage 4 refers to free perforation with fecal contamination of the peritoneal cavity.

TABLE 7-1. ANTIBIOTIC TREATMENT FOR DIVERTICULITIS

Outpatient or Inpatient Status	Antibiotic and Dosage (Adjust Dosages Based on Renal Function)
Outpatient, 7–14 d oral medication	Metronidazole, 500 mg PO every 8 h *and* Ciprofloxacin, 500 mg PO every 12 h *or* Levofloxacin, 500 mg PO once a day *or* Clindamycin, 300 mg PO every 6 h *or* Trimethoprim–sulfamethoxazole DS, one tablet PO every 12 h Amoxicillin–clavulanate, 875 mg PO every 12 h Moxifloxacin, 400 mg PO once a day
Inpatient, moderate-to-severe disease	Ampicillin–sulbactam, 3 g IV every 6 h *or* Piperacillin–tazobactam, 3.35 g IV every 6 h, or 4.5 g IV every 8 h *or* Ertapenem, 1 g IV once a day *or* Ticarcillin–clavulanate, 3.1 g IV every 6 h *or* Moxifloxacin, 400 mg IV once a day Metronidazole, 500 mg IV every 6 h *and* Levofloxacin, 750 mg IV once a day *or* Ciprofloxacin, 400 mg IV every 12 h
Intensive care unit patient, very severe disease	Imipenem, 500 mg IV every 6 h *or* Meropenem, 1 g IV every 8 h *or* Doripenem, 500 mg IV every 8 h (each infusion given over 1 h) Ampicillin, 2 g IV every 6 h *and* Metronidazole, 500 mg IV every 6 h *and* Gentamicin, 2 mg/kg IV as initial dose, then 1.7 mg/kg every 8 h

Reproduced from Graham A. Diverticulitis. In: Tintinalli JE, Stapczynski JS, Ma OJ, Cline DM, Cydulka RK, Meckler GD (eds). *Tintinalli's Emergency Medicine: A Comprehensive Study Guide*, 7th edition. New York: McGraw-Hill; 2011:580. Copyright © The McGraw-Hill Companies, Inc. All rights reserved.

7-35. **The answer is D** (Chapter 86). Neoplasms are by far the most common cause of large bowel obstruction. Colonic obstruction is almost never caused by hernia or surgical adhesions. Adhesions and hernias are common causes for small bowel obstruction in the elderly, whereas carcinoma is the most likely cause of large bowel obstruction in the elderly because of the increased likelihood of cancer as people age.

7-36. **The answer is D** (Chapter 36). In the ED, flat and upright abdominal radiographs and upright chest x-ray or a lateral decubitus view can be used to screen for bowel obstruction, severe constipation, or free air. Plain x-rays can also localize the site to large or small bowel. However, if clinical suspicion for obstruction is strong, a CT scan is the diagnostic method of choice in the ED. If intravenous contrast cannot be used because of renal insufficiency or contrast allergy, oral contrast alone may provide sufficient diagnostic information. Oral and intravenous contrast-enhanced CT can delineate partial or complete bowel obstruction, distinguish partial small bowel obstruction from ileus, and differentiate strangulated from simple small bowel obstruction.

7-37. **The answer is C** (Chapter 87). Seventy-five percent of all hernias occur in the inguinal region making it the most common form of hernia, with two-thirds of these being of the indirect type. Although there is a clear male predilection, inguinal hernias are also the most common hernias in women.

7-38. **The answer is D** (Chapter 87). This patient reveals signs of an incarcerated hernia. If the hernia is incarcerated, but the patient does not yet show signs of strangulation, then try one or two attempts at reduction in the ED. Steps for hernia reduction include (1) NPO status in case reduction attempts are unsuccessful, (2) adequate IV narcotic analgesia, (3) proper positioning with the patient supine in mild Trendelenburg position, and (4) apply cold packs to the hernia site to reduce swelling and make reduction attempts easier. Grasp and elongate the hernia neck with one hand, and with the other hand, apply firm, steady pressure to the distal part of the hernia. Applying pressure on the most distal part of the hernia can cause bulging of the neck and prevent reduction. If the hernia is exquisitely tender and is associated with systemic signs and symptoms, such as intestinal obstruction, toxic appearance, peritonitis, or meets sepsis criteria, then assume hernia strangulation. Consult general surgery immediately.

7-39. **The answer is B** (Chapter 87). A hernia is reducible when the hernia sac itself is soft and easy to replace back through the hernia neck defect. A hernia is incarcerated when it is firm, often painful, and nonreducible by direct manual pressure. Strangulation develops as a consequence of incarceration and implies impairment of blood flow (arterial, venous, or both). A strangulated hernia presents as severe, exquisite pain at the hernia site, often with signs and symptoms of intestinal obstruction, toxic appearance, and, possibly, skin changes overlying the hernia sac. A strangulated hernia is an acute surgical emergency.

7-40. **The answer is D** (Chapter 87). Bedside ultrasound can be very helpful in the identification of an inguinal hernia if the diagnosis remains in question. One study reported 100% sensitivity and 100% specificity of bedside emergency ultrasound for the diagnosis of groin hernia. Sonography has many advantages but is operator and body habitus dependent. The primary role of ultrasound is the identification of the hernia itself. Other roles include identification of blood flow by color Doppler to exclude strangulation, particularly prior to reduction attempts. Ultrasound is most useful for diagnosis in children and pregnant women. CT is the best radiographic test for diagnosis, and can identify uncommon hernia types (e.g., Spigelian or obturator) and demonstrate incarceration and strangulation.

7-41. **The answer is D** (Chapter 87). Hemorrhoidal bleeding is usually limited, with the blood being found on the surface of the stool, on the toilet tissue, or noted at the end of defecation, dripping into the toilet bowl. When patients describe the passage of blood clots, colonic lesions should be suspected and investigated. Although the most common cause of rectal bleeding is hemorrhoids, other, more serious causes should be investigated.

7-42. **The answer is C** (Chapter 88). An isolated perianal abscess not associated with deeper, perirectal abscesses is generally the only type of anorectal abscess that can be adequately treated in the ED. Treatment of perianal abscesses is incision and drainage. All perirectal abscesses (supralevator, intersphincteric, and complicated ischiorectal) should be drained in the operating room.

7-43. **The answer is D** (Chapter 88). External hemorrhoidal hematoma formation is usually self-limiting with resolution in 1 week. Therapy for thrombosed external hemorrhoids depends on the severity of symptoms. If the thrombosis has been present for more than 48 hours, the swelling has started to shrink, is not tense, and the pain is tolerable, the patient may be treated with sitz baths and bulk laxatives. Suppositories, which are placed proximal to the anorectal ring, are of no help. If, on the other hand, the thrombosis is acute, has lasted less than 48 hours, and is extremely painful, significant relief can be provided by clot excision. Excision should not be performed in the ED on immunocompromised patients, children, pregnant women, patients with portal hypertension, and those who are anticoagulated or have a coagulopathy.

7-44. **The answer is B** (Chapter 89). Nasogastric tube placement is confirmed by epigastric auscultation of air insufflated through the tube, aspiration of visually recognizable GI secretions, or pH testing of aspirates (pH <6 indicates gastric placement).

7-45. **The answer is D** (Chapter 89). Large-volume therapeutic paracentesis is a lengthy procedure associated with complications such as hyponatremia, renal impairment, persistent leakage, and encephalopathy. A purse-string suture can be placed to minimize leakage. Recheck the patient in 30 minutes to identify persistent leakage or an increase in symptoms to suggest a complication. Patients with large-volume paracentesis should be monitored for hypotension after the procedure. Cover the puncture site with a dry dressing for 48 hours.

7-46. **The answer is A** (Chapter 90). Potential complications of colonoscopy include hemorrhage, perforation, retroperitoneal abscess, pneumoscrotum, pneumothorax, volvulus, postcolonoscopy distention, splenic rupture, appendicitis, bacteremia, and infection. Hemorrhage is the most common complication and can be secondary to polypectomy, biopsies, laceration of the mucosa by the instrument, or tearing of the mesentery or spleen. If the bleeding is intraluminal, the patient will develop rectal bleeding. Patients with mesenteric or splenic injury will present with signs of intra-abdominal bleeding. Treatment of intraluminal bleeding depends on the magnitude of hemorrhage. Intra-abdominal bleeding requires emergency laparotomy. Colon perforation with pneumoperitoneum usually is evident immediately but can take several hours to manifest. Perforation is usually secondary to intrinsic disease of the colon (e.g., diverticulitis) or to vigorous manipulation during the procedure. Most patients will require immediate laparotomy, but in some patients presenting late (1–2 days later) without signs of peritonitis, hospital observation may be appropriate.

7-47. **The answer is C** (Chapter 90). A common complication of the Roux-en-Y gastric bypass is dumping syndrome, which can occur either right after the meal (early) or 2–4 hours later (late). Dumping symptoms occur when the pylorus is bypassed or removed. The hyperosmolar chyme contents of the stomach are dumped into the jejunum, resulting in rapid influx of extracellular fluid and an autonomic response. Patients experience nausea, epigastric discomfort, palpitations, colicky abdominal pain, diaphoresis, and, in some cases, dizziness and syncope. Patients with early dumping symptoms experience diarrhea, whereas those with late dumping symptoms, 2–4 hours postprandially, usually do not. The late dumping syndrome is believed to be due to a reactive hypoglycemia. The mainstay of treatment is dietary modification; eating small, dry meals; and separating solids from liquids. In refractory cases, pyloroplasty can be tried. Most patients with dumping syndrome do not require admission.

7-48. **The answer is A** (Chapter 90). Fever is a common postoperative complaint. The "five W's": *wind* (atelectasis or pneumonia), *water* (urinary tract infection), *wound*, *walking* (deep vein thrombosis), and *wonder drugs* (drug fever or pseudomembranous colitis) are a common way to think about the potential etiologies of postoperative fever. Atelectasis is a common cause of fever during the initial 24 hours. Other early postoperative causes of fever are necrotizing streptococcal and clostridial infections.

Gynecologic and Obstetric Emergencies
Questions

8-1. A 39-year-old female presents to the emergency department (ED) with persistent vaginal bleeding for 3 weeks. She normally has regular periods, but she has not had a period in the 2 months prior to this bleeding. She denies abdominal pain and states she is soaking about four pads per day. Her vitals are normal, her pregnancy test is negative, and her hematocrit is 40. Which of the following is the most appropriate next step in management?

(A) Acetaminophen 600 mg every 6 hours
(B) Follow up with her gynecologist in 2 weeks
(C) Intravenous estrogen
(D) Progesterone 10 mg/day for 10 days
(E) STAT pelvic ultrasound

8-2. A 64-year-old female presents to the ED with vaginal bleeding for 4 days. She denies abdominal pain and describes the bleeding as light. Her vital signs are normal and exam confirms trace blood in the vaginal vault. Her hematocrit is stable and an ultrasound does not show a cause for her symptoms. Which of the following is the most appropriate next step in management?

(A) Abdominal CT scan
(B) Follow up with her primary care doctor for her routine physical exam
(C) No further care is warranted
(D) Progesterone 10 mg/day for 10 days
(E) Referral to a gynecologist for endometrial biopsy

8-3. Regarding ovarian torsion, which of the following statements is correct?

(A) Drugs that stimulate ovulation are a risk factor for ovarian torsion.
(B) If a patient has vague, bilateral lower abdominal pain, ovarian torsion is extremely unlikely.
(C) Ovarian torsion most commonly occurs on the left side.
(D) Pelvic ultrasound is highly reliable for the evaluation of ovarian torsion.
(E) Pregnancy is not a risk factor for ovarian torsion.

8-4. A 16-year-old female with history of ovarian cysts presents with right lower quadrant pain for 3 hours that started after dance class. She states she has been seen for similar pain in the past and was told it was from an ovarian cyst. Her human chorionic gonadotropin (hCG) is negative and her pelvic exam is remarkable for right adnexal tenderness to palpation. Which of the following is the most appropriate next step in ED management?

(A) Obtain a gynecology consult in the ED
(B) Obtain a pelvic ultrasound
(C) Obtain vaginal swabs for gonorrhea and chlamydia
(D) Prescribe ibuprofen 600 mg three times a day for pain and outpatient referral to a gynecologist
(E) Prescribe oral contraceptives to manage symptoms

8-5. Which of the following factors is a major risk factor for ectopic pregnancy?

(A) Depression

(B) History of ovarian cysts

(C) Low socioeconomic class

(D) Use of assisted reproduction techniques

(E) Young maternal age

8-6. A 35-year-old female G1P0 presents with right lower abdominal pain and vaginal bleeding described as spotting for the last 3 hours. Her last menstrual period was 5 weeks ago and she had a positive pregnancy test at home 2 days ago. She and her husband underwent in vitro fertilization for this pregnancy. hCG is 6000 mIU/mL and she is Rh positive. ED bedside ultrasound confirms an intrauterine pregnancy. The next most appropriate step in management is:

(A) Administer Rhogam 50 MIU IM

(B) Congratulate her on her pregnancy and provide reassurance

(C) Discharge home with the diagnosis of threatened abortion and obstetric follow-up in 2 days

(D) Obtain a formal ultrasound

(E) Obtain urgent obstetric consult for a laparoscopy

8-7. A 23-year-old female presents with lower abdominal cramping and vaginally bleeding for 2 days. Her last menstrual period was 6 weeks ago. Her hCG is 2000 mIU/mL and she is Rh positive. A transvaginal ultrasound shows no intrauterine pregnancy. Which of the following is the next best step in management?

(A) Administer Rhogam 50 MIU IM

(B) Discharge home with ectopic precautions and obstetric follow-up in 2 days for a repeat hCG

(C) Have her return to ED the next day for a repeat ultrasound and hCG

(D) Obtain an obstetric consult in the ED

(E) Schedule her an appointment with an obstetrician and follow up ultrasound in 1 week

8-8. A 32-year-old female presents to the ED with severe lower abdominal pain. She cannot remember when her last menstrual period was because she is irregular. Physical exam reveals a pale female with a blood pressure of 80/50 and heart rate of 120. Her physical exam is remarkable for left lower quadrant tenderness. Her urine hCG is positive (Figure 8-1). Bedside ultrasound is performed. Which of the following is the next best step in management?

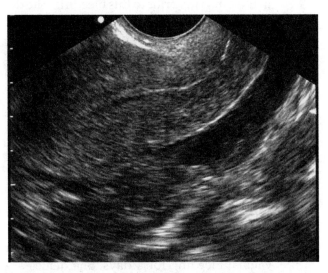

Figure 8-1. Reproduced with permission from Ma OJ, Mateer JR, Blaivas M: *Emergency Ultrasound*, 2nd Edition. Copyright © 2008 The McGraw-Hill Companies, Inc.

(A) Obtain a formal pelvic ultrasound

(B) Obtain a noncontrast abdominal CT scan

(C) Obtain a serum hCG

(D) Obtain a serum progesterone level

(E) STAT OB/GYN consult

8-9. Regarding the use of methotrexate for ectopic pregnancy, which of the following statements is true?

  (A) Methotrexate has a higher failure rate with ectopic pregnancies with fetal cardiac activity.

  (B) Patients should be advised to expect moderate-to-severe abdominal pain after methotrexate.

  (C) Patients should undergo immediate laparoscopy if there is no resolution of the ectopic pregnancy following the initial dose of methotrexate.

  (D) There are no absolute contraindication to methotrexate and should be considered first-line therapy for all patients with ectopic pregnancy.

  (E) Vaginal bleeding is the most common adverse effect of methotrexate.

8-10. Regarding the management of chronic medical illness during pregnancy, which of the following statements is true?

  (A) Angiotensin-converting enzyme inhibiters (ACE-Is) are first-line therapy for chronic hypertension in diabetic pregnant women.

  (B) Labetalol and nifedipine are safe in pregnancy for chronic hypertension.

  (C) Pregnant women are at less risk for diabetic ketoacidosis than nonpregnant women because of a higher basal metabolic rate.

  (D) Methimazole is the drug of choice for hyperthyroidism in pregnancy.

  (E) Trimethoprim–sulfonamide is the best choice for treatment of urinary tract infection in pregnant women in their third trimester.

8-11. A 28-year-old female G2P1 at 24 weeks with history of asthma presents to the ED with 3 days of cough and wheezing with shortness of breath. She is speaking full sentences and her oxygen saturation is 92% on room air. Which of the following statements is true?

  (A) Because of the potential vasoconstriction of the uteroplacental circulation, epinephrine should only be used in the most critically ill pregnant patients.

  (B) Most pregnant patients will have worsening of their underlying asthma during the last trimester of pregnancy.

  (C) Peak expiratory flow rates are decreased in pregnancy and, therefore, cannot be reliably used in pregnant patients as a marker of disease severity.

  (D) Steroids should be reserved for the most critically ill pregnant asthma patients.

  (E) Terbutaline is contraindicated during asthma flares in pregnant patients.

8-12. When discussing the risks of radiation and diagnostic tests with pregnant patients, which of the following statements is true?

  (A) Chest CT scanning results in more radiation exposure than ventilation–perfusion scanning for pulmonary embolism.

  (B) Fetal exposure to less than 10 rad does not increase the risk of fetal death, mental defect, or growth retardation.

  (C) Most of the detrimental effects of radiation occur after 15 weeks of gestation.

  (D) Significant radiation exposure during 8–15 weeks may result in decreased neurodevelopment.

  (E) The first 2 weeks of pregnancy are the period of organogenesis and therefore the highest risk period.

8-13. Which of the following is true regarding airway management in pregnancy?

(A) Aspiration risk is decreased in pregnancy.

(B) A respiratory acidosis is normal in pregnancy.

(C) Because of difficult airway anatomy, intubation should be avoided if possible.

(D) Functional residual volume remains unchanged.

(E) Rapid sequence medications, including paralytics, cross the placenta.

8-14. A 30-year-old woman G1P0 at 36 weeks of pregnancy presents to the ED following a motor vehicle collision. Which of the following statements correctly describes a physiologic change in pregnancy that would impact the resuscitation of this patient?

(A) A baseline tachycardia is expected in the last trimester pregnancy.

(B) Blood pressure decreases to a nadir in the third trimester.

(C) Functional residual capacity is increased in pregnancy.

(D) Hematocrit is decreased in pregnancy.

(E) Pregnant women will not efficiently compensate for blood loss because of a decrease in cardiac output.

8-15. Which of the following therapeutic agents is paired with the correct adverse effect in pregnancy?

(A) Aminoglycosides: dysmorphic syndrome

(B) Lithium: ototoxicity

(C) Sulfonamides: neonatal kernicterus

(D) Tetracycline: congenital heart disease

(E) Valproate: fetal teeth and bone abnormalities

8-16. A 24-year-old female G2P1 at 34 weeks of pregnancy presents with progressive dyspnea on exertion. She states she is much more short of breath than with her last pregnancy. She notes a dry cough and bilateral leg swelling but denies fevers and chest pain. Her physical exam is notable for a HR 112, RR 24, and O2 saturation of 94%. Her breath sounds are clear. Which of the following statements is the most appropriate in her management?

(A) Order lower extremity ultrasounds and, if positive for a deep vein thrombosis, start heparin for presumed pulmonary embolism

(B) Obtain a chest radiograph

(C) Order a ventilation perfusion scan

(D) Prescribe Lovenox for a presumptive pulmonary embolism without imaging

(E) Send a D-dimer for the evaluation of pulmonary embolism

8-17. Which of the following statements regarding preeclampsia and eclampsia is correct?

(A) A 34-year-old female G2P1 at 16 weeks, seen in the obstetric office on two consecutive visits with a blood pressure of 150/80, should be classified as mild preeclampsia.

(B) After magnesium, intravenous ACE-Is are the next line therapy for hypertension in eclampsia.

(C) Magnesium should be started in the ED on any patient in the third trimester with a blood pressure greater than 140/90.

(D) Multiparity is a risk factor for preeclampsia.

(E) Subcapsular liver hematoma is a potential complication of Hemolysis, Elevated Liver Enzymes, Low Platelet Count (HELLP) syndrome.

8-18. A 38-year-old African American female G3P2 at 32 weeks with history of pregnancy-induced hypertension presents with sudden onset of severe lower abdominal pain. Which of the following statements is most correct regarding this patient's condition?

(A) Hypertension is the most common risk factor for placental abruption.

(B) Race is not a risk factor associated with placental abruption.

(C) The patient does not need intravenous steroids for fetal lung maturity since she is 32 weeks pregnant.

(D) Tocolytics such as magnesium should be administered as soon as possible.

(E) Ultrasound is sensitive but not specific for placental abruption.

8-19. Which of the following regarding pregnant patients and Emergency Medical Treatment and Active Labor Act (EMTALA) is the most accurate?

(A) An emergency physician may transfer to a facility with obstetric coverage if none is available in the hospital without prior notification of the facility.

(B) If an emergency physician works in a hospital with no obstetric coverage, he or she should not accept ambulances with pregnant patients.

(C) It is an EMTALA violation to transfer a pregnant patient in active labor under any circumstances.

(D) Under EMTALA, stabilization of the patient is equivalent to delivery.

(E) The emergency physician must perform a medical screening exam prior to transfer.

8-20. Which is the first maneuver that should be performed when managing a shoulder dystocia?

(A) Clockwise rotation of the baby's torso (Wood corkscrew)

(B) Delivery of the posterior shoulder

(C) Flexion of the hips (McRoberts maneuver)

(D) Fundal pressure

(E) Suprapubic pressure

8-21. A 26-year-old woman who is 36 weeks pregnant presents after feeling a gush of fluid after her yoga class and is concerned that her water has broken. Which of the following is true regarding confirmation of rupture of membranes?

(A) A digital exam should be performed for confirmation.

(B) Amniotic fluid has a pH of 4.5–5.5 and turns the nitrazine strip yellow.

(C) False-positive tests can occur with the presence of *Trichomonas vaginalis*.

(D) Lubricant should be used during the sterile speculum exam to decrease patient discomfort.

(E) Thick brownish green fluid is a normal finding with uncomplicated rupture of membranes.

8-22. A 34-year-old female at 41 weeks presents in active labor. Bimanual exam reveals a palpable, pulsating cord. The next step in management is:

(A) Carefully reduce the prolapsed cord.

(B) Elevate the presenting fetal part and remain in place as the patient is prepared for surgery.

(C) Give terbutaline to halt uterine contraction and increase blood flow to the fetus.

(D) Place the patient on her left lateral side and apply oxygen.

(E) Start to prep the patient's abdomen for an ED C-section.

8-23. A 23-year-old female 10 weeks pregnant presents with vaginal irritation and a malodorous discharge. Pelvic exam demonstrates a thin gray discharge and the following wet mount is obtained (Figure 8-2). Which of the following statements is correct regarding her diagnosis?

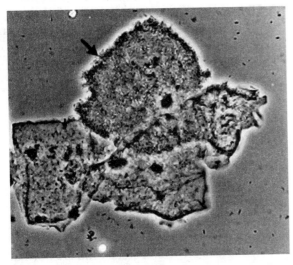

Figure 8-2. Reproduced from Eckert LO: Clinical practice. Acute vulvovaginitis. *N Engl J Med.* 2006;355(12):1244.

(A) Metronidazole 2 g single-dose therapy has the highest efficacy for treatment.

(B) Metronidazole 250 mg three times a day for 7 days is appropriate therapy.

(C) This diagnosis is not associated with spontaneous abortion and preterm rupture of membranes.

(D) This diagnosis is also associated with a vaginal pH <4.5.

(E) Vaginal cultures of Gardnerella confirm the diagnosis.

8-24. Which of the following statements is true regarding vulvovaginitis?

(A) Oral metronidazole is more effective than metronidazole gel for the treatment of *T. vaginalis.*

(B) Patients infected with *T. vaginalis* are not at increased risk for transmission of other infections including HIV and herpes.

(C) Since most males are symptomatic with *T. vaginalis*, male partners do not need to be treated unless symptomatic.

(D) Single-dose oral fluconazole is recommended for pregnant women with vulvovaginal candidiasis.

(E) Treatment of atrophic vaginitis consists of topical progesterone creams.

8-25. An 18-year-old female presents with pain and swelling on her labia. Physical exam findings are remarkable for a tender, fluctuant mass at the 8 o'clock position of her labia minora near the introitus. Which of the following statements is true regarding her diagnosis?

(A) Incision and drainage with packing placed for 2 days is the best treatment option.

(B) Patient should be given intravenous antibiotics and admitted to the hospital.

(C) The culprit glands are normally positioned at 2 and 10 o'clock position.

(D) The infection is usually caused by gonorrhea.

(E) Treatment involves placement of a Word catheter for 4–6 weeks.

8-26. A 21-year-old female presents with lower abdominal pain for 3 days. Her last menstrual period was 1 week ago, she is sexually active with one partner but does not used condoms. Her physical exam includes a temperature of 100.4, heart rate of 112, and blood pressure of 104/45. She is tender to palpation in the right and left lower quadrants. Her bimanual is notable for cervical motion tenderness and right adnexal tenderness. Her hCG is negative. The next best step in management is:

(A) Obtain a noncontrast abdominal/pelvic CT scan.

(B) Obtain a urine analysis.

(C) Obtain a transvaginal ultrasound to evaluate for a tubo-ovarian abscess.

(D) Send cervical cultures and, if positive, start her on antibiotics for pelvic inflammatory disease (PID).

(E) Start her on antibiotics for presumed PID and arrange outpatient follow-up with gynecology.

8-27. A 27-year-old female presents with lower abdominal pain and fever. She is HIV positive with a CD4 count of 700. She has an intrauterine device in place. Her hCG is negative. She is afebrile with a blood pressure of 125/60. Exam demonstrates cervical motion tenderness and adnexal tenderness. Her ultrasound is unremarkable. Which of the following statements is correct regarding her management?

(A) As she is not an adolescent and is not planning on becoming pregnant, discharge home on oral antibiotics for presumed PID.

(B) Due to her HIV status, she should be admitted to the hospital with intravenous antibiotics for presumed PID.

(C) Her intrauterine device does not need to be removed as long as antibiotics are started.

(D) Levaquin with doxycycline is the treatment of choice.

(E) Since her CD4 count is above 200, she can be discharged home on oral antibiotics for presumed PID.

8-28. A 32-year-old female presents 2 weeks postpartum with a painful right breast and chills. She is breastfeeding without difficulty. Her right breast is firm, red, and diffusely tender with no obvious fluctuant mass. Which of the following statements is correct regarding her diagnosis and management?

(A) If the infection fails to respond to the initial antibiotics, intravenous antibiotics should be initiated.

(B) Fluoroquinolones are the treatment of choice.

(C) Most cases are caused by Gram-negative bacteria.

(D) She can continue to breast-feed without interruption.

(E) She should not breast-feed but rather "pump and dump" until the erythema has resolved.

8-29. A 32-year-old female 24 weeks pregnant presents very concerned because she is occasionally incontinent of small amounts of urine. She notices it is worse when she coughs. Which of the following statements is true regarding her diagnosis?

(A) She has overflow incontinence.

(B) She has urge incontinence.

(C) She should be treated for a presumptive urinary tract infection.

(D) This likely occurs because intra-abdominal pressure is lower than intraurethral pressure.

(E) Treatment includes Kegel exercises.

8-30. A 30-year-old female presents 2 days postdilatation and curettage for a missed abortion at 12 weeks. Her physical exam is notable for fever 102°F, heart rate of 110, blood pressure of 120/80. Her pelvic exam is notable for a closed os with firm, tender uterus. What is the next appropriate step in her management?

(A) Obtain an upright chest x-ray to evaluate for free air.

(B) Obtain an ultrasound to evaluate for retained products of conception.

(C) Rhogam 300 MIU IM.

(D) Start oral trimethoprim/ sulfamethoxazole for likely staph infection.

(E) STAT gynecology consult for concern of uterine perforation.

Gynecologic and Obstetric Emergencies
Answers and Explanations

8-1. **The answer is D** (Chapter 99). Ovulatory dysfunctional uterine bleeding can be treated with oral contraceptives, nonsteroidal anti-inflammatory drugs (NSAIDs), or progesterone. The progesterone will decrease the number of available estrogen receptors and can be given 10 mg daily for 10 days. In nonpregnancy patients, ultrasound can be helpful to determine the size of the uterine and the characteristics of the endometrium but, since she is not pregnant and is hemodynamically stable, it can be deferred for outpatient evaluation. Intravenous estrogen can be used in the ED management of life-threatening hemorrhage in the nonpregnancy patient. Although this patient will need follow-up, C is the answer given the duration of bleeding. NSAIDs, not acetaminophen, are helpful in dysfunctional uterine bleeding by reducing blood flow and reducing dysmenorrhea.

8-2. **The answer is E** (Chapter 99). Endometrial cancer must be considered in any woman with abnormal vaginal bleeding who is older than 35, or any woman younger than 35 with risk factors for endometrial cancer. Referral for endometrial biopsy is warranted. Abdominal CT scan is not indicated since she has no abdominal pain. A routine physical exam would not be appropriate follow-up given the risk for cancer. The patient does not need progesterone since she has minimal bleeding and is hemodynamically stable.

8-3. **The answer is A** (Chapter 100). Risk factors for developing ovarian torsion include preg-

nancy, the presence of a large ovarian cyst or mass, and chemical induction of ovulation. Ultrasound is often the first imaging modality to evaluate torsion but should not be relied upon to rule out the diagnosis when clinical suspicion is high. Although patients classically present with severe unilateral pain, atypical presentations of ovarian torsion are common and patients may present with bilateral, mild, or intermittent pain.

8-4. **The answer is B** (Chapter 100). The patient is at risk of ovarian torsion given the history of ovarian cyst and pain that started after exercise; therefore, an ultrasound should be performed in the ED. Ultrasound with Doppler sonography is the primary imaging modality for suspected ovarian torsion. Ibuprofen and oral contraception can be used to treat dysfunctional uterine bleeding and dysmenorrhea. Culture swabs would be indicated if the patient had purulent discharge and cervical motion tenderness.

8-5. **The answer is D** (Chapter 101). The following are major risk factors for ectopic pregnancy: assisted reproduction techniques, PID, history of tubal surgery, use if an intrauterine device, and previous ectopic pregnancy. Young maternal age and low socioeconomic class are risk factors associated with postpartum endometritis. Ovarian cysts are a risk factor for ovarian torsion.

8-6. **The answer is D** (Chapter 101). Since this patient underwent in vitro fertilization, a formal ultrasound should be obtained to evaluate for a heterotopic pregnancy. In this population of patients, heterotopic pregnancy should be considered in symptomatic patients even when a bedside ultrasound demonstrates an intrauterine pregnancy. Rhogam is not indicated since the patient is Rh positive. Laparoscopy is used for patients with suspected ectopic pregnancy and a nondiagnostic ultrasound.

8-7. **The answer is D** (Chapter 101). An obstetrician should be consulted for concern of an ectopic pregnancy with a hCG above the discriminatory zone and an empty uterus on transvaginal ultrasound. The discriminatory zone for transvaginal ultrasound is 1500 mIU/mL and transabdominal is 6000 mIU/mL. The patient should not be discharged without obstetric evaluation given her high risk for an ectopic pregnancy. Rhogam is not indicated since the patient is Rh positive.

8-8. **The answer is E** (Chapter 101). The ultrasound shows an empty uterus with free fluid in the cul-de-sac concerning for a ruptured ectopic pregnancy. Since the patient is unstable, she needs a STAT obstetric consult for possible laparotomy before a formal ultrasound is obtained. While a serum hCG should be obtained, it should not delay an obstetric consult. An abdominal CT scan is not useful in the evaluation of an ectopic pregnancy. Serum progesterone may help differentiate an early normal from a pathologic pregnancy but is not readily available and not indicated in the unstable patient.

8-9. **The answer is A** (Chapter 101). Factors associated with a higher failure rate for methotrexate treatment include larger tubal diameter, higher initial serum hCG level, severe abdominal pain, and fetal cardiac activity. The most common side effect of methotrexate is abdominal pain followed by flatulence and stomatitis. Lower abdominal pain lasting up to 12 hours is common 3–7 days after methotrexate treatment and is thought to be secondary to methotrexate-induced tubal abortion or tubal distention due to hematoma formation. Moderate-to-severe pain warrants evaluation with an ultrasound and blood count for concern of ongoing rupture or hemoperitoneum. Methotrexate should not be used in a hemodynamically unstable patient. If the hCG is greater than 5000 mIU/mL, multiple dose methotrexate may be needed, and there is a higher failure rate of the therapy.

8-10. **The answer is B** (Chapter 102). During pregnancy, labetalol and nifedipine are safe to use in the management of chronic hypertension. ACE-Is should be avoided in pregnancy because of teratogenic effects and intrauterine growth retardation. Ketosis occurs more rapidly and at lower glucose level in pregnancy compared with nonpregnancy; therefore, any pregnant woman with elevated blood sugar and who is ill appearing should be evaluated for diabetic ketoacidosis. Propylthiouracil is the first-line treatment for hyperthyroidism in pregnancy; methimazole may be used as an alternative if patients develop a pruritic rash. Sulfonamide should not be used in the third trimester because of concern of kernicterus in the infant.

8-11. **The answer is A** (Chapter 102). Epinephrine may cause vasoconstriction of the uteroplacental circulation; therefore, it should only be used in severely ill asthmatic patients. Peak expiratory flow rates are not altered in pregnancy and should be used to guide therapy and need for admission. Terbutaline and steroids are considered safe in pregnancy and may be used if clinically indicated. In general, during pregnancy, asthma follows a rule of one-thirds: about one-third of the patients have improvement, one-third of the patients worsen, and one-third of the patients have their asthma symptoms remain the same.

8-12. **The answer is D** (Chapter 102). Significant radiation exposure during 8–15 weeks may result in decreased neurodevelopment including a small head size. Chest CT results in less radiation exposure (0.02–0.1 rad) than ventilation and perfusion scan (0.215 rad) for pulmonary embolism. The first 8 weeks of pregnancy is the period of organogenesis. Fetal exposure to less than 5 rad does not increase the risk of fetal death, mental defect, or growth retardation.

8-13. **The answer is E** (Chapter 103). Because pregnant women are at increased risk for aspiration and more prone to hypoxia due to decreased oxygen reserves, early intubation is recommended in the critically ill or seriously injured pregnant woman. Rapid sequence intubation is the first-line method used. These medications do cross the placenta, but are generally well tolerated by the fetus. Weight gain and fluid retention are two reasons the intubation can be more technically difficult in a pregnant patient. Progesterone stimulates an increased respiratory drive in pregnancy producing a respiratory alkalosis. Functional residual volume is decreased because of a rise in the level of the diaphragm.

8-14. **The answer is D** (Chapter 103). In pregnancy, there is an increase in blood volume and a smaller increase in red blood cell mass leading to a dilutional anemia and a drop in the hematocrit. Cardiac output is increased by 30–40% in pregnancy. Many respiratory changes occur during pregnancy. The minute ventilation, tidal volume, and respiratory rate increase during pregnancy resulting in a decreased functional residual capacity and a slight respiratory alkalosis. Blood pressure decreases to a nadir in the second trimester.

8-15. **The answer is C** (Chapter 103). Sulfonamides may cause neonatal kernicterus at near term. Valproate and other antiseizure medications have been associated with dysmorphic syndrome. Lithium can cause congenital heart disease specifically Ebstein's anomaly. Aminoglycosides are associated with ototoxicity. Tetracyclines can cause fetal teeth and bone abnormalities.

8-16. **The answer is B** (Chapter 104). Pregnant women with severe dyspnea should be evaluated for pneumonia, congestive heart failure, and pulmonary embolism. In this situation, a chest x-ray should not be withheld because of fear of radiation exposure to the fetus. The use of D-dimer in pregnant patients remains controversial but is likely to be elevated in the second and third trimester; therefore, it is not a useful test for pulmonary embolism. If a pregnant patient has a deep vein thrombosis on ultrasound and shortness of breath, she could be started on heparin for presumed pulmonary embolism, but, in this scenario, a chest x-ray should be performed for concern of congestive heart failure. While both Lovenox and heparin are safe in pregnancy because they do not cross the placenta, these medications should not be started without imaging or high clinical suspicion for thrombosis given the potential complication of bleeding and the need to guide the duration of therapy.

8-17. **The answer is E** (Chapter 104). Subcapsular liver hematoma is a potential life-threatening complication of HELLP. If the patient is hemodynamically stable, the hematoma can be diagnosed by CT scan, or, if the patient is unstable and rupture is suspected, bedside ultrasound may be helpful. Diagnostic criteria for preeclampsia include gestation greater than 20 weeks, systolic blood pressure ≥140 or diastolic ≥90 on two occasions at least 6 hours apart, and proteinuria >0.3 g in 24-hour period. Edema is no longer part of the criteria. Because this patient is only 16 weeks pregnant, she is considered to have chronic hypertension. In addition to diabetes, hypertension, multiple gestations, and obesity, nulliparity is a risk factor for preeclampsia. Magnesium should be started on pregnant women who meet the criteria for severe preeclampsia, have evidence of HELLP syndrome, or have seizures after 20 weeks of gestation or within 4 weeks postpartum. ACE-Is are contraindicated in pregnancy because of toxic effects on the fetus. Methyldopa, labetalol, hydralazine, and nifedipine are safe to use in pregnancy.

8-18. **The answer is A** (Chapter 104). Hypertension is the most common risk factor for placental abruption. Trauma, smoking, advanced maternal age, African American race, and cocaine use are other risk factors. Ultrasound is specific but not sensitive for the detection of a retroplacental clot. Antenatal administration of corticosteroids before 34 weeks, not 32 weeks, of gestation speeds lung maturity and decreases the incidence of intraventricular hemorrhage and necrotizing enterocolitis. Tocolytics, like magnesium, may be considered in preterm rupture of membranes but not in placental abruption.

8-19.   **The answer is E** (Chapter 104). With regard to the EMTALA, emergency physicians should approach pregnant patients in the same fashion as all ED patients. A screening exam must be done, and the patient must be stabilized as much as possible at the current facility. This does not necessarily mean delivery. When a patient is to be transferred, the transferring physician must certify that a facility and doctor has accepted the patient and that the benefits of transfer outweigh potential risks. If an emergency physician works in a hospital with no obstetric coverage, he or she should be familiar with protocols in place for transfer and equipment available for an emergency delivery.

8-20.   **The answer is C** (Chapter 105). When shoulder dystocia is recognized, the patient's legs should be immediately flexed up to the abdomen with the legs held by the patient or assistant known as the McRoberts maneuver. Next suprapubic pressure should be applied to disimpact the anterior shoulder from the pubic symphysis. Fundal pressure should never be applied because it will further impact the shoulder on the pelvic rim. If McRoberts maneuver and suprapubic pressure do not work, the Wood corkscrew maneuver can be performed by grasping the posterior scapula and rotating the infant's torso 180 degrees to rotate the posterior shoulder into the anterior position to deliver the shoulder. If this fails, the physician may try to deliver the posterior shoulder.

8-21.   **The answer is C** (Chapter 105). Amniotic fluid has a pH of 7.0–7.4 and will turn nitrazine paper blue. False-positive tests can occur with blood, lubricant, the presence of *T. vaginalis*, semen, or cervical mucus. Once membranes have broken, digital examination should be avoided because there is an increased risk of infection after even a single digital examination. Thick brownish green fluid is not a normal finding in amniotic fluid and is consistent with meconium. This should alert the physician of possible fetal complications from meconium aspiration.

8-22.   **The answer is B** (Chapter 105). In the event of a prolapsed cord, the examiner should not remove his/her hand and should elevate the fetal presenting part to decrease compression of the cord. The examiner's hand should remain in place as the patient is prepared for surgery. A prolapsed cord should never be reduced. Placing the patient on her left side and applying oxygen may increase maternal blood flow and help during decelerations but is not as essential as relieving pressure on the cord.

8-23.   **The answer is B** (Chapter 106). Since bacterial vaginosis has been associated with spontaneous abortion, preterm labor, and premature rupture of membranes, pregnant women should be treated with metronidazole 250 mg PO three times a day for 7 days. Metronidazole 2 g single-dose therapy has the lowest efficacy; therefore, it should not be used in pregnant patients. The diagnosis of bacterial vaginosis is associated with a vaginal pH >4.5; thin, gray discharge; clue cells; and a positive whiff test. Cultures of Gardnerella are not useful since it is also found in normal vaginal flora.

8-24.   **The answer is A** (Chapter 106). Because the trichomonads infect the urethra and glands, metronidazole gel is less effective than oral metronidazole and is not recommended for the treatment of trichomonas. Trichomonas is associated with increased risk of transmission of herpes, HIV, and human papillomavirus. Up to 90% of men with trichomonas are asymptomatic, but they should be treated if they have had a known exposure. Since oral fluconazole is a class C drug, topical therapy is recommended for pregnant women with vulvovaginal candidiasis. Treatment of atrophic vaginitis includes topical estrogens not progesterone creams.

8-25. **The answer is E** (Chapter 106). Bartholin glands are located in the labia minora and drain into the posterior vestibule at 4 and 8 o'clock positions. Obstruction of a gland can lead to abscess formation. Bartholin gland abscess should be treated with incision and drainage with a Word catheter left in place for 4–6 weeks to prevent reoccurrence. Intravenous antibiotics and hospital admission are usually not indicated once the abscess had been drained. The infection is usually polymicrobial although has been associated with gonorrhea and chlamydia.

8-26. **The answer is C** (Chapter 107). Women with suspected PID and asymmetric pelvic findings should have an ultrasound to evaluate for tubo-ovarian abscess. CT and MRI can be used to evaluate for PID and exclude other causes for pain, but, in this case, ultrasound is the more appropriate imaging modality. Antibiotics and outpatient follow-up may be appropriate for hemodynamically stable patients with PID, but admission is required for all patients with tubo-ovarian abscess. If a patient has a history and clinically findings concerning for PID, antibiotics should be started immediately before cervical cultures return.

8-27. **The answer is B** (Chapter 107). Patients with PID should be admitted if they are pregnant, fail to respond to outpatient therapy, are unable to tolerate or comply with outpatient therapy, have severe toxicity, tubo-ovarian abscess, or HIV infection irrespective of their CD4 count. Parenteral treatment includes cefoxitin plus doxycycline or clindamycin plus gentamicin. Due to emerging resistant, fluoroquinolones are not longer recommended to treat gonorrhea. Intrauterine devices should be removed after antibiotics are started.

8-28. **The answer is D** (Chapter 108). Mastitis is treated with frequent breast emptying, analgesia, and anti-staphylococcal penicillin or cephalosporin plus Bactrim if methicillin-resistant staphylococcus aureus (MRSA) is a concern. There is no need to interrupt breast-feeding with mastitis. Fluoroquinolones are not used for the treatment of mastitis. If an infection fails to respond to antibiotics, an abscess should be suspected and an ultrasound and surgical consult should be obtained for incision and drainage or needle aspiration.

8-29. **The answer is D** (Chapter 109). Stress incontinence occurs when intra-abdominal pressure exceeds intraurethral pressure in the absence of bladder contractions. This type of incontinence is associated with pregnancy, multiparity, menopause, and chronic cough. The nonsurgical treatment includes Kegel exercises, estrogen, and alpha-adrenergic medications. Overflow incontinence is the continuous leakage from impaired detrusor muscle contractility or bladder outlet obstruction. Urge incontinence is related to uninhibited bladder contractions often the result of interstitial cystitis. Although all urinary tract infections, including asymptomatic bacteruria, should be treated in pregnant women, a urinalysis and culture should be performed before antibiotics are started.

8-30. **The answer is B** (Chapter 109). Complications of dilatation and curettage include uterine rupture, retained products of conception, and postabortal endometritis. When postabortal endometritis is suspected with fever and tender uterus, an ultrasound should be performed to look for retained products of conceptions. Rhogam is indicated if the patient is Rh negative and should be given at the time of the dilatation and curettage. Most uterine perforations occur at the time of surgery and are asymptomatic. Delayed presentations of uterine perforation include abdominal pain and shock that would warrant a STAT gynecologic consult.

Hematologic Disorders
Questions

9-1. In the evaluation of a patient with anemia, which of the following is TRUE?

(A) Altered mental status is never attributable to anemia.

(B) Folate deficiency causes microcytic anemia.

(C) Mean corpuscular hemoglobin concentration (MCHC) is a direct measure of bone marrow activity.

(D) Patients with slowly developing anemia may have no complaints even with a hemoglobin concentration as low as 5g/dL.

(E) Serum ferritin is the most useful test in the diagnosis of thalassemia.

9-2. A 67-year-old man presents to the emergency department complaining of weakness. On examination, his blood pressure is 88/46 mm Hg and his heart rate is 89 beats/min. He is pale, and his rectal examination reveals melena. Laboratory studies are remarkable for a hemoglobin of 5.5g/dL. What is the most appropriate initial step in the management of this patient?

(A) Infusion of an inotrope

(B) Infusion of a proton pump inhibitor

(C) Infusion of erythropoietin

(D) Infusion of iron

(E) Infusion of packed red blood cells (PRBCs)

9-3. A 23-year-old man presents to the emergency department with persistent bleeding after cutting himself while shaving. Which of the following is TRUE?

(A) D-dimer is lowered in disseminated intravascular coagulation.

(B) Elevated prothrombin time suggests a problem with the extrinsic and/or common coagulation pathways.

(C) Normal platelet count excludes platelets as a cause for bleeding.

(D) Warfarin causes prolongation of the activated partial thromboplastin time.

(E) Protein C is dependent on vitamin E.

9-4. At what platelet count level does the risk for spontaneous bleeding become significant?

(A) <10–$20,000/mm^3$

(B) 20–$30,000/mm^3$

(C) 30–$40,000/mm^3$

(D) 40–$50,000/mm^3$

(E) 50–$60,000/mm^3$

9-5. Which of the following is the most common sign of idiopathic thrombocytopenic purpura?

(A) Epistaxis

(B) Gingival bleeding

(C) Hematochezia

(D) Petechiae

(E) Subconjunctival hemorrhage

9-6. A 21-year-old man with idiopathic thrombocytopenic purpura presents to the emergency department for care of a cut to his face he sustained while shaving. His vital signs are normal, and the examination reveals bleeding from a small abrasion to his left cheek. Laboratory studies reveal a platelet count of 56,000/mm^3. What is the appropriate management for this patient?

(A) Cryoprecipitate infusion

(B) Direct pressure

(C) Oral steroids

(D) Platelet infusion

(E) Polyclonal antibody infusion

9-7. A 24-year-old woman presents for the second time to your emergency department with the complaint unilateral lower leg swelling and pain. Similar to year ago, the patient is found to have a deep venous thrombosis—this time of the opposite leg. On further questioning, you discover that both of her siblings have also had a lower extremity deep vein thrombosis without a clear cause. What is the most common heritable hypercoagulable disorder?

(A) Antithrombin deficiency

(B) Factor V Leiden mutation

(C) Protein C deficiency

(D) Protein S deficiency

(E) Prothrombin gene mutation

9-8. A 66-year-old man presents to the emergency department complaining of unilateral leg swelling and pain. On review of his hospital records, you discover that the patient was treated with prophylactic subcutaneous heparin during his recent stay for pneumonia. His vital signs are normal, and the physical examination is only notable for a swelling and tenderness of the left lower leg. Laboratory studies reveal a platelet count of 43,000/mm^3. At discharge 2 weeks ago, the platelet count was 209,000/mm^3. You suspect that the patient may have heparin-induced thrombocytopenia (HIT). Which of the following is TRUE?

(A) Clinicians should suspect HIT when the platelet count has dropped 25% after exposure to heparin products.

(B) Definitive laboratory testing for HIT is easy.

(C) HIT occurs in 10% of patients treated with heparin products.

(D) Patients with HIT are prone to thromboembolic events.

(E) Treatment with low-molecular-weight heparin should be continued in patients suspected of having HIT.

9-9. A 19-year-old man with hemophilia A is brought into the emergency department for evaluation of unresponsiveness after a fall down six steps today. His blood pressure is 187/101 mm Hg, his heart rate is 46 beats/min—otherwise his vital signs are within normal limits. His Glasgow Coma Score is 6. Paramedics brought him in intubated with full spinal immobilization. After the primary and secondary surveys, which of the following is the next most appropriate step in the management of this patients?

(A) Computed tomography (CT) of the brain

(B) Consultation of a neurosurgeon

(C) Nicardipene

(D) Recombinant factor VIII

(E) Recombinant factor IX

9-10. In terms of the hemophilia A and B and von Willebrand disease (vWD), which of the following is TRUE?

(A) Bruising is an uncommon manifestation of vWD.

(B) Cryoprecipitate is the treatment of choice for types II and III vWD.

(C) Hemophilia A and B predominantly affects girls and women.

(D) Hemophilia B is caused by a deficiency of factor VIII.

(E) Prothrombin time is elevated in patients with hemophilia A.

9-11.   An 81-year-old man with metastatic prostate cancer presents to the emergency department complaining of fever. He tells you that he last received chemotherapy 6 days ago at another facility. He takes no medications other than the chemotherapy. His vital signs are normal with the exception of his temperature that measures 39.1°C. The physical examination is unremarkable, except for chronic vertebral tenderness. He has no indwelling catheters. Laboratory studies reveal an absolute neutrophil count of 400/mm^3. His chest radiograph and urine analysis are normal. After obtaining blood and urine cultures, what is the best empiric antibiotic regimen?

(A) Amikacin

(B) Amoxicillin/clavulanate

(C) Ceftriaxone

(D) Imipenem/cilastatin

(E) Vancomycin

9-12.   A 36-year-old woman with metastatic breast cancer presents to the emergency department complaining of confusion, abdominal pain, nausea, and vomiting. Your evaluation reveals a serum calcium level of 17 mg/dL as the cause for her symptoms. Which of the following is TRUE regarding hypercalcemia of malignancy?

(A) Clinical presentation is more attributable to the calcium level than to the rate of rise of the calcium level.

(B) Furosemide is the first-line treatment of hypercalcemia of malignancy.

(C) Hypercalcemia is a rare complication of cancer.

(D) Hypovolemia and dehydration account for many of the nonspecific symptoms.

(E) Steroids are contraindicated in the treatment of cancer-related hypercalcemia.

9-13.   In considering emergency complications of cancer, which of the following is TRUE?

(A) Cancer patients with back pain should undergo spinal imaging.

(B) Demeclocycline is the treatment of choice for cancer patients with hyponatremia from inappropriate antidiuretic hormone secretion.

(C) Electrical alternans is a common electrocardiographic finding in patients with malignant pericardial effusion.

(D) Hypokalemia is frequent laboratory abnormality associated with tumor lysis syndrome.

(E) Thromboembolism is the leading cause of death in cancer patients.

9-14.   A 29-year-old African American man with sickle cell disease presents to the emergency department complaining of bilateral elbow and lower leg pain. These symptoms are typical of his pain crises. Which of the following complications is the leading cause of death in patients with sickle cell disease?

(A) Acute chest syndrome

(B) Aplastic crisis

(C) Bacteremia

(D) Hypersplenism

(E) Stroke

9-15. A 45-year-old Asian man presents to the emergency department complaining of progressive shortness of breath and fatigue. A smear of her blood is shown below (Figure 9-1). Which of the following is TRUE regarding the patient's likely diagnosis?

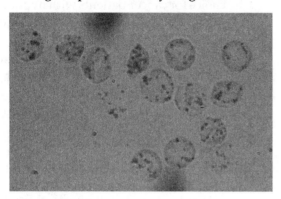

Figure 9-1. Reproduced with permission from Lichtman M, Beutler E, Kaushansky K, et al: *Williams Hematology*, 7th Edition. Copyright © 2006 The McGraw-Hill Companies, Inc.

(A) Caucasians are predominantly affected.

(B) It is inherited in an autosomal-dominant fashion.

(C) It is caused by a rare enzyme deficiency.

(D) There are three clinical variants of this disease.

(E) Trimethoprim–sulfamethoxazole can trigger a flare of this disease.

9-16. A 19-year-old woman, struck by a car, is brought to your emergency department. Her vital signs are as follows: blood pressure 65/palpation; pulse 144 beats/min; respirations 34 breaths/min; and pulse oximetry 99% by face mask. Physical examination reveals full spinal immobilization, a Glasgow coma score of 12, and a traumatic amputation of her left lower extremity with uncontrolled bleeding. In the resuscitation of this patient, you administer 13 units of PRBCs and several units of fresh frozen plasma (FFP) and platelets. Which of the following is TRUE?

(A) Each unit of PRBCs should raise the hemoglobin concentration by 5 g/dL.

(B) Hypercalcemia may result from the transfusion of large quantities of PRBCs.

(C) *Staphylococcus aureus* is the most likely bacterium to be transmitted during a blood transfusion.

(D) Transfusing more than 20 units of PRBCs in a 24-hour period constitutes a massive transfusion.

(E) Transfusion-related acute lung injury is usually caused by the transfusion of FFP and/or platelets.

9-17. A 67-year-old man with a history of atrial fibrillation for which he takes warfarin presents to the emergency department with a small bleeding abrasion after shaving. His vital signs are normal. International normalized ratio (INR) is 10. Which of the following represents proper management of this patient?

(A) Direct pressure alone

(B) Direct pressure and holding warfarin

(C) Direct pressure, holding warfarin and oral vitamin K

(D) Direct pressure, holding warfarin, oral vitamin K and FFP

(E) Direct pressure, holding warfarin, intravenous vitamin K and FFP

9-18. A mother brings her 7-year-old boy into the emergency department for evaluation of fatigue and easy bruising. The mother also reports that her child has had diarrhea (sometimes bloody) for about 1 week. Her vital signs are normal, except for a mild tachycardia. The physical examination is notable for three medium-sized bruises over her lower extremities. Laboratory data reveals a platelet count of 62,000/mm^3, a hematocrit of 20%, and a serum creatinine of 1.2. Which of the following is TRUE regarding her likely diagnosis?

(A) Administration of antibiotics in the treatment of the causative organism is absolutely contraindicated.

(B) Atypical forms of this disease are only caused by infections.

(C) Onset of this disease typically occurs immediately after ingestion of the causative bacterium.

(D) The typical form of this disease is most commonly caused by *Salmonella species*.

(E) This is the most common cause of preventable acute renal failure in childhood.

Hematologic Disorders
Answers and Explanations

9-1. **The answer is D** (Chapter 226). Anemia that develops over a long period of time may present with almost no symptoms. Rapidly developing, severe anemia can present with altered sensorium. Folate and vitamin B_{12} deficiencies cause macrocytic anemia. The MCHC is a measure of hemoglobin concentration in the average red blood cell. Serum ferritin is the most useful test for the diagnosis of iron deficiency anemia.

9-2. **The answer is E** (Chapter 226). Although all of these interventions may be appropriate at some point in the care of this patient, infusion of PRBCs is the first best step. The patient described in this scenario has a hemodynamically unstable gastrointestinal bleed and requires prompt transfusion of blood to address this and his acute anemia.

9-3. **The answer is B** (Chapter 227). Basic laboratory evaluation of the bleeding patient should include a complete blood count, prothrombin time, and activated partial thromboplastin time. Having said this, there are many other laboratory tests that can be performed to evaluate the cause for bleeding. The prothrombin time is a measure of the function of the extrinsic and common coagulation pathways. Although a patient may have a normal platelets, the platelets may not have normal function. Treatment with coumadin causes a delay in the prothrombin time. The D-dimer is elevated in a number of disease states, including in disseminated intravascular coagulation. Finally, protein S is a vitamin D-dependent protein.

9-4. **The answer is A** (Chapter 228). The risk for spontaneous bleeding, particularly within the brain, is much increased as the platelet count falls below the $10,000–20,000/mm^3$ range. Clinicians should consider transfusion of platelets, even in the asymptomatic patient, when the platelet level falls below $10,000/mm^3$.

9-5. **The answer is D** (Chapter 228). Epistaxis, gingival bleeding, hematochezia, and subconjunctival hemorrhage may be seen in a patient with idiopathic thrombocytopenic purpura. Petechiae, however, are the most common physical finding.

9-6. **The answer is B** (Chapter 228). Management of this patient requires only direct pressure, as patients with platelet counts exceeding $50,000/mm^3$ infrequently necessitate other specific treatments. Clinicians should consider steroids in patients with platelet counts between $20,000/mm^3$ and $30,000/mm^3$ or with life-threatening bleeding—neither of which this patient has. Clinicians should strongly consider platelet infusion in patients with life-threatening bleeding and/or a count less than $10,000/mm^3$—again neither of which this patient has. Similarly, infusion of polyclonal antibody should be reserved for patients with a very low platelet count and/or significant or life-threatening bleeding. There is no specific role for cryoprecipitate in the care of the patient with idiopathic thrombocytopenic purpura.

9-7. **The answer is B** (Chapter 229). Factor V Leiden mutation is the most prevalent inherited clotting disorder. It occurs in approximately 5% of American whites, with a much lower rate in other races.

9-8.   The answer is D (Chapter 229). Despite the low platelet count associated with HIT, patients are more prone to clotting as opposed to bleeding. HIT occurs in 0.5–5% of patients treated with heparin products. The diagnosis of HIT should only be considered in patients exposed to heparin products and in whom the platelet count has dropped at least 50%. All heparin products, including Lovenox®, should be stopped in patients suspected of having HIT. Definitive laboratory testing is challenging. Test with high specificity are complex and only done in a few centers. Widely available immunologic assays have a lower specificity.

9-9.   The answer is D (Chapter 230). Any patient with hemophilia who presents with a new headache, lateralizing neurologic signs, decreased level of consciousness, and/or head trauma requires immediate factor replacement followed by CT of the brain. This patient has hemophilia A and therefore requires an infusion of factor VIII—not factor IX. Surely consultation of a neurosurgeon will be required once the bleeding is addressed. The patient's hypertension and bradycardia are signs of increased intracranial pressure—known as the Cushing response. This is primarily addressed by treating the underlying cause (in this case, intracranial bleeding).

9-10.   The answer is B (Chapter 230). Cryoprecipitate is the treatment of choice for patients with types II and III vWD. Patients with type I vWD are treated initially with desmopressin. Patients with vWD often present with mucocutaneous bleeding, including easy bruising. Hemophilia A and B are X-linked diseases, therefore affects boys and men more. Hemophilia A is caused by a deficiency in factor VIII, and hemophilia B is caused by a deficiency of factor IX. Hemophilia A and B can cause prolongation of the activated partial thromboplastin time—a measure of

intrinsic pathway function. They do not affect the prothrombin time.

9-11.   The answer is D (Chapter 235). Imipenem/ cilastatin is indicated as monotherapy for cancer patients with neutropenic fever. Amikacin is indicated only as a second antimicrobial in the treatment of febrile neutropenia. Ceftriaxone is not indicated as monotherapy in the treatment of cancer patients with febrile neutropenia, as it does not cover pseudomonas. Vancomycin may be added to another antimicrobial in the treatment of neutropenic fever in patients at increased risked for gram-positive sepsis (e.g., those with indwelling catheters). Amoxicillin/clavulanate, when combined with ciprofloxacin, can be used to treat cancer patients with neutropenic fever in the outpatient setting.

9-12.   The answer is D (Chapter 235). Many of the vague symptoms attributable to hypercalcemia of malignancy are caused by hypovolemia and dehydration, and as such, saline infusion is the mainstay of treatment. How patients present has more to do with the rate of rise of the serum calcium level than the absolute serum calcium concentration. Hypercalcemia is not an infrequent complication, occurring in upward of 30% of patients with advanced cancer. Steroids can be used to treat hypercalcemia, particularly when caused by steroid-sensitive tumors, such as lymphomas and multiple myeloma. Furosemide is no longer routinely recommended in the treatment of cancer-related hypercalcemia, as it has little additive effect to the use of saline alone in patients with normal cardiac and renal function.

9-13.   The answer is A (Chapter 235). Because approximately 80% of patients with malignant spinal cord compression have a prior diagnosis of cancer, back pain in those with a known history of cancer should undergo imaging. Said another way, these patients have spinal column metastases until proven otherwise. Fluid restriction—not demeclocycline—is the mainstay of treatment in nonseizing patients with hyponatremia caused by inappropriate antidiuretic hormone secretion. Although electrical alternans is a classic electrocardiographic finding in patients with malignant pericardial effusion, it is seen rarely. Tumor lysis syndrome is characterized by hyperuricemia, hyperkalemia, hyperphosphatemia, and hypocalcemia. Thromboembolism is the second leading cause of death in cancer patients.

9-14. **The answer is A** (Chapter 231). Acute chest syndrome is the leading cause of death in patients with sickle cell disease. It is also the second most common cause for admission, after vaso-occlusive pain crisis, in patients with sickle cell disease.

9-15. **The answer is E** (Chapter 231). The picture shows Heinz bodies, often seen in patients with glucose-6-phosphate dehydrogenase (G6PD) deficiency. Several medications, including trimethoprim–sulfamethoxazole, can induce acute hemolysis. G6PD deficiency is the most common enzymopathy of red blood cells in humans, affecting more than 400 million people worldwide. All races are affected; however, this disease has mostly been found in persons of African, Asian, and Mediterranean descent. G6PD deficiency is an X-linked disease, affecting mostly boys and men. There are five variants of the disease, as defined by the World Health Organization.

9-16. **The answer is E** (Chapter 233). Transfusion-related acute lung injury occurs infrequently. It is usually caused by the infusion of platelets and/or FFP; it rarely occurs after an infusion of PRBCs alone. Each unit of PRBCS should raise the hemoglobin concentration by 1 g/dL (and the hematocrit by 3%). Citrate, used to preserve PRBCS, may cause hypocalcemia by chelation during a massive transfusion. *Yersinia enterocolitica* is the most likely bacterium to be transmitted during a blood transfusion, as it readily grows in refrigerated blood. The transfusion of at least 10 units of PRBCs with a 24-hour period constitutes a massive transfusion.

9-17. **The answer is C** (Chapter 234). This patient presents with a greatly elevated INR. Despite this, the patient presents with only minor bleeding, and therefore, he does not require factor replacement or intravenous vitamin K. As is always the case, direct pressure to the site of bleeding is necessitated. In addition, the offending agent, in this case warfarin, should be held for at least one or two doses. And it is also recommended that warfarin-treated patients with an INR greater than 9 without significant bleeding receive oral vitamin K therapy.

9-18. **The answer is E** (Chapter 232). This 7-year-old boy has hemolytic uremic syndrome (HUS)—characterized by microangiopathic hemolytic anemia, acute renal failure/insufficiency, and low platelets. HUS is the most common preventable cause of acute renal failure in children. It occurs in a typical and atypical form. The typical form is usually caused by *Escherichia coli* O157:H7. HUS typically manifests itself after about 1 week into a case of infectious diarrhea—not immediately after ingestion of the causative organism. As mentioned earlier, there is also an atypical form of HUS—sometimes caused by bone marrow transplantation or administration of chemotherapy drugs or immunosuppressants. Finally, the use of antibiotics in the treatment of the underlying infection is controversial and should be addressed on a case-by-case basis.

Systemic Infectious Disorders
Questions

10-1. A 24-year-old male presents to your emergency department (ED) complaining of a painful ulcer on his penis for 1 week (Figure 10-1). He denies constitutional symptoms or penile discharge. He reports having unprotected sexual intercourse with a prostitute in Nairobi 2 weeks ago. On exam, you also notice that he has bilateral tender and erythematous inguinal lymphadenopathy. Which of the following is MOST appropriate?

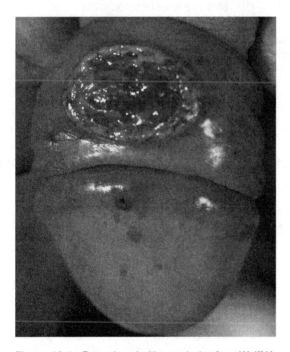

Figure 10-1. Reproduced with permission from Wolff K, Johnson RA: *Fitzpatrick's Color Atlas & Synopsis of Clinical Dermatology*, 6th Edition. Copyright © 2009 The McGraw-Hill Companies, Inc.

(A) Azithromycin by mouth and ceftriaxone 125 mg intramuscularly along with a prescription to give to his partner.

(B) Azithromycin by mouth in a single dose, needle aspiration of lymph nodes, and referral for human immunodeficiency virus (HIV) and syphilis testing.

(C) Acyclovir 400 mg by mouth three times daily for 7 days and report the disease to the Centers for Disease Control and Prevention (CDC).

(D) Benzathine penicillin G 2.4 million units intramuscularly and follow up with public health for repeat serological testing.

(E) Doxycycline by mouth for 21 days, consideration for incision and drainage of lymph nodes, and referral for HIV and syphilis testing.

10-2. A 26-year-old female is complaining of a diffuse rash, as well as fever. Syphilis is on the differential. Which of the following is TRUE of the typical rash of secondary syphilis?

(A) Begins as a symmetrically distributed macular rash on the trunk and flexor surfaces and may extend to involve the palms, soles, and oral mucosa.

(B) Is not associated with systemic symptoms such as fever, fatigue, or myalgia.

(C) May include wart-like lesions known as *condyloma latum* in moist areas of the body that are not infectious.

(D) Typically develops 6–8 months after the appearance of the primary chancre.

(E) Will not resolve without treatment with penicillin.

10-3. A 22-year-old female is complaining of vaginal discomfort and discharge for 2 days. She also complains of mild dysuria. On exam, you notice a thin yellowish discharge, a friable cervix, but no cervical motion or adnexal tenderness. Sodium chloride and potassium hydroxide microscopy slides are negative. What is the MOST likely cause?

(A) *Candida albicans*

(B) *Chlamydia trachomatis*

(C) Human papillomavirus

(D) *Neisseria gonorrhoeae*

(E) *Trichomonas vaginalis*

10-4. A 60-year-old female returns to the ED 3 days after anterior nasal packing for epistaxis. She now complains of fevers, chills, myalgias, and diffuse abdominal pain. Her temperature is 39.2°C, blood pressure is 82/44, and heart rate is 132. She has a diffuse, raised, blanching, erythematous rash that resembles severe sunburn. What is the MOST beneficial course of treatment?

(A) Intravenous access, blood transfusion, leave the nasal packing in place due to likely disseminated intravascular coagulation, and admission.

(B) Intravenous access, fluid resuscitation, administer intravenous antibiotics, remove the nasal packing, and admission.

(C) Intravenous access, fluid resuscitation, epinephrine for anaphylaxis, and admission.

(D) Order a CT scan of the abdomen to evaluate for abscess.

(E) Reassure the patient she has sinusitis and a viral exanthema and discharge home.

10-5. A 40-year-old male with diabetes and chronic alcoholism presents complaining of extreme pain in his left shoulder. He states he may have bumped into a wall 2 days ago, but it did not start hurting until today. His temperature is 39.0°C, blood pressure 88/50, and heart rate 120. He has only mild erythema and swelling on his left shoulder. However, his exam is significant for severe pain of his left shoulder with decreased range of motion. The pain appears out of proportion to your exam. He has a noticeably diffuse erythroderma. His white blood cell count is 20,000 with 40% bands. What is the MOST critical step in treatment?

(A) Bedside incision and drainage and discharge on oral antibiotics

(B) CT scan with intravenous contrast of the left upper extremity

(C) Immediate surgical consultation

(D) Intravenous antibiotics

(E) Intravenous benzodiazepines

10-6. A 45-year-old male with end-stage renal disease presents to the ED with 2 days of fever up to 39.0°C. His initial blood pressure is 74/40 and his heart rate is 130. There is a dialysis catheter in his right internal jugular vein. There is mild erythema around the site but no frank pus. His last dialysis was 3 days ago. What intervention is necessary for definitive treatment of this infection?

(A) Catheter removal

(B) Emergent dialysis

(C) Intravenous fluids

(D) Levofloxacin 750 mg intravenously

(E) Vancomycin 1 g intravenously

10-7. A 58-year-old male presents complaining of pain, swelling, and redness to his right lower extremity that has progressed over 4 days. He was seen by his primary care physician 2 days ago and was prescribed cephalexin. His temperature is 38.3°C, blood pressure is 140/82, heart rate is 118, and respiratory rate is 16. A fingerstick glucose is 140. The white blood cell count is 18,000 cells/mm³. His right lower extremity has a strong dorsalis pedis pulse and is depicted below (Figure 10-2). Which of the following is the MOST appropriate antimicrobial treatment?

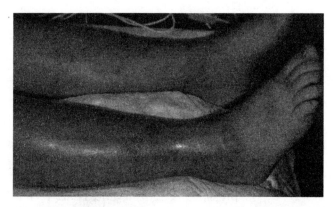

Figure 10-2. Reproduced with permission from Knoop KJ, Stack LB, Storrow AB, Thurman RJ: *The Atlas of Emergency Medicine*, 3rd Edition. Copyright © 2010 The McGraw-Hill Companies, Inc. Photo contributor: Lawrence B. Stack, MD.

(A) Cefazolin intravenously

(B) Ciprofloxacin by mouth

(C) Clindamycin intravenously

(D) Trimethoprim/sulfamethoxazole by mouth

(E) Vancomycin intravenously

10-8. A 30-year-old female comes to the ED complaining of pelvic pain and discharge. She acknowledges multiple sexual partners in the previous month. On exam, there is a tender and fluctuant 2-cm mass located on the medial labia minora with mild overlying erythema at the 4 o'clock position. There is also a thin, yellowish discharge. What is the MOST appropriate management?

(A) Incision of the abscess with placement of a Word catheter and treatment with ceftriaxone, doxycycline, and metronidazole.

(B) Incision of the abscess with placement of a Word catheter and treatment with cephalexin and metronidazole.

(C) Incision and drainage without packing and Sitz baths at home.

(D) Incision and drainage with iodoform gauze and treatment with cephalexin and metronidazole.

(E) Marsupialization of the abscess and referral to gynecology for biopsy.

10-9. A 40-year-old male with a history of end-stage liver disease presents with fever, swelling, and extreme leg pain. He sustained a minor abrasions to the area 2 days prior while swimming in the Gulf of Mexico. His temperature is 39.0°C, blood pressure is 94/50, and his heart rate is 122. His right leg is severely swollen with bullous skin lesions (Figure 10-3). What is the MOST likely pathogen?

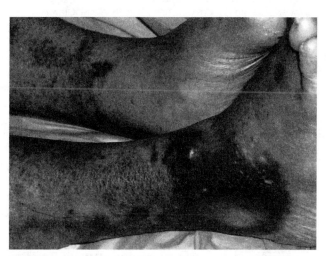

Figure 10-3. Reproduced with permission from Goldsmith LA, Katz SI, Gilchrest BA, Paller AS, Leffell DJ, Wolff K: *Fitzpatrick's Dermatology in General Medicine*, 8th Edition. Copyright © 2012 The McGraw-Hill Companies, Inc.

(A) *Aeromonas* species

(B) *Clostridium* species

(C) *Erysipelothrix rhusiopathiae*

(D) *Staphylococcus epidermidis*

(E) *Vibrio vulnificus*

10-10. A 26-year-old male presents to the ED with 3 days of malaise and the painful rash depicted in Figure 10-4. In addition to treating with antiviral agents, what further testing should be considered in this patient?

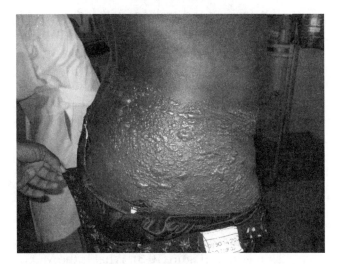

Figure 10-4. Reproduced with permission from Knoop KJ, Stack LB, Storrow AB, Thurman RJ: *The Atlas of Emergency Medicine*, 3rd Edition. Copyright © 2010 The McGraw-Hill Companies, Inc. Photo contributor: John Omara, MD.

(A) Aspiration of a vesicle for viral culture

(B) HIV testing

(C) Punch biopsy for histology and cytology

(D) Skin scraping for KOH prep

(E) Swab of an unroofed vesicle for Tzanck smear

10-11. A 14-year-old otherwise healthy Caucasian female presents to the ED with fever and altered mental status. Per her mother, she has been complaining of a progressive headache for 2 days, has had trouble walking, and has vomited multiple times. The patient has a temperature of 39.2°C. She is disoriented and agitated, and responds only to painful stimuli. No rash is detected. You initiate treatment. A CT scan of the brain does not show any focal lesions. In addition to bacterial meningitis, what other diagnosis and therapy should you consider?

(A) Brain abscess and consult neurosurgery for drainage

(B) Coccidiomycosis meningitis and treatment with IV amphotericin

(C) Cryptococcal meningitis and treatment with IV fluconazole

(D) HSV encephalitis and treatment with IV acyclovir

(E) Toxoplasmosis and treatment with pyrimethamine PO

10-12. A 30-year-old G1P0 female at 34 weeks of gestation presents complaining of a rash for 2 days. There are papules, vesicles, and crusted lesions on her torso and face. When queried, she denies all childhood immunizations. What concern do you have for this patient?

(A) Bioterrorism

(B) Congenital deformity

(C) Meningococcemia

(D) No concerns

(E) Pneumonia

10-13. A 16-year-old male presents complaining of fever, fatigue, and sore throat for the previous 2 days. His temperature is 102.1°C, blood pressure is 120/80, and heart rate is 98. On exam, you notice mild tonsillar erythema and significant exudates. He also has diffuse lymphadenopathy and a prominent spleen. A complete blood cell count is within the normal range but shows a lymphocytosis with atypical lymphocytes. What is the proper treatment?

(A) Acyclovir

(B) Amoxicillin

(C) Antipyretics and avoidance of contact sports for 4 weeks

(D) Blood cultures, broad-spectrum antibiotics, and admission

(E) Dexamethasone

10-14. What is the MOST common cause of serious opportunistic viral disease in patients with advanced AIDS?

(A) Cytomegalovirus

(B) Herpes simple virus

(C) Influenza virus

(D) Human papillomavirus

(E) Varicella zoster virus

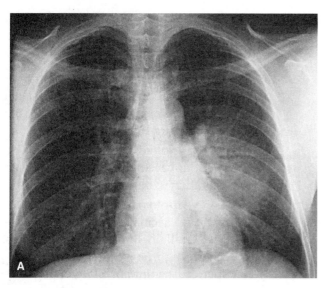
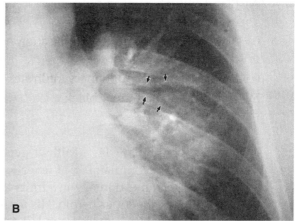

Figure 10-5. Reproduced with permission from Schwartz DT: *Emergency Radiology: Case Studies.* Copyright © 2008 The McGraw-Hill Companies, Inc.

10-15. A 35-year-old male with AIDS presents complaining of fever and a productive cough for 1 day. His last known CD4 count 1 month ago was 350. The following chest radiograph was obtained (Figure 10-5). What is the MOST likely diagnosis?

(A) Cryptococcus neoformans pneumonia

(B) Disseminated *Mycobacterium avium* complex

(C) *Pneumocystis carinii* pneumonia

(D) Pulmonary tuberculosis

(E) *Streptococcus pneumoniae*

10-16. Which of the following is the highest risk exposure and supports three-drug postexposure prophylaxis (PEP) against HIV?

(A) A police officer who was spit in the eyes by an otherwise healthy male who is refusing testing

(B) A male who tested negative for HIV 6 months ago who last had anal intercourse 5 days ago and is worried the condom broke

(C) A nurse who was vomited in the face by an HIV patient with CD4 count of 600

(D) A resident who was stuck with a hollow-bore needle after performing a thoracentesis on a patient with disseminated *M. avium* complex

(E) A gynecology resident who was splashed in the eyes with amniotic fluid from a woman with a known low viral load of HIV

10-17. A 44-year-old female with AIDS presents complaining of pain when she swallows, but is able to tolerate liquids and solids. The pain radiates down her chest. She appears nontoxic. On exam, you notice a white plaque on her tongue and oropharynx that is easily scraped off. Her CD4 count is 100. What is the MOST appropriate treatment?

(A) Acyclovir

(B) Fluconazole

(C) Ganciclovir

(D) Immediate endoscopy

(E) Proton pump inhibitor

10-18. Which pathogen is the MOST common cause of infective endocarditis in the industrialized world?

(A) *Bartonella* spp.

(B) *Eikenella corrodens*

(C) *Enterococcus* spp.

(D) *Staphylococcus aureus*

(E) *Streptococcus viridans*

10-19. Which of the following is likely to have right-sided endocarditis?

(A) Blood cultures positive for streptococci in an injection drug user

(B) Native-valve disease in a noninjection drug user

(C) Multiple bilateral pulmonary infiltrates

(D) New left bundle-branch block

(E) Pulmonary edema

10-20. A 23-year-old previously healthy male presents to the ED complaining of fever for 4 days. On further questioning, he admits to regularly using intravenous heroin. His temperature is 38.9°C, blood pressure is 110/60, and heart rate is 110. He appears ill. He has a sister with systemic lupus erythematosus. The rest of his exam appears nonfocal. What is the MOST appropriate management?

(A) Erythrocyte sedimentation rate and antinuclear antibody

(B) Reassure patient it is a viral syndrome and discharge home

(C) Three blood cultures from separate sites, antibiotics, and admit

(D) Thyroid function assessment

(E) Urine drug screen

10-21. A 74-year-old diabetic patient is brought in by ambulance because of intermittent fever and malaise for the previous 2 weeks. Upon further questioning, you learn he underwent a transurethral resection of the prostate 1 month ago. He has a diastolic decrescendo murmur on exam. You suspect bacterial endocarditis. Which pathogen is classically associated with this history?

(A) *Cardiobacterium* spp.

(B) *Enterococcus* spp.

(C) *Escherichia coli*

(D) *S. aureus*

(E) *S. viridans*

10-22. Which of the following patients would MOST likely benefit from tetanus immunoglobulin (TIG)?

(A) A 30-year-old male who underwent the full vaccination series with last booster 4 years ago who has an open Grade 3 tibia fracture after a dirt bike crash.

(B) A 44-year-old diabetic woman with no previous vaccinations with a small 1-cm laceration while washing a kitchen knife.

(C) A 45-year-old male who completed the primary vaccinations series but developed Guillain–Barré after his last booster 15 years ago, now presenting with an open crush injury of bilateral thighs.

(D) A 52-year-old farmer who completed the primary vaccination series but no booster in over 10 years who has a large jagged laceration to his shin due to farm equipment.

(E) A 60-year-old male who completed the vaccination series but has not had a booster in over 10 years who lacerated his finger while cutting carrots.

10-23. You are volunteering in Haiti in the ED and see a patient who appears to be seizing. He is a 30-year-old male who is brought in by his family because of jaw pain and muscle spasms. You also notice many small abscesses with central necrosis on his upper extremities. He is arching his back, flexing his arms, clenching his fists, and extending his lower extremities, but appears to be awake and in pain. What complication should you anticipate?

(A) Death unless treated with rabies immunoglobulin

(B) Laryngospasm and arrest of respiration

(C) Overwhelming sepsis unless treated with penicillin

(D) Permanent central nervous system injury

(E) Spread by respiratory droplets

10-24. A 33-year-old intoxicated male presents to the ED 2 hours after being bit by a raccoon he was trying to feed while hiking. He states, "the raccoon did not appear rabid." It retreated back into the woods and is unavailable. He has a small puncture wound proximal to his right thumb. What is the proper treatment?

(A) Cleanse the wound with soap and water and administer both rabies vaccine and human rabies immunoglobulin (HRIG) directly into the wound.

(B) Cleanse the wound with soap and water, administer as much HRIG as possible directly into the wound with remaining in the right deltoid, and administer rabies vaccine into the left deltoid.

(C) Irrigate the wound with high-pressure normal saline, administer HRIG directly into the wound with remaining into the right gluteus, and administer rabies vaccine into the left gluteus.

(D) Scrub the wound with povidone-iodine, administer HRIG into the left deltoid, and follow up with public health for vaccination.

(E) Scrub the wound with povidone-iodine and discharge home with amoxicillin/clavulanate.

10-25. What type of nonbite exposure is highest risk and may require PEP for rabies?

(A) Close contact with a bat in a confined space
(B) Dry scratch from a stray cat
(C) Petting a wild dog
(D) Sprayed by a skunk
(E) Stepping in raccoon feces

10-26. A 40-year-old male presents complaining of intermittent fever, myalgias, and malaise for 8 days. The patient informs you that he had returned from India 6 months ago and had a similar illness diagnosed as malaria that was treated with chloroquine. What process is MOST likely?

(A) Dengue fever
(B) Influenza virus after successful treatment of malaria
(C) Recrudescence of *Plasmodium falciparum*
(D) Relapse of *P. falciparum*
(E) Relapse of *P. vivax*

10-27. A 68-year-old female is brought in by EMS for fever for 4 days. She was found altered by her husband today who called 911. You learn that she just returned from a trip to Africa, and went on a safari in Tanzania. She had used chloroquine for prophylaxis. She was seen in the ED 2 days earlier and diagnosed with a viral syndrome. She is hypoglycemic but her mental status does not improve with therapy. You intubate her due to altered mental status and respiratory distress. She is pale and jaundiced. She does not have a rash. In addition to treating for possible bacterial meningitis, what else is crucial to her care?

(A) Await results of a single thin and thick smear before initiating additional therapy.
(B) Ensure health care workers treating the patient receive prophylaxis for meningococcemia.
(C) Start quinidine and doxycycline intravenously and contact the CDC for possible artesunate therapy.
(D) Send the cerebrospinal fluid for encephalitis panel.
(E) Test for HIV.

10-28. Which of the following supports the use of antibiotics for diarrhea?

   (A) Bloody diarrhea and fever for 3 days in a 42-year-old female returning from South America.

   (B) A 9-year-old female with confirmed enterohemorrhagic *E. coli* 0157:H7.

   (C) An 11-year-old boy with frequent watery stools for 1 day with moderate decreased skin turgor.

   (D) A 68-year-old female with multiple episodes of watery diarrhea, vomiting, and diffuse blanching erythema after eating fresh tuna.

   (E) An otherwise healthy 17-year-old male with 2 days of diarrhea after swimming in a lake.

10-29. You volunteered to be a physician for a Mediterranean cruise and are enjoying your much deserved vacation until the third day when dozens of patients and cruise members present to you complaining of nausea, vomiting, and nonbloody diarrhea. Which of the following is the MOST likely culprit?

   (A) Rotavirus

   (B) Norovirus

   (C) Ciguatera

   (D) Enterotoxigenic *E. coli*

   (E) Shigellosis

10-30. A 60-year-old female is brought by EMS from home complaining of fever and malaise for 2 days. Upon further questioning, she also complains of feeling confused with a severe headache, muscle aches, and nausea with vomiting. She visited her sister in South Carolina 4 days ago. On exam, she does not appear to have nuchal rigidity; her lungs are clear to auscultation, and her abdomen nontender. However, you notice a petechial rash on her wrists and ankles. Her temperature is 39.0°C, blood pressure is 90/50, heart rate is 120. Preliminary lab results show neutropenia, thrombocytopenia, and hyponatremia. You consider meningococcemia, but what else should you suspect and treat?

   (A) Babesiosis

   (B) Brucellosis

   (C) Rocky Mountain spotted fever (RMSF)

   (D) Tick-borne relapsing fever

   (E) Tularemia

10-31. A 53-year-old patient is seen in the ED complaining of fever and headache for 2 days. One month ago, he took his family on vacation to eastern Massachusetts. Two weeks ago, he was seen by his primary care provider for the rash depicted in Figure 10-6. He was treated with doxycycline for 21 days. His temperature is 38.5°C. There is no rash. Which of the following is the MOST likely explanation for his current symptoms?

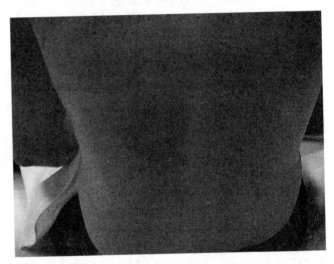

Figure 10-6. Reproduced from Snyder SB, Thurman RJ: Images in emergency medicine. Erythema migrans in Tennessee. *Ann Emerg Med.* 2005;46(3):224. Photo contributor: Shannon B. Snyder, MD.

   (A) Anaplasmosis

   (B) Babesiosis

   (C) Colorado tick fever

   (D) Ehrlichiosis

   (E) Secondary syphilis

10-32. A 9-year-old male from Connecticut presents to the ED with a 1-day history of bilateral facial nerve palsy that involves the forehead. Upon further questioning, he recalls a nonpruritic, nonpainful rash 2 months ago for which he did not tell his mother or seek treatment. What is the MOST likely pathogen?

(A) *Borrelia burgdorferi*
(B) *Chlamydophila psittaci*
(C) *Pasteurella multocida*
(D) *Rickettsia rickettsii*
(E) *Yersinia pestis*

10-33. Which travel-related disease can still be commonly acquired despite proper vaccination?

(A) Hepatitis A
(B) Hepatitis B
(C) Rabies
(D) Typhoid fever
(E) Yellow fever

10-34. Which of the following infections that may be seen in a returning traveler is paired with the correct exposure?

(A) Amebiasis and percutaneous inoculation through intact skin
(B) Chagas disease and tick bite
(C) Cysticercosis and uncooked beef
(D) Leptospirosis and freshwater
(E) Schistosomiasis and uncooked pork

10-35. A nurse informs you that a mother has brought her child in with the following rash (Figure 10-7). What kind of precautions should be taken to decrease the risk of disease spread?

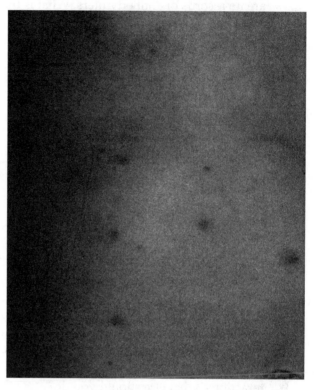

Figure 10-7. Reproduced with permission from Wolff K, Johnson RA: *Fitzpatrick's Color Atlas & Synopsis of Clinical Dermatology*, 6th Edition. Copyright © 2009 The McGraw-Hill Companies, Inc.

(A) Airborne
(B) Contact
(C) Droplet
(D) None
(E) Universal

10-36. An intern experiences a needlestick after attempting to place a central line in a septic patient. The source patient has liver cancer from chronic hepatitis B. The intern received the vaccination series for hepatitis B, but there are no records of antibody titers. What is the proper course of action?

(A) If the source is positive for hepatitis B core antigen (HBcAg), test the intern for HBsAg. If inadequate, treat with vaccine booster.

(B) No treatment is necessary; the intern has received proper vaccination.

(C) Test the intern for anti-HBs. If adequate, give only hepatitis B immune globulin (HBIG).

(D) Test the intern for anti-HBs. If inadequate, treat with HBIG and vaccine booster.

(E) Treat the intern with HBIG.

10-37. A 60-year-old female with diabetes, congestive heart failure, and atrial fibrillation is diagnosed with a urinary tract infection. She is on multiple medications. You plan to prescribe ciprofloxacin, but due to drug–drug interactions, what else should you do?

(A) Ensure close follow-up to recheck her prothrombin time while on warfarin.

(B) Hold her digoxin due to prolonged QT and risk for torsades de pointes.

(C) Hold her furosemide to decrease the risk of ototoxicity.

(D) Increase her glyburide due to hyperglycemia.

(E) Recommend that she continues her antacids to decrease the risk of gastritis.

10-38. You have a high suspicion of malaria caused by *P. falciparum* in a toxic appearing patient. You initiate therapy with intravenous quinidine. Which of the following is a complication of therapy?

(A) Hemolysis in the setting of glucose-6-phosphate dehydrogenase deficiency.

(B) Hyperglycemia.

(C) Methemoglobinemia.

(D) None, it is relatively safe therapy.

(E) Prolonged QT syndrome.

10-39. Which of the following mandates antiretroviral therapy in an HIV + patient?

(A) Acute retroviral syndrome

(B) CD4+ T cell count of 450

(C) Diarrheal illness due to shigellosis

(D) Pregnancy

(E) Tertiary syphilis

10-40. A 32-year-old male with AIDS presents with diarrhea for the past 4 days. He denies travel or recent antibiotics. He is afebrile and his blood pressure is 100/50 and heart rate is 120. His is negative for fecal blood. His last known CD4 count was 26. If this patient has the most common cause of diarrhea in AIDS patients, what treatment is likely to be most beneficial?

(A) Azithromycin

(B) Ciprofloxacin

(C) Highly active antiretroviral therapy

(D) Metronidazole

(E) Nitazoxanide

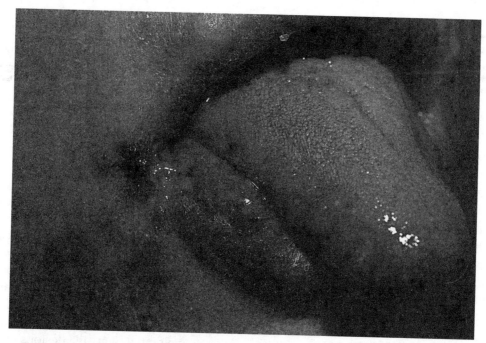

Figure 10-8. Reproduced with permission from Wolff K, Johnson RA: *Fitzpatrick's Color Atlas & Synopsis of Clinical Dermatology*, 6th Edition. Copyright © 2009 The McGraw-Hill Companies, Inc.

10-41. What is the most likely cause of this lesion (Figure 10-8)?

(A) A primary infection with coxsackie A virus

(B) A primary infection with herpes simplex virus (HSV) type 1

(C) A primary infection with HSV type 2

(D) A reactivation of HSV type 1 or type 2 from the trigeminal ganglion

(E) Infectious mononucleosis caused by the Epstein–Barr virus (EBV)

10-42. You are treating an obtunded 72-year-old female for severe sepsis due to pneumonia. You have administered 3 L normal saline and broad-spectrum antibiotics. After performing endotracheal intubation, you place a central venous oxygen saturation catheter and arterial line in preparation for early goal directed therapy. The patient's blood pressure is now 88/34, central venous pressure is 11 mm Hg, and venous oxygen saturation is 66%. Lab values are not yet available. What is the MOST appropriate next step?

(A) Administer 1 L normal saline intravenously.

(B) Begin infusion of dobutamine 0.5–1.0 µg/kg/min IV.

(C) Begin infusion of norepinephrine 5 µg/min IV.

(D) No further actions, the endpoints of early goal directed therapy have been met.

(E) Transfuse 2 units packed red blood cells.

Systemic Infectious Disorders
Answers and Explanations

10-1. The answer is B (Chapter 144). Ulcerative genital lesions are usually due to herpes simplex, syphilis, or chancroid. The epidemiology of sexually transmitted infections is important in the evaluation and thus a travel history should be obtained. Chancroid is rare in the United States and other developed countries. However, in developing countries, it is extremely common. Chancroid, caused by *Haemophilus ducreyi*, typically presents as a painful papule that forms an ulcer on a friable base with a yellow-gray necrotic exudate. After 1–2 weeks, painful bilateral inguinal lymphadenopathy (buboes) can develop that may require incision and drainage or needle aspiration to prevent fistula formation. First-line treatment is azithromycin 1 gm by mouth in a single dose. Chancroid is also a prominent cofactor for transmission of HIV, and patients diagnosed with chancroid should also be screened for other communicable diseases. Sexual partners should be instructed to receive an examination and treatment. Single-dose azithromycin and ceftriaxone intramuscularly will treat urethritis or cervicitis. Herpes can be differentiated from chancroid by the smaller, depressed ulcerations without a preceding papule, as well as the presence of systemic symptoms. While many STDs are reportable, herpes is not. Penicillin is the treatment for syphilis. The chancre of syphilis can be differentiated from chancroid by its painless character. Doxycycline for 21 days is the treatment for the painless chancre caused by Lymphogranuloma Venereum.

10-2. The answer is A (Chapter 144). The rash of secondary syphilis typically occurs 4–6 weeks after the initial infection. It develops as nonpruritic, rough, red or reddish brown macules on the trunk and flexor areas and often extends to the palms, soles, and oral mucosa. The involvement of the palms and soles is an important diagnostic clue to secondary syphilis. Moist areas, especially the vulva and scrotum, may develop flat, wart-like lesions known as condyloma latum; these lesions are extremely infectious. Secondary syphilis is often associated with systemic symptoms. The rash will resolve without treatment, but the disease may progress to latent disease and possibly tertiary syphilis. Intramuscular benzathine penicillin remains the treatment of choice.

10-3. The answer is B (Chapter 144). The most common sexually transmitted disease, and also the most common cause of cervicitis/urethritis, is *C. trachomatis*. This is followed by *N. gonorrhoeae*, which usually has a much more profuse, purulent discharge than *C. trachomatis*. Given high rates of coinfection, patients are often empirically treated for both infections. Uncomplicated *C. trachomatis* is treated with either azithromycin 1 g single dose or doxycycline 100 mg twice daily for 7 days. Uncomplicated *N. gonorrhoeae* cervicitis/urethritis is treated with ceftriaxone 125 mg intramuscularly. Single-dose azithromycin 2 g is an alternative. Fluoroquinolones are no longer recommended due to high rates of resistance. Sodium chloride microscopy is used to detect *T. vaginalis* or clue cells suggestive of bacterial vaginosis. Trichomonads are motile and therefore detectable for approximately 10–20 minutes after plating. *T. vaginalis* should be a consideration when first-line treatment for urethritis fails in male patients. Potassium hydroxide microscopy is utilized for hyphae of *C. albicans*. Human papillomavirus causes genital warts and is known to lead to cervical cancer. Other less common causes of urethritis are *Ureaplasma urealyticum*, *Mycoplasma genitalium*, HSV, and adenovirus.

10-4. **The answer is B** (Chapter 145). The presentation is strongly suggestive for toxic shock syndrome (TSS). Menstrual causes of TSS have decreased since the withdrawal of highly absorbent tampons. Nonmenstrual causes of TSS include wound infections, mastitis, respiratory infections following viral pneumonia, and enterocolitis. Additionally, nasal packing has been associated with *S. aureus* invasion. The diffuse rash is known as erythroderma. Patients may experience massive vasodilation and cardiac dysfunction, requiring profound fluid resuscitation. The history and the erythroderma are not consistent with anaphylaxis. Vague, diffuse abdominal pain is characteristic of the disease, and while investigation may be indicated, the nasal packing is a likely source and a CT is not initially indicated. Erythroderma is not consistent with a viral exanthem. Vancomycin plus clindamycin is an appropriate antibiotic regimen for staphylococcal TSS. Although patients may develop bleeding complications due to thrombocytopenia, the nasal packing must be removed, as it is the source of the disease.

10-5. **The answer is C** (Chapter 145). This patient has a presentation suggestive for streptococcal TSS with necrotizing fasciitis. Both diabetes and chronic alcoholism are associated with more severe disease. Immediate surgical consultation is prudent for both diagnosis and treatment. Necrotizing soft-tissue infections carry an extremely high mortality. Earlier operative treatment involving debridement, fasciotomy, and even amputation improves outcomes. Broad-spectrum intravenous antibiotics and fluid resuscitation are indicated. Imaging with a CT scan or MRI may be useful in patients who are not critically ill and in whom the diagnosis is not certain. It would only delay definitive care in this case. The patient is showing signs of sepsis and cannot be treated with bedside incision and drainage. Streptococcal TSS is often associated with severe infection and blood cultures are often positive. However, intravenous antibiotics cannot substitute for emergent surgical debridement. Alcohol withdrawal may eventually be a concern, but is not currently.

10-6. **The answer is A** (Chapter 146). This patient has characteristics suggestive of severe sepsis. Source control is a key component of successful therapy in sepsis. Definitive treatment of sepsis would be removal of the nidus of infection if feasible. Patients receiving dialysis through temporary external catheters are at higher risk for bacteremia than those with AV fistulas. Coagulase-negative staphylococcus and *S. aureus* comprise the majority of infections. Enterococcus and enteric gram-negative organisms must also be considered. While this patient should receive fluid resuscitation and antimicrobial therapy, this patient is unlikely to recover without removal of the source of infection. It would be prudent to assess this patient's chemistry panel, but it is more likely that he is suffering from sepsis than dialyzable conditions such as uremia or hyperkalemia.

10-7. **The answer is E** (Chapter 147). The patient is presenting with cellulitis and has failed outpatient therapy with an oral beta-lactam. He is also showing signs of systemic toxicity and should likely be hospitalized for parenteral therapy. A patient that warrants hospitalization should receive therapy for methicillin-resistant *S. aureus* (MRSA) and *Streptococcus pyogenes*. Vancomycin would be an ideal agent. Alternative choices may be linezolid or daptomycin. MRSA with resistance to clindamycin is high in some communities and should not be relied on for severe soft-tissue infections. Trimethoprim/sulfamethoxazole would provide adequate coverage for MRSA in a patient stable for outpatient treatment. However, it has minimal activity against

S. pyogenes and should not be sole therapy. Cefazolin and other beta-lactam antibiotics are appropriate treatment for streptococcus and methicillin-sensitive *S. aureus* cellulitis, but treatment of severe disease should cover MRSA. MRSA in many communities develops rapid resistance to ciprofloxacin, and it should not be first-line treatment.

10-8. **The answer is A** (Chapter 147). Appropriate treatment in the ED for a Bartholin gland abscess is incision with placement of a Word catheter. Use of the Word catheter promotes fistula formation and decreases the rate of reformation. Antibiotics can be added as clinically necessary. Cephalexin plus metronidazole has been standard therapy if a sexually transmitted disease is not suspected, as the infection is typically polymicrobial vaginal flora. There have been reports of MRSA causing vaginal infections and thus there is a trend toward obtaining cultures. Although less common, both *N. gonorrhoeae* and *C. trachomatis* can each cause a Bartholin gland abscess. If clinical suspicion is high for sexually transmitted disease, treatment should be the typical regimen for cervicitis plus metronidazole. A Bartholin gland abscess in perimenopausal women may require biopsy due to a higher relationship with carcinoma. Simple incision and drainage with iodoform gauze packing has a high rate of discomfort and recurrent abscess formation. Marsupialization involves an elliptical incision and suturing usually performed by a gynecologist.

10-9. **The answer is E** (Chapter 147). *V. vulnificus* and *Vibrio parahaemolyticus* are the major bacteria associated with soft-tissue infections after exposure to seawater. Cases are predominantly found along the Gulf Coast, but can be seen on both the East and West Coasts as well. *V. vulnificus* often involves bullous lesions and should be suspected when the presentation suggests necrotizing fasciitis. It is often an aggressive process, especially in patients with liver disease, end-stage renal disease, or other immunosuppression. Aggres-

sive resuscitation is warranted as patients tend to have cardiovascular collapse. History of exposure to seawater is important, as the antibiotic of choice, doxycycline, is not typically used for necrotizing fasciitis and septicemia. As with all necrotizing wounds, consultation for surgical debridement is prudent. *Aeromonas* is associated with freshwater exposure. Wounds due to *Clostridium* are less common due to improved hygiene. *E. rhusiopathiae* is related to contaminated meat or fish exposure. Immunocompromised patients are at risk for *S. epidermidis* deep space infections.

10-10. **The answer is B** (Chapters 148 and 149). Herpes zoster is a reactivation of latent infection with the varicella zoster virus. The papulovesicular rash typically has a unilateral, dermatomal distribution that does not cross the midline, and at most may involve two to three contiguous dermatomal segments. It is predominantly a disease of older patient populations due to waning cell immunity. Zoster in younger patients, or lesions involving multiple noncontiguous dermatomes, should raise suspicion for an immunocompromised state. Testing this patient for HIV is prudent. The diagnosis of zoster is typically made on clinical grounds. Viral culture may be warranted in severe disseminated disease or when the diagnosis is uncertain, but would not apply to this case. In a typical presentation of zoster, a biopsy would not add to the case. A Tzanck smear may reveal giant cells with multiple nuclei but cannot differentiate between varicella-zoster and other herpes viruses and is not useful.

10-11. **The answer is D** (Chapter 148). The presentation of HSV encephalitis can closely mirror bacterial meningitis and must be considered in any patient who presents with fever, altered mental status, and focal neurologic signs. HSV encephalitis can represent a primary infection or a reactivation and may occur in normal immunocompetent hosts. It has a predilection for the medial temporal and inferior frontal lobes. Factors leading to encephalitis are largely unknown. The proper treatment is intravenous acyclovir, and even with treatment, survivors have a high rate of persistent neurological deficits. Dosing should be reduced in patients with renal dysfunction at baseline. Space-occupying lesions should be ruled out by CT scan prior to lumbar puncture in a patient with focal neurologic signs. Brain abscess could present with seizure and signs of cerebral edema, but would typically be apparent on CT scan. Coccidiomycosis, cryptococcosis, and toxoplasmosis typically invade the CNS in the setting of immunosuppression. Furthermore, the proper first-line treatment for CNS cryptococcal disease would be with amphotericin.

10-12. **The answer is E** (Chapter 148). The description is classic for chickenpox caused by the varicella zoster virus. Pregnant women are typically screened for antibodies due to a higher rate of complications. Chickenpox in the first or second trimester may lead to congenital embryopathy. Disease in the third trimester does not typically affect the fetus, but has a much higher rate of serious pulmonary complications in the mother. Smallpox has been eradicated through global vaccination, but has resurfaced as a potential biochemical weapon. Clinically, the lesions of smallpox tend to be uniform (either all vesicles or all pustules), as opposed to the variable stages of lesions seen in chickenpox. Additionally, the lesions in smallpox are denser peripherally and include the palms and soles. The rash of meningococcemia is initially petechial. As the disease progresses, it may become purpuric with central necrosis, and patients demonstrate severe systemic toxicity.

10-13. **The answer is C** (Chapter 148). This presentation is suggestive of infectious mononucleosis caused by EBV. Treatment is usually supportive and rarely requires admission. Patients may develop splenomegaly, and should be advised to avoid contact sports for at least 4 weeks to avoid splenic rupture. Acyclovir is active against EBV, but is only effective against oral hairy leukoplakia in HIV. Amoxicillin can be used for streptococcal pharyngitis, but when mistakenly used for EBV will cause a diffuse morbilliform rash. The patient does not have signs of sepsis, is not at risk for endocarditis, and has a presentation classic for EBV and does not warrant hospitalization. Dexamethasone is often utilized in streptococcal pharyngitis, but increased complications are noted in the setting of EBV. It should be avoided unless the patient has airway compromise.

10-14. **The answer is A** (Chapter 149). While HSV, human papillomavirus, and varicella-zoster virus all have a higher prevalence and a tendency for disseminated disease in HIV-infected individuals, cytomegalovirus is the most common. It can establish itself in many organ systems and becomes a serious risk with CD4+ T cell counts below 50. It is the most serious and common ocular opportunistic infection causing blindness. Gastrointestinal, pulmonary, and central nervous system disseminated disease also occur.

10-15. **The answer is E** (Chapter 149). In order to provide appropriate care to patients with HIV, it is critical to have an understanding of diseases relative to the absolute CD4+ T cell count. Patients with CD4 counts above 500 typically will develop febrile illnesses similar to the general population. A patient with a CD4 count between 200 and 500, who presents with fever, is most likely to have a bacterial mediated pulmonary infection, and *S. pneumoniae* is the most common cause. However, tuberculosis is also dramatically increased at this CD4 level, often without the classic radiographic findings of upper lobe involvement or cavitary lesions. It may be prudent to place this patient in respiratory isolation until ruled out by acid-fast bacilli stain and sputum culture. *Pneumocystis jirovecii* pneumonia is the most common opportunistic pathogen in AIDS patients. It becomes the primary consideration with fever or shortness of breath and CD4 count below 200. Although less likely, cryptococcal pneumonia is also a consideration, and may be included in the workup. Disseminated *M. avium* complex typically occurs when the CD4 count is below 100. Symptoms are typically fever and night sweats and may include malaise, diarrhea, and weight loss.

10-16. **The answer is D.** (Chapters 149 and 157). Basis for treatment and the regimen depends upon the mechanism of exposure and the disease state of the source. Risks for seroconversion include deep injury, visible blood on the device, previous needle placement in a vein or an artery, and a source with late-stage HIV infection or high viral load. Specific advice is available through a national hotline. Low-risk exposure to an unknown source does not support treatment. Two-drug PEP is utilized in low-risk exposure to low-risk patients (those with low viral loads and asymptomatic HIV), and three-drug PEP is advised with high-risk exposure to low-risk patients and any significant exposure to a high-risk source (end-stage AIDS or high viral load). Unless saliva or vomit contains blood, each is unlikely to cause transmission. Blood, semen, and vaginal secretions, along with pleural, peritoneal, and amniotic fluid, all can harbor and transmit HIV. Nonoccupational PEP is traditionally recommended only for high-risk exposure within the previous 72 hours. Treatment outside 72 hours is at the discretion of the physician.

10-17. **The answer is B** (Chapter 149). Odynophagia with a CD4 count fewer than 100 and oral thrust strongly suggests esophageal candidiasis. If the patient can tolerate oral therapy, fluconazole is the first-line treatment. Endoscopy is reserved for treatment failure or atypical presentation. Cytomegalovirus and HSV are diagnosed by endoscopy, and are treated with ganciclovir and acyclovir, respectively. Patients with HIV can have esophagitis due to reflux, but in this setting, empiric treatment for candidiasis is the most appropriate.

10-18. **The answer is D** (Chapter 150). Streptococci and staphylococci account for up to 90% of all cases of infective endocarditis. There has gradually been a change in the microbiology of infective endocarditis and currently *S. aureus* is thought to be the most common pathogen of native-valve endocarditis in both injection drug users and nonusers. Enterococcus and coagulase-negative staphylococcus are the next most common after staphylococcus and streptococci. The rest of the cases in noninjection drug users are usually attributable to the HACEK group, *Bartonella* species, and *Coxiella burnetti.*

10-19. **The answer is C** (Chapter 150). Patients with right-sided endocarditis often have septic pulmonary emboli. They can present with chest pain, hemoptysis, and dyspnea. Right-sided endocarditis is more likely in injection drug users infected with *S. aureus*, malformed right-sided valves, prosthetic right-sided valves, and bilateral pulmonary infiltrates suggesting septic emboli. Streptococcus and enterococcus both have a predilection for left-sided endocarditis even in injection drug users. Pulmonary edema suggests a left-sided lesion, as do all other embolic phenomena, unless the patient has a large septal defect.

10-20. **The answer is C** (Chapter 150). Ten to fifteen percent of injection drug users who develop fever have endocarditis. The high rate of disease supports a workup. The absence of a discernable murmur, especially in a noisy ED, does not negate the diagnosis of endocarditis. This patient may have another reason for fever, but given the risks of disease, strong consideration should be made for admission and antibiotic therapy in a febrile and toxic injection drug user. Although it is unfortunate that his sister has systemic lupus erythematosus, this family history is less likely to have anything to do with the patient's clinical presentation.

10-21. **The answer is B** (Chapter 150). Enterococcus endocarditis is associated with manipulation of the lower gastrointestinal or genitourinary tract, and is increased among diabetics. It has a propensity for infecting abnormal left-sided valves. Underlying senile aortic stenosis develops with age and can be a risk factor for endocarditis during bacteremia.

10-22. **The answer is C** (Chapter 151). TIG is indicated for nonminor wounds in a patient who had less than three tetanus toxoid doses. It is not necessary for clean, minor wounds, even with an incomplete vaccination series. TIG is typically not necessary for major wounds if the primary vaccination series has been completed. TIG may be considered in patients who should receive tetanus toxoid (Td or Tdap) based on time since last booster but who have a contraindication to toxoid administration. Contraindications include Guillain–Barré syndrome within 6 weeks of tetanus toxoid, previous Arthus reaction within 10 years, current moderate illness, or unstable neurologic condition.

10-23. **The answer is B** (Chapter 151). This classic description of muscular rigidity is highly suggestive of tetanus. Initial symptoms may be described as jaw pain, dysphagia, or generalized muscular rigidity or cramping. This can progress to generalized spasticity as described, and can lead to rhabdomyolysis and lactic acidosis. It can involve laryngospasm and can lead to respiratory arrest. Early attention to airway management is prudent, as nearly two-thirds of cases require intubation. Tetanus may eventually lead to infectious complications due to a protracted course, but it does not typically involve overwhelming sepsis early in the disease. Although the central nervous system is involved, permanent injury can be avoided if hypoxia is adverted. Person-to-person transmission of tetanus does not occur. The presentation of rabies involves mental status changes, hyperactivity, and may include paralysis rather than spasticity. It is typically fatal even with immunoglobulin administration after development of the disease. Of note, this presentation also mirrors strychnine poisoning, which can be a contaminant in heroin or cocaine. Treatment for strychnine is supportive.

10-24. **The answer is B** (Chapter 152). It is critical to know the indications for PEP for rabies, as the goal is disease prevention (Table 152–5). Once a patient shows signs of rabies, it is almost always uniformly fatal. PEP in nonimmunized individuals largely depends on the animal and route of exposure. Raccoons, skunks, foxes, bats, and many other large terrestrial carnivores are regarded as rabid unless direct animal testing proves negative. Bites from healthy dogs, cats, and ferrets do not need prophylaxis if the animal can be observed for 10 days and it does not exhibit signs of rabies. Treatment begins with immediate, thorough cleansing with soap and water, as the virus is highly lipophilic. HRIG should be injected directly into the wound without compromising tissue integrity, and any remaining is injected into the ipsilateral deltoid. The rabies vaccine should always be injected into the deltoid on the opposite side of the body to avoid neutralization by HRIG. Failure rates have been associated with gluteal injection and should be avoided. Current guidelines suggest giving 4 or 5 doses of HRIG depending on the patient's immune status.

10-25. **The answer is A** (Chapter 152). The most cases of rabies in the United States are bat related. The risk of rabies following exposure to a bat may be underestimated since the wounds inflicted from a bite may be perceived as insignificant. Current guidelines suggest treatment when a person is not absolutely sure a bite did not occur. Such is the case when a bat is found with a sleeping person, unattended infant, mentally disabled person, or intoxicated person. Raccoons, skunks, and foxes are all considered rabid unless proven otherwise, but the virus is only transmitted through saliva. The virus replicates in the salivary gland of infected animals and is transmitted through nonintact skin or mucous membranes. Dry wounds, such as a scratch from a claw, can be considered noninfectious.

10-26. **The answer is E** (Chapter 153). Malaria caused by *P. vivax* is typically successfully treated by chloroquine. However, both

P. vivax and *Plasmodium ovale* develop an exoerythrocytic phase known as a hypnozoite that lays dormant in the liver. Chloroquine is not active against the hypnozoite form, and therefore most patients diagnosed with *P. vivax* are also treated with primaquine. Without primaquine treatment, patients may have a relapse of infection after reactivation of the hypnozoite form. *P. falciparum* does not have a hypnozoite form. Recent illness with malaria should heighten suspicion, even after treatment, and symptoms should not be quickly attributed to an influenza-type illness. Fever in a returning traveler after 14 days essentially rules out the diagnosis of dengue fever. Recrudescence refers to a reappearance of malaria in days or weeks after apparently successful treatment, typically due to treatment failure of *P. falciparum*.

10-27. **The answer is C** (Chapters 153 and 156). Suspicion for malaria must be high in a febrile patient who has recently traveled to a malarial zone, even if chemoprophylaxis was used. Chloroquine is inappropriate chemoprophylaxis for travel to Africa. The manifestation of *P. falciparum* is often more severe and the progression of the disease is much more rapid in a nonimmune host. The early disease process can mirror an influenza-type illness with fever, malaise, myalgia, and headache. The classic cyclical pattern of fever is often absent in *P. falciparum* infection. As the disease progresses, it may manifest in any organ system. Cerebral malaria is marked by coma, seizures, or focal neurologic signs. Jaundice develops through hemolysis, hepatocellular injury, and cholestasis. Respiratory distress, renal failure, lactic acidosis, and disseminated intravascular coagulation can also all develop. The diagnosis of *P. falciparum* is made by observing small ring forms with double-chromatin knobs within the erythrocyte on thin and thick blood smears. Absence in one sample does not exclude the disease and should not preclude immediate treatment when suspicion is high. Smears should be continued twice daily for 2–3 days. Ideal treatment for *P. falciparum* is with an artemesin-based derivative. The only intravenous derivative available in the United States is artesunate, which is only available through the CDC. Therapy should begin immediately with quinidine and doxycycline. The CDC should be contacted for artesunate therapy for severe disease or if antimalarial agents are not available at one's hospital. HIV infection can lead to more severe manifestation of malaria, but immediate testing is not necessary. This patient should receive a lumbar puncture after a CT scan to rule out bacterial meningitis and viral encephalitis, but it is not the critical step in the management of this patient. Chemoprophylaxis is typically given for exposure to respiratory droplets from a patient with infection due to *Neisseria meningitidis* or *Haemophilus influenzae*.

10-28. **The answer is A** (Chapter 154). Initial therapy in the majority of patients with foodborne illness focuses on treating dehydration. Occasionally, patients will benefit from antibacterial therapy. Patients with bloody diarrhea and fever often have invasive infections and may benefit from antibiotics. The caveat to treatment lies in the similarity of enterohemorrhagic *E. coli* 0157 (EHEC) to *shigella*. It produces a shiga-like toxin and may have similar symptoms. EHEC typically has an antecedent watery diarrhea for 2 days that develops into bloody diarrhea, as opposed to the more immediate and very frequent bloody diarrhea of shigellosis. Patients with EHEC also tend to be afebrile. Differentiation may be prudent as antibiotics during EHEC infection have a high correlation with hemolytic–uremic syndrome. Frequent nonbloody stools for less than 1 day are more likely due to rotavirus or noroviruses. Both may lead to severe dehydration necessitating intravenous therapy, but neither is abated by antibiotics. Diarrhea associated with vomiting and flushing suggests scombroid, which is best treated with antihistamines. Diarrhea after recreational freshwater exposure is often due to *cryptosporidium*. It is typically a self-terminating disease without complications in immunocompetent individuals. However, consideration for *Giardia lamblia* may be indicated.

10-29. **The answer is B** (Chapter 154). Outbreaks of viral gastroenteritis are most likely due to norovirus. In addition to the consumption of contaminated food and water, noroviruses are easily transmitted person to person. Rotavirus is a major cause of diarrheal illness in infants and children. Ciguatera toxin comes from infected reef fish such as barracuda. Symptoms typically are neurologic and they include paresthesias, hypesthesias, and reversal of hot/cold sensation. Enterotoxigenic *E. coli* is the most common cause of traveler's diarrhea but is typically not associated with outbreaks on cruise ships. *Shigella* infections are often associated with fever and bloody diarrhea.

10-30. **The answer is C** (Chapter 155). RMSF is a disseminated infection with *R. rickettsii*. The presentation of RMSF may closely resemble disseminated meningococcemia and the untreated mortality rate of RMSF is 5–10%. The petechial rash of RMSF tends to begin on the wrists and ankles and spreads centrally while the converse is typical for meningococcemia. There are unfortunately no rapid tests that can aid in diagnosis in the ED. Diagnosis is by clinical suspicion and treatment should not be delayed. Any organ system can be affected. Factors suggesting RMSF may include rash (although absent in 10–15% of cases), history of tick bite, laboratory abnormalities as in this patient, or travel to areas populated by the Ixodes deer tick (most cases are in the southeastern United States, but are occasionally seen in California and Arizona). Babesiosis is transmitted by the Ixodes tick (same as Lyme disease), and is a protozoal illness that clinically resembles malaria. Brucellosis is a difficult diagnosis. The most common symptoms are fever and malaise, and it can infect any organ system. Exposure to unpasteurized milk or animals, especially cattle, or a prolonged febrile illness should heighten suspicion. Tick-borne relapsing fever is a *Borrelia* spirochete-mediated disease that typically involves an eschar at the site of the tick bite and presents as alternating febrile and afebrile episodes along with myalgia, arthralgia, abdominal pain, and malaise. Tularemia

is transmitted by the same Dermacentor tick species as RMSF. The most common form of the disease involves ulceration at the site of tick bite along with painful regional adenopathy.

10-31. **The answer is B** (Chapter 155). Erythema migrans, a well-defined macular rash, often with central clearing, is usually diagnostic of Lyme disease. It is the most common vector-borne zoonotic disease in the United States and occurs predominantly in the northeastern and north central United States, but has been reported in all continental 48 states. Lyme disease is transmitted by the *Ixodes scapularis* deer tick, which also is the vector for both babesiosis and anaplasmosis. The patient's symptoms are most likely the result of a coinfection with *Babesia* that occurred at the same time the patient was infected with Lyme disease. While anaplasmosis, which may present as an influenza-type illness, is treated by the same regimen of doxycycline, babesiosis is not. Babesiosis is often asymptomatic, but when present closely mimics malaria. It is diagnosed by a Wright or Giemsa-stained peripheral blood smear that demonstrates intraerythrocytic parasites (ring forms with a central pallor), known as the Maltese cross. Treatment is atovaquone plus azithromycin. The vector for Colorado tick fever is the wood tick, *Dermacentor andersoni*, and treatment is mainly supportive. Ehrlichiosis is transmitted by the lone star tick *Amblyomma americanum*. It typically presents as an influenza-type illness 1–2 weeks after tick bite, but in a minority of patients can progress to renal failure, respiratory failure, and encephalitis. Treatment is with doxycycline. Secondary syphilis presents with nonpruritic, rough, red or reddish brown macules on the trunk and flexor areas and often extends to the palms and soles.

10-32. **The answer is A** (Chapter 155). Lyme disease, caused by *B. burgdorferi* can infect anyone, but it has a significant bimodal expression from 5 to 9 years and 50 to 54 years of age. The second stage of Lyme disease usually occurs days to 6 months after the primary infection.

It involves fever, adenopathy, arthritis, atrioventricular nodal block, malaise, and cranial nerve palsies. The most common cranial nerve affected is the facial nerve (7th), and it can be bilateral. The rash of erythema migrans is not always present, so a careful travel history and antecedent rash is prudent with any child presenting with a peripheral facial nerve (7th) palsy. *C. psittaci* is the agent that causes psittacosis, an avian to human zoonosis that most commonly presents with fever, malaise, and pulmonary symptoms. *P. multocida* is implicated in soft tissue infections developing from cat and dog bites. *R. rickettsii* is the pathogen responsible for RMSF. *Y. pestis* causes both pneumonic and bubonic plague.

10-33. **The answer is D** (Chapter 156). Vaccination history is extremely important when discerning the cause of an illness in anyone, let alone an immigrant or returning traveler. The vaccinations for hepatitis A and B and yellow fever are very effective and nearly 100% effective if neutralizing antibodies are present. Rabies vaccination requires multiple doses and requires further management after an exposure, but, if following the guidelines, is also extremely effective. The vaccine for typhoid fever is highly recommended, as it is widely prevalent in the developing world and is easily transmitted by contamination of food with feces or urine. However, the vaccine is only 75% effective.

10-34. **The answer is D** (Chapter 156). Obtaining a detailed travel history is tantamount to deciphering disease in a returning traveler. Key aspects are destination, adherence to chemoprophylaxis, immunization history, rural or remote travel, eating uncooked meats or vegetables, freshwater exposure, and insect bites. Leptospirosis, also known as mud fever, occurs after exposure to freshwater and has been seen in adventure travelers and triathletes. Patients abruptly develop high fever, myalgias, hepatitis, and often a subconjunctival injection. This can progress to meningitis, renal failure, and respiratory failure. Amebiasis is a protozoal disease transmitted by the fecal-oral route. Complications include

dysentery and invasive extraintestinal disease, most commonly amebic liver abscess. Chagas disease is transmitted through the bite of the reduviid bug. After biting, it deposits its feces nearby, and the victim autoinoculates after rubbing the wound. Cysticercosis is a widespread global disease that is transmitted through undercooked pork. It can infest almost any tissue and is the leading cause of adult-onset seizures worldwide. In schistosomiasis, a freshwater fluke penetrates intact skin and begins a complex life cycle that can lead to both localized and systemic disease.

10-35. **The answer is A** (Chapter 156). Varicella, or chickenpox, is a very common illness of childhood (although rates are decreasing with vaccine utilization), and is highly contagious. It is spread through respiratory secretions and disease control is actually through airborne precautions, as the virus is able to remain suspended in air and can be dispersed over a long distance. This requires placing the patient in a monitored negative air pressure room with at least 6 air changes per hour with air discharged outdoors or through a filtration system. Other diseases that mandate airborne precautions include measles and tuberculosis. Droplet precautions are for diseases also spread through the respiratory route, but spread is usually limited to direct contact with nasal or respiratory secretions. This requires personnel to use special fit masks when within 3 feet of the patient when exposed to secretions. A simple mask may be placed on the patient during transport to decrease droplet spread. Notable diseases spread by droplets include respiratory viruses, such as novel H1N1, *H. influenzae*, *Neisseria*, and *Streptococcus*. Universal precautions, also known as standard precautions, include hand washing after patient care, use of gloves, masks and/or gowns when handling fluids or exposed to secretions, and proper disposal of contaminated equipment.

10-36. **The answer is D** (Chapter 157). Management for possible hepatitis B after bodily fluid exposure is guided by the hepatitis B status of the source and the response to vaccination in the person exposed. Documentation of antibody to hepatitis B surface antigen (anti-HBs) >10 mIU/mL demonstrates a proper response to the vaccine and signifies immunity. No intervention is necessary if exposed. However, if the exposed is unvaccinated or the response to vaccine unknown, then testing begins with the source. Ability to transmit hepatitis B is demonstrated by the presence of hepatitis B surface antigen (HBsAg). Exposure to an HBsAg positive source without proper vaccination requires both HBIG and the primary vaccination series. Exposure without proper response to the vaccine requires HBIG and vaccination booster or a second dose of HBIG in follow-up. Treatment should be within the first 24 hours.

10-37. **The answer is A** (Chapter 158). An awareness of drug–drug interactions is critical to limiting iatrogenic injury. Antibiotics are among the most common medications prescribed by emergency physicians, and so knowledge of the potential complications is prudent. Ciprofloxacin, a commonly used fluoroquinolone for urinary tract infections, is typically a well-tolerated medication, but it has many interactions to consider. Ciprofloxacin is a known inhibitor of cytochrome P450 and can enhance the activity of many other medications. This list includes some that have a narrow therapeutic index, such as warfarin and theophylline. The interaction with warfarin is not consistent or predictable. Doses do not need to be initially adjusted, but the prothrombin time should be followed closely. Fluoroquinolones also can cause QT prolongation that is usually clinically insignificant. However, patients with prolonged QT, or who also take amiodarone, procainamide, sotalol, or another drug that may prolong the QT interval, have a small but increased risk of torsades de pointes when also taking a fluoroquinolone. There have been case reports detailing prolonged hypoglycemia due to concomitant use of a fluoroquinolone while taking an oral sulfonylurea, such as glyburide. Absorption of fluoroquinolones, as well as the tetracyclines, is inhibited by coingestion of divalent cations. Patients should avoid taking iron, calcium, or antacids at the same time as fluoroquinolones. Furosemide has an increased rate of ototoxicity when taken along with aminoglycosides.

10-38. **The answer is E** (Chapter 153). Quinidine is a class 1A antiarrhythmic. Cardiac sodium channel blockade can lead to prolonged QT syndrome, and all patients receiving quinidine intravenously must be on cardiac monitor. Quinidine and especially quinine cause a hyperinsulinemia that can cause profound hypoglycemia, in addition to that caused by *P. falciparum* itself. Primaquine causes massive hemolysis in patients with glucose-6 phosphate deficiency. Both chloroquine and primaquine can cause methemoglobinemia. Artemesin-derived antimalarial agents are relatively safe and more effective but are currently only available as artesunate through Centers for Disease Control supplies only.

10-39. **The answer is D** (Chapter 149). Antiretroviral therapy is indicated after an AIDS-defining illness, CD4 count under 350, pregnancy, HIV-associated nephropathy, and hepatitis B virus coinfection requiring treatment. Acute retroviral syndrome occurs outside the window for PEP and requires further workup prior to initiating antiretroviral therapy. While shigellosis and tertiary syphilis may occur more frequently in patients with HIV, they are not AIDS-defining illnesses.

10-40. **The answer is C** (Chapter 154). Cryptosporidium rarely causes serious disease in normal hosts, but may cause protracted disease in AIDS and often warrants hospitalization due to dehydration and malabsorption. Nitazoxanide and azithromycin are effective against cryptosporidium, but neither affects a cure with a CD4 count below 100. The most effective therapy is highly active antiretroviral therapy, and symptoms generally subside when the CD4 count is above 100. Ciprofloxacin is effective therapy for most typical bacterial pathogens. Metronidazole is active against *Giardia*, *Entamoeba*, and *Clostridium difficile*.

10-41. **The answer is B** (Chapter 148). Gingivostomatitis and pharyngitis are the typical primary manifestations of HSV type 1. Although HSV-2 can cause similar disease, HSV-1 is much more likely to cause oral lesions. Reactivation of HSV-1 from the trigeminal ganglion typically presents as orolabial lesions. HSV-2 is believed to reside in the sacral ganglion and represents as genital lesions. EBV causes infectious mononucleosis.

10-42. **The answer is C** (Chapter 146). Early goal directed therapy in severe sepsis is guided by an algorithmic approach (Figure 10–9). After initial supplemental oxygen or intubation, fluid resuscitation, and broad-spectrum antibiotics, patients must be repeatedly reassessed for response to therapy. Target values include a mean arterial pressure >65 mm Hg, central venous pressure of 8 mm Hg, venous oxygen saturation of 70%, and urine output >0.5 mL/kg/hr. This patient demonstrates persistent hypoperfusion after initial fluid resuscitation with a mean arterial pressure of 52 mm Hg (mean arterial pressure is approximated by diastolic plus one-third of the pulse pressure). Although many patients have large fluid deficits, a central venous pressure of 11 mm Hg suggests adequate resuscitation. The next step in management is inotropic support, and norepinephrine or dopamine is the typical agent of choice for initial management. Dobutamine may be used in select settings with invasive monitoring, but typically not until after dopamine administration. The patient should be transfused until the hematocrit is greater than 30%, but would not be indiscriminately transfused unless anemia and severe blood loss were obvious.

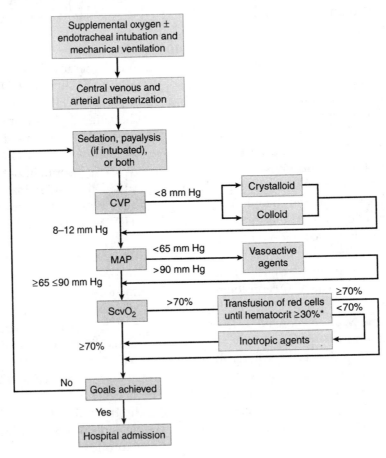

Figure 10-9.

CHAPTER 11

Musculoskeletal Disorders
Questions

11-1. A 27-year-old female without significant past medical history arrives in the emergency department complaining of neck pain. She reports being a seatbelted passenger in a parked car that was struck from behind at a low rate of speed about 12 hours prior to arrival. The patient felt fine at the time of the accident, but has now developed neck pain and stiffness. She denies any focal numbness or weakness, and denies any other injuries. A physical exam reveals tender paracervical muscles, but does not reveal any midline tenderness to palpation, and her neurologic examination is normal. The patient does report pain on the contralateral side of the neck when turning her head from side to side and a decreased range of motion secondary to pain. What is the MOST appropriate next diagnostic or therapeutic intervention?

(A) Place the patient in a cervical collar and obtain plain radiographs of the cervical spine.

(B) Place the patient in a semirigid collar and advise follow-up with her primary care physician in 2 weeks.

(C) Place the patient in a cervical collar and backboard, and obtain plain radiographs of the cervical, thoracic, and lumbar spine.

(D) Place the patient in a cervical collar and obtain an MRI scan to assess for ligamentous injury.

(E) Prescribe analgesics and muscle relaxants, and advise the patient to maintain motion as usual and avoid activities that produce pain.

11-2. Which of the following patients with back pain is LEAST likely to be at risk for serious disease?

(A) 26-year-old male ejected from his motorcycle at highway speeds reporting acute lumbar pain.

(B) 30-year-old male with a history of injection drug use reporting fever and saddle anesthesia.

(C) 45-year-old male with nonradiating lumbar pain after lifting a couch.

(D) 65-year-old female with history of breast cancer reporting midthoracic pain for several weeks that is worse at night.

(E) 73-year-old male with history of smoking, hypercholesterolemia, and coronary artery disease with complaint of sudden onset of severe back pain.

11-3. A 52-year-old male without significant past medical history reports mild lumbar pain and sharp shooting pain extending below his left knee for the last 2 weeks. He also reports some tingling along the lateral aspect of his left thigh. He does not remember any specific etiology for his symptoms, but does report lifting heavy objects at work. Physical examination reveals a positive straight leg raise test, and paresthesias along his left lateral thigh, but no weakness. The presence of which of the following history or physical exam findings would indicate that an emergent MRI is the appropriate next step?

(A) A positive crossed straight leg test.

(B) All patients with back pain and sensory symptoms should receive an emergent MRI.

(C) No relief of symptoms with nonsteroidal anti-inflammatory drugs (NSAIDs).

(D) Pain in the gluteal area with performance of the straight leg raise test.

(E) Poor tone on rectal exam.

11-4. What is the MOST common finding in cauda equina syndrome?

(A) Abnormal results on straight leg raising

(B) Gait difficulty

(C) Sensory deficit over the buttocks, posterosuperior thighs, and perineal region

(D) Urinary retention with or without overflow incontinence

(E) Weakness or stiffness in the lower extremities

11-5. A 36-year-old male presents to the emergency department reporting aching in his right shoulder for 6 weeks. The patient works as a house painter, and denies any known trauma. He reports this pain occurs at night and is causing him insomnia. He also reports that holding a paintbrush over his head causes an exacerbation of his symptoms. He denies any numbness, but does endorse some shoulder stiffness with the pain. On physical exam, the patient has both active and passive full range of motion, and moderate pain with rotator cuff strength testing. He is noted to have tenderness over the rotator cuff insertion at the lateral aspect of the proximal humerus. Which of the following therapeutic actions is NOT recommended for treatment of this condition?

(A) Cryotherapy for 15 minutes three to four times per day

(B) Gentle range of motion exercises

(C) Medication to reduce pain and inflammation

(D) Minimize overhead activities and avoid aggravating activities

(E) Shoulder immobilization until orthopedic follow-up in 2 weeks

11-6. What is the MOST common source of pain referred to the shoulder?

(A) Brachial plexus injury

(B) Cervical spine

(C) Diaphragmatic irritation from intra-abdominal bleeding or hollow viscous perforation

(D) Myocardial infarction

(E) Thoracic outlet syndrome

11-7. A patient abducts his arm to 90° and forward flexes it to 30° with the thumb pointed down. Pain or weakness against resistance (continued abduction) in this position suggests injury to what structure in the shoulder?

(A) Biceps tendon

(B) Coracoacromial ligament

(C) Deltoid muscle

(D) Humeral head

(E) Supraspinatus tendon

11-8. A 55-year-old female with insulin-dependent diabetes arrives in the emergency department complaining of right knee pain. The patient reports she underwent an uncomplicated right knee osteotomy approximately 3 months ago secondary to severe arthritis. She denies recent trauma, but does report that she has had elevated blood glucose levels for the past week. On exam, the patient is found to have a diffusely tender knee with decreased range of motion secondary to pain. Which of the following diagnostic modalities available in the emergency department is preferred to confirm your suspicion that the patient has developed osteomyelitis?

(A) Bone biopsy
(B) Bone density scan
(C) Plain radiographs of the hip and knee
(D) MRI of the knee
(E) Ultrasound of the knee

11-9. A 32-year-old male with a history of active participation in long distance running for several years reports a 1-month history of right anterior knee pain. He reports the pain was gradual in onset and nonradiating. He reports he is sure he has a torn meniscus, although does not remember any particular traumatic incident. Which of the following history or physical exam findings would suggest that patellofemoral syndrome is the cause of his symptoms rather than a meniscal or ligamentous injury?

(A) Knee gives out or buckles intermittently
(B) Pain on palpation of the joint line
(C) Popping sensation or sound at the onset of pain
(D) Recurrent effusion after activity
(E) Relief of pain when lifting the patella away from the knee joint while passively bending and straightening the knee

11-10. Which of the following systemic rheumatologic diseases is the MOST likely to require an intensive care unit (ICU) admission?

(A) Polymyositis/dermatomyositis
(B) Rheumatoid arthritis
(C) Systemic lupus erythematosus
(D) Systemic sclerosis (scleroderma)
(E) Wegener granulomatosis

11-11. Patients with which of the following systemic rheumatic diseases have the highest relative risk of atherosclerosis?

(A) Ankylosing spondylitis
(B) Antiphospholipid syndrome
(C) Psoriatic arthritis
(D) Rheumatoid arthritis
(E) Systemic lupus erythematosus

11-12. An 8-year-old previously healthy male presents to the emergency department complaining of rash on the lower extremities and buttock, bilateral knee pain with mild lower extremity edema, intermittent colicky abdominal pain, and vomiting. The patient's parents report he had a viral upper respiratory infection 10 days before the current symptoms began. On exam, the patient is noted to have palpable purpura and bilateral knee arthralgias. His laboratory exam is notable only for a moderate thrombocytosis and leukocytosis. Which of the following is NOT a serious complication associated with this disease (Figure 11-1)?

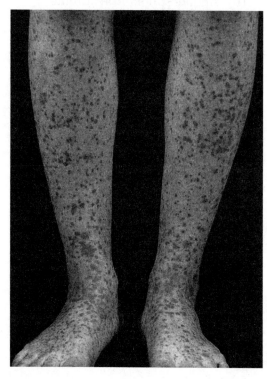

Figure 11-1. Reproduced with permission from Wolff K, Johnson RA: *Fitzpatrick's Color Atlas & Synopsis of Clinical Dermatology*, 6th Edition. Copyright © 2009 The McGraw-Hill Companies, Inc.

(A) Acute pericarditis

(B) Intussusception

(C) Orchitis

(D) Pulmonary alveolar hemorrhage

(E) Rapidly progressive glomerulonephropathy

11-13. A 26-year-old male presents to the emergency department with left ring finger pain and swelling for 36 hours. The patient reports he was at work on a construction site 2 days ago and punctured his ring finger with a staple gun, but removed the staple immediately. He reports subsequent swelling and pain in the left ring finger. The patient's hand appears in this picture. Which of the following physical exam findings is NOT considered one of the cardinal signs of flexor tenosynovitis (Figure 11-2)?

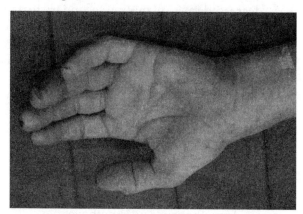

Figure 11-2. Reproduced with permission from Brunicardi FC, Anderson DK, Billiar TR, Dunn DL, Hunter JG, Matthews JB, Pollock RE: *Schwartz's Principles of Surgery*, 9th Edition. Copyright © 2010 The McGraw-Hill Companies, Inc.

(A) Flexed posture of the involved digit at rest to minimize pain

(B) Identification of a puncture wound over the flexor surface of the finger

(C) Intense pain with passive extension

(D) Symmetric finger swelling along the length of the tendon sheath

(E) Tenderness over the entire length of the flexor tendon sheath

11-14. What are the MOST common organisms responsible for superficial cellulitis of the hand?

(A) *Eikenella corrodens* and *Pasteurella multocida*

(B) *Fusobacterium nucleatum* and *Prevotella melaninogenica*

(C) *Staphylococcus aureus* (predominantly methicillin resistant) and *Streptococcus pyogenes*

(D) *Streptococcus anginosus* and *S. aureus* (predominantly methicillin resistant)

(E) *S. pyogenes* and *Mycobacterium*

11-15. A 37-year-old female presents to the emergency department reporting burning and itching on the lateral distal surface of her right index finger. The patient works as a dental hygienist, and noticed the development of erythema and bullous vesicles in the area 24 hours ago. The patient denies any history of trauma or difficulty with range of motion. On exam, the area is tender and erythematous with slight induration, but does not appear to be tense or fluctuant. Bullous vesicles are present. The finger is immobilized and elevated, and the patient is given pain medication. What is the MOST appropriate treatment for this infection?

(A) Acyclovir 400 mg three times daily for 10 days

(B) Amoxicillin–clavulanate 875/125 mg twice daily for 5 days

(C) Incision and drainage of the affected area followed by trimethoprim/sulfamethoxazole (TMP/SMX) double strength 1–2 tabs twice per day for 7–10 days

(D) Trimethoprim/sulfamethoxazole (TMP/SMX) double strength 1–2 tabs twice per day for 7–10 days

(E) Trimethoprim/sulfamethoxazole (TMP/SMX) double strength 1–2 tabs twice per day for 7–10 days plus cephalexin 500 mg for 7–10 days

11-16. A 22-year-old unmarried male reports a recent history of joint pain involving his ankles, knees, and left elbow over the past 4 days. He now reports the development of severe pain and swelling only in the right knee over the last 5 hours. He denies any recent trauma or significant past medical history, but does report having multiple sexual partners. On exam, the affected knee has a moderate effusion, is erythematous, and warm to the touch. The patient is very resistant to active or passive movement of the knee secondary to pain. The patient undergoes arthrocentesis and the joint fluid is remarkable for 35,000 white blood cells (WBC/mL), 92% polymorphonuclear leukocytes (PMNs), and no

crystals. What is the MOST likely etiology of the patient's symptoms?

(A) Gonococcal septic arthritis

(B) Gout

(C) Lyme disease

(D) Rheumatic fever

(E) Systemic lupus erythematosus

11-17. A 50-year-old male presents to the emergency department reporting left knee pain that developed over the last 6 hours. He denies any acute injury to the knee and states that he has had similar symptoms in the past, but has not previously sought treatment. The patient reports a history of hypertension and mild renal insufficiency, and has had a change in his medications in the last 10 days. On exam, the knee is hot, swollen, and tender to the touch. The patient can range the joint, but movement is limited secondary to pain. Arthrocentesis is performed and reveals the presence of uric acid crystals, and no organisms on Gram stain. Which of the following medications is the MOST appropriate for treating this patient's condition?

(A) Ceftriaxone plus vancomycin

(B) Colchicine

(C) Imipenem

(D) Indomethacin

(E) Oxycodone

11-18. A 47-year-old male reports knee pain and swelling for 3 days. The joint appears to have a large effusion, and the decision is made to perform arthrocentesis in the emergency department. Which of the following is NOT a contraindication or relative contraindication to joint aspiration?

(A) Aspiration before factor replacement in patients with hemophilia

(B) Cellulitis or impetigo on the skin overlying the joint

(C) Coagulopathy

(D) Presence of a prosthetic joint

(E) Trauma associated effusion

11-19. Which of the following is NOT a cause of onychocryptosis?

(A) Bony deformities

(B) Improper nail trimming

(C) Recurrent calluses

(D) Tight footwear

(E) Using sharp tools to clean the nail gutters

11-20. A 38-year-old female mail carrier reports 3 weeks of heel pain on the plantar surface of her right foot. She denies trauma, but does report that she has taken over a larger delivery route in the last 2 months and has nearly doubled the amount of walking she does. She reports the pain is worse after getting up in the morning and after her daily walking route. Physical exam is notable for point tenderness at the anterior medical aspect of the calcaneus, and the pain and tenderness increase when the toes are dorsiflexed. Which of the following short-term treatment options should NOT be undertaken in the emergency department?

(A) Advise the patient that rest and ice will improve her symptoms.

(B) Advise the patient to obtain heel and arch support shoe inserts.

(C) Give the patient a corticosteroid injection.

(D) Prescribe a short course of NSAIDs.

(E) Teach the patient plantar and Achilles tendon stretching exercise.

11-21. A 63-year-old female presents to the emergency department reporting a deep and achy left-sided neck pain for a few days; patient reports she now has sharp burning pain in her posterior upper arm, dorsal forearm, and middle finger. Today the patient noticed that her arm feels weaker and became concerned. She denies any known trauma, chest pain, or other focal neurologic symptoms. On physical exam, she is found to have a decreased triceps reflex in the left arm and decreased sensation to light touch on her distal dorsal forearm. The patient also reports her symptoms increase when her neck is extended, and decrease when her neck is flexed. The patient undergoes an MRI exam in the emergency department and is found to have a herniated cervical disk. What cervical root is responsible for causing this patient's symptoms?

(A) C2

(B) C5

(C) C6

(D) C7

(E) C8

11-22. A 59-year-old female reports 3 months of lumbar pain that awakens her from sleep and has been unrelenting despite using NSAID and narcotic analgesics left over from her recent surgery. She had a lumbar fusion requiring the placement of several plates and screws about 4 months ago, and had an uncomplicated recovery. She denies fever, but does report some intermittent diaphoresis associated with exacerbations of her pain at night. On physical exam, the patient has a well-healed surgical scar without any erythema, but has significant point tenderness over her vertebral bodies in that area. Her neurologic exam is normal. Which of the following is TRUE regarding the diagnosis and treatment of vertebral osteomyelitis?

(A) Administering antibiotics before obtaining a bone biopsy may result in negative culture results from the biopsy.

(B) An erythrocyte sedimentation rate is only elevated about 50% of the time.

(C) Blood cultures are rarely positive in vertebral osteomyelitis.

(D) Plain radiographs will be normal, so all patients suspected to have vertebral osteomyelitis will require an MRI for diagnosis.

(E) The classic triad of vertebral osteomyelitis is fever, severe back pain, and neurological deficits.

Musculoskeletal Disorders
Answers and Explanations

11-1. **The answer is E** (Chapter 276). Whiplash injury results from sudden acceleration–deceleration trauma, and patients typically complain of neck pain and stiffness that is often delayed for a number of hours after the injury occurs. The NEXUS criteria can be followed to determine if these patients require cervical spine imaging. In patients with a normal neurologic exam and no midline tenderness to palpation, no cervical imaging is required. Patients with simple neck pain without radiculopathy or myelopathy do not require immobilization and may be treated conservatively with analgesics and muscle relaxants. These patients should be advised to maintain motion as tolerated and encouraged to follow up with their primary care physician to determine the need for physical or manual therapies.

11-2. **The answer is C** (Chapter 276). Risk factors for serious disease in both neck and back pain are similar (see Table 276-1). Concerns for serious diseases include tumor, infection, epidural compression, fracture, congenital anomaly (in pediatric patients), nerve root impingement or disk herniation, and intra-abdominal processes such as pancreatitis and abdominal aortic aneurysm. The patients in all of the answer choices except C have historical features or symptoms that are concerning for serious illness including trauma, injection drug use, focal neurologic complaints, a history of cancer, pain that is worse at night, and pain indicative of a possible intra-abdominal process such as an abdominal aortic aneurysm. The patient described in answer choice C does not have any of these risk factors and is unlikely to be at risk for serious illness.

11-3. **The answer is E** (Chapter 276). This patient has sciatica, which is present in 95% of patients with a symptomatic herniated disk. More than 95% of disk herniations occur at L4-L5 or L5-S1, causing radicular pain that extends below the knee in the dermatomal distribution of the nerve root. A positive straight leg raise test should generate radicular symptoms in the affected leg that radiate below the knee. A straight leg raise test that produces back pain, gluteal pain, or hamstring pain when the leg is raised is not a positive test. A positive crossed straight leg raise test elicits radicular symptoms in the affected leg when the asymptomatic leg is lifted. The treatment of patients with a herniated disk is similar to that of patients with nonspecific back pain; however, NSAIDs are less effective in treating the radicular symptoms of sciatica than they are in treating nonspecific back pain. Sciatica can also be caused by anything that compresses or impinges on spinal nerve roots, cauda equina, or the spinal cord. If the patient has no risk factors in the history and physical exam for serious disease, there is no indication for performing emergent imaging in the emergency department. It is recommended that patients with severe or rapidly progressive neurologic deficits (in this case, decreased rectal tone on exam) receive emergent imaging (MRI preferred).

11-4. **The answer is D** (Chapter 276). The most common finding in cauda equina syndrome is urinary retention with or without overflow incontinence. This finding is 90% sensitive and about 95% specific. Abnormal results on straight leg raising, gait difficulty, saddle anesthesia, and weakness or stiffness in the lower extremities are other common findings in cauda equina syndrome. A decrease in rectal tone occurs in 60–80% of cases.

11-5. **The answer is E** (Chapter 277). This patient has impingement syndrome, and the goal of treatment is to reduce pain and inflammation, and prevent progression of the process. The patient may be offered a sling for brief periods of support, but complete immobilization should be avoided to minimize loss of motion. Patients should be encouraged to engage in gentle range of motion exercises, use medication to reduce pain and inflammation, apply ice to provide analgesia and decrease inflammation, and avoid overhead motion or aggravating activities. Patients may also benefit from strengthening and stretching exercises performed under the supervision of a physical therapist, and local corticosteroid injections (should be performed by orthopedist or primary care physician). Patients should follow up with an orthopedist or their primary care physician within 1–2 weeks.

11-6. **The answer is B** (Chapter 277). Shoulder pain is usually caused by problems local to the shoulder joint, but is a site of referred pain for some serious conditions such as myocardial infarction and diaphragmatic irritation from intra-abdominal bleeding or hollow viscous perforation. Other extrinsic causes of shoulder pain include brachial plexus injuries, axillary artery thrombosis, suprascapular nerve injury, thoracic outlet syndrome, Pancoast tumor, and other thoracoabdominal disorders. The most common source of referred pain is from the neck. Degenerative disease of the cervical spine, degenerative disk disease, and a herniated cervical disk may present with shoulder pain.

11-7. **The answer is E** (Chapter 277). The supraspinatus muscle originates on the posterior and superior aspect of the scapula, passes beneath the acromion, and inserts on the

great tuberosity of the humeral head. It initiates arm elevation and abducts the shoulder. Abducting the patient's arm to 90 degrees and forward flexing it to 30 degrees with the patient's thumb pointing down isolates the supraspinatus muscle. This manuever is used to test its strength. Pain or weakness against resistance to continued abduction in the position demonstrated suggests injury to the supraspinatus ranging from impingement syndrome to a rotator cuff tear. The supraspinatus is the most commonly injured tendon of the rotator cuff.

11-8. **The answer is D** (Chapter 278). MRI is the preferred imaging modality for patients in whom the diagnosis of osteomyelitis is a concern, with approximately 95% sensitivity. Plain radiographs are normal early in the course, but later will show bone demineralization, periosteal elevation, and late lytic lesions. Bone density scanning is used for the detection of osteoporosis and is not a modality used for diagnosis in the emergency department setting. A bone biopsy performed by an orthopedic surgeon will be required to confirm the diagnosis, along with debridement of infected/dead bone.

11-9. **The answer is E** (Chapter 278). Patellofemoral syndrome or Runner's knee is a major cause of anterior knee pain and is typically caused by overuse, abnormal patellar tracking as it moves in the patellar groove (more common in females), or focal trauma. The pain associated with this syndrome is gradual in onset, nonradiating, and usually unilateral. Treatment is conservative with NSAIDs, rest, heat, and an emphasis on strengthening and physical therapy. Meniscal injuries are suggested by the presence of pain on palpation of the joint line, a popping sensation after activity, and a recurrent effusion after activity. A sensation of the knee buckling or giving out is generally due to pain and may represent patellar subluxation, ligamentous injury, or joint instability.

11-10. **The answer is B** (Chapter 279). Rheumatoid arthritis is the most common rheumatic disease requiring ICU admission. Infection is the leading cause for the ICU admission, followed by rheumatic disease flare. Rheumatoid arthritis is a chronic, systemic inflammatory disorder with symmetrical and potentially destructive arthritis. Complications seen in rheumatoid arthritis include airway obstruction, obliterative bronchiolitis, acute respiratory failure, acute coronary syndrome, heart failure, thoracic aortic dissection, arrhythmias and conduction disturbances, subluxation of the atlantoaxial joints, bowel ischemia and perforation, septic arthritis, and scleritis. The other systemic diseases listed in the answer choices may also cause a variety of extra-articular manifestations that can result in serious morbidity and mortality, but do not as commonly require ICU admission as complications associated with rheumatoid arthritis.

11-11. **The answer is E** (Chapter 279). Based on epidemiological, clinical, laboratory, and experimental data, several systemic rheumatic diseases promote accelerated coronary atherosclerosis. The relative risks for atherosclerosis vary from 1.6 in ankylosing spondylitis and psoriatic arthritis to 6.0 in systemic lupus erythematosus. Coronary atherosclerosis is a major cause of cardiac mortality in young patients with systemic lupus erythematosus, and the risk of acute myocardial infarction in premenopausal women is increased up to 50-fold compared with women without lupus. Patients with rheumatoid arthritis have a higher risk than nonaffected patients of unrecognized acute myocardial infarction and sudden death, and are less likely to undergo invasive evaluation and treatment.

11-12. **The answer is A** (Chapter 279). This patient has Henoch–Schonlein purpura, a systemic vasculitis associated with IgA deposition that generally occurs in children. It is characterized by palpable purpura, arthritis/arthralgias, interstitial lung disease, abdominal pain, and renal impairment (more likely in adults). Serious complications associated with this usually self-limited dis-

ease include respiratory failure and alveolar hemorrhage, seizures, intracranial bleeding, gastrointestinal hemorrhage, bowel ischemia or perforation, acute pancreatitis, intussusception, rapidly progressive glomerulonephropathy, and orchitis. Henoch–Schonlein purpura is not associated with cardiovascular complications seen in other systemic rheumatologic diseases.

11-13. **The answer is B** (Chapter 280). Flexor tenosynovitis is a surgical emergency and failure to diagnose and treat flexor tenosynovitis will lead to loss of function of the digit. The diagnosis is clinical, and is made by recognizing the four classical findings described by Kanavel. These include tenderness over the entire length of the flexor tendon sheath, symmetric finger swelling along the length of the tendon sheath, intense pain with passive extension, and a flexed posture of the involved digit at rest to minimize pain. The underlying infection is usually associated with penetrating trauma of the affected area, but the patient may be unaware of injury. Treatment with parenteral antibiotics should be started immediately because infection can spread rapidly through deep fascial planes. The hand should be immobilized and elevated and a hand surgeon should be consulted in the emergency department.

11-14. **The answer is C** (Chapter 280). The most common organisms associated with superficial cellulitis of the hand are *S. aureus* (predominantly methicillin resistant) and *S. pyogenes*. In most US cities, community-associated methicillin-resistant *S. aureus* (MRSA) is the most common organism cultured from all skin and soft tissue infections in emergency departments, including 43–73% of hand infections. Therefore, in cases where the presence of MRSA cannot be identified or ruled out clinically, consider treating cellulitis with two antibiotics, a beta-lactam antibiotic and a MRSA-specific antibiotic. Human bites are typically polymicrobial and common pathogens include *S. anginosus* (52%), *F. nucleatum* (32%), *E. corrodens* (30%), and *P. melaninogenica* (22%). Cat and dog bites may harbor *P. multocida* and patients with diabetes or acquired immunodeficiency syndrome may harbor atypical infections caused by *Mycobacterium* or *Candida albicans*.

11-15. **The answer is A** (Chapter 280). Antiviral agents such as acyclovir may shorten the duration of a herpetic whitlow infection. This infection is usually self-limited, although recurrent infections are common. Health care professionals are at high risk for this infection and care should be taken to wear gloves whenever contact with saliva is possible. If there is any doubt concerning the diagnosis of herpetic whitlow, a vesicle may be unroofed and the drainage fluid may be used for a Tzanck smear to confirm the diagnosis. Antibiotics are not effective in the treatment of viral infections, and incision and drainage of a herpetic whitlow may result in a secondary bacterial infection and a prolonged failure to heal.

11-16. **The answer is A** (Chapter 281). Gonococcal arthritis is the most common cause of septic arthritis in adolescents and young adults. There is usually a prodromal period in which migratory arthritis and tenosynovitis occur before pain and swelling settles on one septic joint. Synovial fluid analysis of septic joints will reveal a markedly elevated (>25,000) white blood cell count (WBC/μL) and >90% PMNs, as well as the absence of crystals. Gout, Lyme disease, systemic lupus erythematosus, and rheumatic fever will all demonstrate a lower percentage of PMNs (see Table 281-4).

11-17. **The answer is E** (Chapter 281). Gout is the most common form of inflammatory joint disease in men older than age 40, and an acute attack often follows trauma, surgery, a significant illness, or a change in medication. The finding of uric acid crystals in synovial fluid establishes the diagnosis of gout, and although a concordant septic joint is rare, it may occur. The absence of bacteria on Gram stain can help clarify the diagnosis. Antibiotics are not indicated in the treatment of inflammatory arthritis in the absence of bacterial infection. Traditionally, gout or pseudogout is treated with NSAIDs; however, this patient has a history of renal insufficiency and should not receive NSAIDs. Colchicine is an alternative agent used to treat crystal-induced synovitis, but is only appropriate for patients with normal renal and hepatic function. The most appropriate medication for this patient with renal insufficiency is a narcotic analgesic for pain relief. Once acute symptoms have resolved, long-term control may be achieved with reduction or elimination of gout-inducing agents (diuretics, aspirin, or cyclosporine).

11-18. **The answer is E** (Chapter 281). The skin overlying joints should be free of cellulitis or impetigo in order to avoid contamination of the joint space during arthrocentesis. Other relative contraindications to joint aspiration are coagulopathy, hemarthrosis in hemophiliac patients before factor replacement, and the presence of a prosthetic joint. However, if the concern for septic arthritis is very high, arthrocentesis may be performed in these settings. A history of trauma is not a contraindication to arthrocentesis, and aspiration of very large traumatic effusions will provide pain relief and increase range of motion.

11-19. **The answer is C** (Chapter 282). Normal nail function requires a small space between the nail and the lateral nail folds. An ingrown toenail occurs when irritation of the tissue surrounding the nail causes overgrowth obliterating that space. Causes of ingrown toenails include improper nail trimming, using sharp tools to clean the nail gutters, tight footwear, rotated digits, and bony deformities. Onychocryptosis (ingrown toenail) is characterized by inflammation, swelling, or infection of the medial or lateral aspect of the toenail, and the great toe is the most commonly affected. Calluses are caused by pressure or irritation that results in focal hyperkeratotic lesions of the skin of the foot, and are protective. They should not be treated if they are not painful, and they are not a cause of ingrown toenails.

11-20. **The answer is C** (Chapter 282). Plantar fasciitis is the most common cause of heel pain and is usually a result of overuse. The symptom of plantar fasciitis is pain on the plantar surface of the foot, and is worse after waking up and after physical activity. Plantar fasciitis is generally a self-limited disease and 80% of cases resolve spontaneously within 12 months. Short-term treatment consists of rest, ice, NSAIDs, heel and arch support shoe inserts, taping or strapping of the foot, and dorsiflexion night splints. Plantar and Achilles tendon stretching exercises are also helpful. Corticosteroid injections can also provide short-term benefit, but are associated with plantar fascia rupture and should not be performed in the emergency department. Patients should be referred to a podiatrist, orthopedist, or primary care physician for follow-up care.

11-21. **The answer is D** (Chapter 276). The levels most commonly involved in cervical disk herniation are C5-C6 (C6 root) and C6-C7 (C7 root). C6 root compression accounts for 20% of cases, and C7 root compression accounts for 70% of disk herniation. The symptoms of an acute cervical disk prolapse include neck pain, pain referred to the shoulder and along the medial scapular border, and dermatome and dysesthesia in the spinal root distribution to the shoulder and arm. Motor signs include fasciculation, atrophy and weakness in the dermatome distribution of the spinal root, and loss of deep tendon reflexes. Cervical compression of the C7 root causes pain in the neck, posterior arm, dorsum of the proximal forearm, chest, medial third of the scapula, and middle finger. It also causes sensory abnormalities in the middle finger or forearm, motor weakness in the triceps and pronator teres, and reduced triceps reflex. Cervical compression of C2, C5, C6,

or C8 will cause pain, sensory abnormalities, motor weakness, and altered deep tendon reflexes along different distributions (see Table 276-3).

11-22. **The answer is A** (Chapter 276). Risk factors for vertebral osteomyelitis include immunocompromised states, recent invasive procedures, spinal implants and devices, injection drug use, and skin abscesses. On physical exam, about half of the patients with vertebral osteomyelitis will have a fever and vertebral body tenderness to percussion. The white blood cell count may be normal, but the erythrocyte sedimentation rate is almost universally elevated. Blood cultures are positive in approximately 40% of patients with vertebral osteomyelitis. Most patients with vertebral osteomyelitis have prolonged symptoms, and many have had pain for more than 3 months. In osteomyelitis, plain radiographs are normal until bone demineralizes, which can take from 2 to 8 weeks. Given the prolonged length of most patients' symptoms, plain radiographs can demonstrate abnormalities consistent with vertebral osteomyelitis. The most common radiographic abnormalities are bony destruction, irregularity of vertebral end plates, and disk space narrowing. The treatment for vertebral osteomyelitis is primarily medical with a 6-week course of intravenous antibiotics followed by a 4–8-week course of oral antibiotics. Before starting antibiotics in the emergency department, a spine surgeon should be consulted because antibiotics may result in negative culture results from a bone biopsy. The triad of fever, severe back pain, and neurologic deficits is associated with spinal epidural abscess, not vertebral osteomyelitis, although this classic triad is only present in 13% of patients.

CHAPTER 12

Nervous System Disorders
Questions

12-1. An 80-year-old woman with a history of atrial fibrillation presents with sudden-onset headache, vomiting, and somnolence. She takes warfarin. Her blood pressure is 160/90. She is sleepy but easily arousable and answers questions appropriately. She has moderate left-sided weakness and numbness and ignores the nurse standing to her left. Head CT shows a right intracerebral hemorrhage. The INR is 1.9. Which of the following actions is most likely to reduce this patient's mortality?

(A) Administering aspirin
(B) Administering fresh frozen plasma and vitamin K
(C) Intubation for airway protection
(D) Lowering the blood pressure
(E) Therapeutic hypothermia

12-2. A 35-year-old man complains of progressive facial numbness, ear pain, and dizziness for the past 2 days. The salient neurologic findings are shown in Figure 12-1. The rest of the neurologic exam, including facial sensation, is normal. Hearing is diminished on the left, and vertigo is induced when the patient turns his head quickly to the left. Grouped vesicles on an erythematous base are seen on the left anterior tongue and in the left external auditory canal. What is the diagnosis?

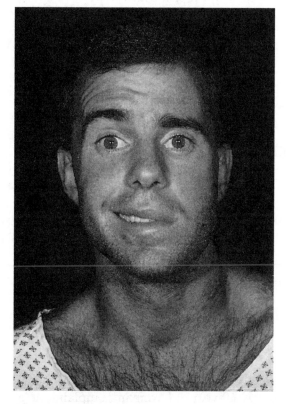

Figure 12-1. Reproduced with permission from Knoop KJ, Stack LB, Storrow AB, Thurman RJ: *The Atlas of Emergency Medicine*, 3rd Edition. Copyright © 2010 The McGraw-Hill Companies, Inc. Photo contributor: Frank Birinyi, MD.

(A) Bell palsy
(B) Otitis externa
(C) Otitis media with mastoiditis
(D) Ramsay Hunt syndrome
(E) Right middle cerebral artery stroke

12-3. A 50-year-old woman complains of a severe headache that started suddenly 18 hours ago while she was running on a treadmill. Initially it affected only the back of her head and neck but is now diffuse. She is nauseated. She had a similar headache, though milder, a couple of weeks ago, and while she gets headaches on occasion, this one feels different and is more severe. She has hypertension and is a smoker. Vital signs and physical exam are normal. Head CT is normal. What is the most appropriate next step?

(A) Admission for overnight observation

(B) Carotid ultrasound

(C) Confront the patient about secondary gain

(D) Lumbar puncture

(E) Pain control and discharge

12-4. A 19-year-old man is brought to the ED by paramedics for a generalized tonic–clonic seizure. He was given rectal diazepam gel en route with no effect. His glucose level in the ambulance was 105 mg/dL. He has now been seizing for 10 minutes and an IV has been placed. What is the treatment of choice?

(A) Intravenous dextrose

(B) Intravenous fosphenytoin

(C) Intravenous lorazepam

(D) Intravenous phenobarbital

(E) Rectal diazepam

12-5. A 60-year-old woman complains of a few weeks of paroxysms of severe electric shock–like pain on her left face that last a few seconds at a time. Physical examination is normal, though when you test light touch sensation on her left face she feels an attack of pain. What is the best initial treatment for this condition?

(A) Carbamazepine

(B) Gabapentin

(C) Hydrocodone/acetaminophen

(D) Ibuprofen

(E) Valproic acid

12-6. What cerebrospinal fluid (CSF) finding is most diagnostic of subarachnoid hemorrhage (SAH)?

(A) Elevated opening pressure

(B) Greater than 50 red blood cells (RBCs)/ microliter in tube no. 1

(C) High white blood cell count (WBC)

(D) Low glucose

(E) Xanthochromia

12-7. A 40-year-old previously healthy man is brought to the ED by his wife because he has been confused for the past 2 days. She says he has been forgetful and has difficulty speaking. The patient only complains that his "head hurts" and generally answers questions with one or two words. On exam, his temperature is 38.3°C, he is disoriented, has mild photophobia and meningismus, and moderate aphasia with an otherwise nonfocal neurologic exam. Ceftriaxone is given. A head CT is normal. Lumbar puncture reveals 150 WBCs/hpf (55% lymphocytes and 45% neutrophils) and 100 RBCs/hpf in tube no. 4. What is the most appropriate step at this time?

(A) Acyclovir

(B) Ampicillin

(C) Dexamethasone

(D) Neurosurgery consultation

(E) Therapeutic hypothermia

12-8. A 72-year-old woman awoke at 6 AM with great difficulty speaking or moving the right side of her body. She arrives in the ED by ambulance at 6:45 AM. Her husband corroborates the history and says she was normal last night when she went to sleep. Physical exam shows moderate right-sided weakness and sensory loss and aphasia. Blood pressure is 140/90. Head CT shows signs of an early left middle cerebral artery stroke, no bleeding. Glucose, platelets, and coagulation studies are normal. She has no risk factors for bleeding. It is now 7:30 AM. What is the most appropriate treatment at this time?

(A) Aspirin

(B) Heparin

(C) Nimodipine

(D) Norepinephrine

(E) Thrombolysis

12-9. A 22-year-old motorcyclist is involved in a moderate speed crash. He complains of severe neck pain and inability to move his arms or legs. On exam, he has mid-cervical spine tenderness as well as paralysis and loss of sensation of his upper and lower extremities. Testing of which of the following would be most useful in distinguishing between complete or partial spinal cord injury?

(A) Maximum inspiratory force

(B) Pain and temperature sensation in the upper extremities

(C) Reflexes

(D) Sensation at the angle of the mandible

(E) Sensation in the perineum

12-10. A 77-year-old man is brought in by his family for unusual behavior. He has been confused and paranoid for a couple of days, repeatedly claiming that the neighbors are poisoning him. He is worse at night and is sleeping irregularly. He has a history of schizophrenia, diabetes, and benign prostatic hyperplasia. At triage the patient was disoriented to time and place and answered questions nonsensically. Vital signs are as follows: temperature 37.9°C, blood pressure 110/85, heart rate 105, respiratory rate 18, oxygen saturation 98% on room air. On exam, he is oriented to self, place, and year and answers some questions appropriately but has difficulty paying attention and occasionally nods off to sleep. He complains, "my penis is on fire." What is the most likely explanation for the change in his mental status?

(A) Delirium

(B) Dementia

(C) Mania

(D) Paranoid personality disorder

(E) Psychosis

12-11. Which of the following would be atypical for a migraine headache?

(A) Duration >12 hours

(B) Severe pain

(C) Sudden onset

(D) Unilateral

(E) Vomiting

12-12. A 36-year-old man presents with right neck pain that started while he was wrestling with his dog 2 days ago. Today he also has a right-sided frontotemporal headache and complains that he can hear his heartbeat ringing in his right ear. Vital signs are normal. There is no evidence of head or neck trauma. Neurologic exam shows the abnormalities of the right eye seen in Figure 12-2. What is the most likely diagnosis?

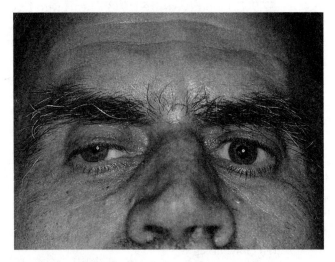

Figure 12-2. Reproduced with permission from Knoop KJ, Stack LB, Storrow AB, Thurman RJ: *The Atlas of Emergency Medicine*, 3rd Edition. Copyright © 2010 The McGraw-Hill Companies, Inc. Photo contributor: Frank Birinyi, MD.

(A) Carotid artery dissection

(B) Right third cranial nerve palsy

(C) Severe neck strain

(D) Temporal arteritis

(E) Vertebral artery dissection

12-13. A 27-year-old man complains of abdominal cramps and vomiting for 1 day. He has also had double vision and difficulty swallowing for about 12 hours. His symptoms started gradually and have progressed. He has a history of multiple skin abscesses from injection drug use, and he continues to inject heroin regularly. On physical exam, he has a low-grade fever and appears somewhat weak. He

has ptosis, cannot seem to hold his head up straight, his speech is garbled, and he drools on occasion. His pupils are dilated and respond minimally to light, and he complains of diplopia when looking in any one direction for more than a few seconds. His extremity strength and sensation as well as reflexes are normal. His abdomen is soft and nontender, though he has suprapubic fullness and discomfort. He has large ulcerating tender wound on his right thigh without surrounding redness. What is the most appropriate next step?

(A) Antibiotics

(B) Antitoxin

(C) CT of the head

(D) Edrophonium (Tensilon)

(E) Steroids

12-14. A young woman with a history of autoimmune diseases complains of new-onset weakness. You are considering myasthenia gravis. Examination of which of the following is most likely to help confirm this diagnosis?

(A) Distal lower extremities

(B) Eyes

(C) Gait

(D) Reflexes

(E) Vibratory sense

12-15. A 63-year-old man complains that he suddenly lost vision in his left eye. On neurologic exam, visual acuity is 20/20 bilaterally and there is a left homonymous hemianopsia. The remainder of the exam is normal. What vessel is most likely occluded?

(A) Left central retinal artery

(B) Left posterior cerebral artery

(C) Right anterior cerebral artery

(D) Right middle cerebral artery

(E) Right posterior cerebral artery

12-16. A 46-year-old woman with a history of diabetes and palpitations presents with sudden vertigo, loss of balance, inability to walk, and vomiting. Neurologic exam reveals severe limb and truncal ataxia, with the patient falling to the left when she sits at the edge of the bed. Emergent MRI shows a large left cerebellar infarction and mild hydrocephalus. Besides arranging for admission to the intensive care unit, what is an important step in the management of this patient?

(A) Carotid ultrasound

(B) Heparin

(C) Maintaining the patient in Trendelenburg position

(D) Neurosurgery consultation

(E) Thrombolysis

12-17. A 68-year-old woman complains of paresthesias of the legs and progressive difficulty walking over the last couple of weeks. She is a vegan with no medical problems. On exam the patient is thin. Her cranial nerves, strength, and light touch sensation are normal. Muscle tone is normal and there is no tremor. She performs the finger-to-nose and rapid alternating movement tests normally. When she walks she looks down at her feet, has a wide-based gait, and slaps her feet down with each step. When the patient stands with eyes closed she is very unsteady; with eyes open she is steady. What is most likely location of the lesion?

(A) Basal ganglia

(B) Cerebellum

(C) Cerebral cortex

(D) Posterior column of the spinal cord

(E) Thalamus

12-18. Noncontrast CT of the head is most sensitive for SAH how long after the onset of bleeding?

(A) Less than 12 hours

(B) 12–23 hours

(C) 24–71 hours

(D) 3–7 days

(E) 7–14 days

12-19. A 30-year-old office manager complains of a gradual-onset headache that started yesterday and is now severe. He is covering his eyes with a blanket to avoid the room lights. He has no medical history and no drug allergies. His temperature is 38.5°C and he has nuchal rigidity. His mental status and neurologic examination are normal, as is the fundoscopic exam. The charge nurse asks you to attend to two trauma patients. What is the most appropriate sequence of orders for this patient?

(A) Ceftriaxone 2 g IV → head CT → set up for lumbar puncture (LP)

(B) Ceftriaxone 2 g IV → set up for LP

(C) Head CT → set up for LP → Ceftriaxone 2 g IV after CSF obtained

(D) Set up for LP → Ceftriaxone 2 g IV after CSF obtained

(E) Set up for LP (no order for antibiotics until CSF studies confirm bacterial meningitis)

12-20. A 26-year-old woman complains of a gradual-onset diffuse headache that started a few weeks ago. It is worse when she awakens in the morning and is better after prolonged sitting or standing. She has had transient episodes of blurry vision for a few days, and today she has double vision. On examination the patient is moderately obese. Visual acuity is normal. She is unable to abduct either eye. The fundoscopic exam is shown in Figure 12-3. Head CT is normal. What do you expect to find on LP?

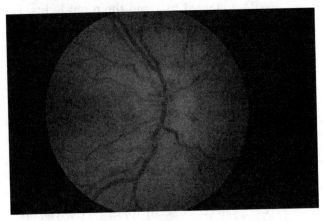

Figure 12-3. Reproduced with permission from Knoop KJ, Stack LB, Storrow AB, Thurman RJ: *The Atlas of Emergency Medicine*, 3rd Edition. Copyright © 2010 The McGraw-Hill Companies, Inc. Photo contributor: Department of Ophthalmology, Naval Medical Center, Portsmouth, VA.

(A) High opening pressure

(B) High protein level

(C) High RBC

(D) High WBC

(E) Low glucose

12-21. A 25-year-old man is brought to the ED by his partner, who complains that the patient is "out of it." The partner describes episodes in which the patient claims to smell and hear things that aren't there, complains that people are out to get him, then smacks his lips for about a minute and doesn't interact. Finally he begins responding again but remains confused for several minutes before becoming normal. What is the diagnosis?

(A) Complex partial seizure

(B) Lysergic acid diethylamide (LSD) abuse

(C) Schizophrenia

(D) Simple partial seizure

(E) Tourette syndrome

12-22. A 35-year-old woman complains of trouble walking that started gradually 1 week ago and has worsened. Today she has double vision as well. Three weeks ago she had a severe diarrheal illness with fevers. She has no medical history, takes no medications, and denies alcohol or drug abuse. On exam she has ophthalmoplegia, ataxia, absent reflexes, and minimal symmetric weakness in her lower extremities. Mental status is normal. There are no visible ticks on a thorough skin exam. CSF analysis reveals normal cell counts and elevated protein level. What is the diagnosis?

(A) Guillain–Barré syndrome, Miller-Fisher variant

(B) Myasthenia gravis

(C) Multiple sclerosis (MS)

(D) Tick paralysis

(E) Wernicke's encephalopathy

12-23. An 83-year-old woman presents with 30 minutes of left-sided weakness that started suddenly while she was on the phone. On exam, her blood pressure is 200/110, she has moderate weakness on her left face and left upper extremity, and she only pays attention to you if you are standing to her right. CT of the head is normal. Glucose, platelets, and coagulation studies are normal. By history she has no risk factors for bleeding. What is the most appropriate management?

(A) Aspirin, no lowering of blood pressure

(B) Careful lowering of blood pressure, aspirin

(C) Careful lowering of blood pressure followed by thrombolysis

(D) Careful lowering of blood pressure, no thrombolysis

(E) Thrombolysis, no lowering of blood pressure

12-24. Which of the following increases the risk of post-LP headache?

(A) Patient moving her legs while spinal needle is in subarachnoid space

(B) Patient sitting up within 1 hour of completion of the procedure

(C) Replacing the stylet before removing the spinal needle

(D) Using a cutting (Quincke) spinal needle

(E) Using a small (22-gauge) spinal needle

12-25. A 72-year-old man complains of the sudden onset of vertigo and a hoarse voice 2 hours ago. He has history of hypertension, diabetes mellitus, and gout. On neurologic examination, he has ptosis of the left eye, numbness on his left face, poor palatal rise on the left, a hoarse voice, numbness on his right upper and lower extremities, and dysmetria on left-sided finger-nose testing. What is the diagnosis?

(A) Cerebellar stroke

(B) Left middle cerebral artery stroke

(C) Multiple sclerosis

(D) Perilymph fistula

(E) Wallenberg's (lateral medullary) syndrome

12-26. A 32-year-old woman presents after a first-time seizure in which her left arm became stiff and then shook for 2 minutes while she stared blankly. She feels normal now and denies any recent illnesses or unusual symptoms. She emigrated from Mexico 2 years ago, has no medical history and no family history of seizures, and she denies drug use. Her vital signs and physical exam are normal. MRI is shown in Figure 12-4. What is the most likely cause of her seizure?

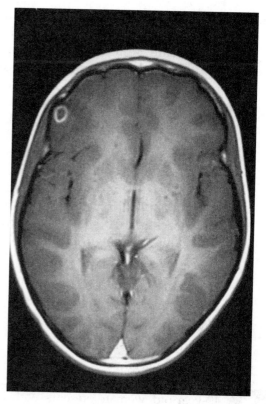

Figure 12-4. Reproduced with permission from Shah BR, Lucchesi M: *Atlas of Pediatric Emergency Medicine.* Copyright © 2006 The McGraw-Hill Companies, Inc.

(A) Brain tumor

(B) Cocaine abuse

(C) Hyponatremia

(D) Primary epilepsy

(E) Worms in her brain

12-27. Both Wernicke encephalopathy and normal pressure hydrocephalus present with what abnormality?

(A) Ataxia

(B) Headache

(C) Mydriasis

(D) Ophthalmoplegia

(E) Urinary incontinence

12-28. A 28-year-old woman complains of gradual-onset double vision and a lazy left hand. The latter has made it difficult for her to type or even button her clothes unless she looks at the hand. She has no medical history other than a 1-month episode of near-blindness of her right eye as a teenager in Canada. Exam reveals that the patient is unable to adduct either eye beyond midline during horizontal gaze. Strength and reflexes are normal, including in the left hand. Light touch and proprioception are diminished in the left hand. When her neck is flexed, she develops an electrical shooting pain down her spine. What is the most likely diagnosis?

(A) Amyotrophic lateral sclerosis

(B) Central cord syndrome

(C) Conversion disorder

(D) Multiple sclerosis

(E) Myasthenia gravis

12-29. A 40-year-old woman presents with acute weakness. On exam she appears tired but nontoxic. After a careful neurologic examination, your differential diagnosis includes myasthenia gravis, Guillain–Barré syndrome, and less likely botulism. In addition to specific testing to elucidate the diagnosis, which of the following is a critical management step in the ED?

(A) Central venous pressure monitoring

(B) Empiric steroids

(C) Measurement of forced vital capacity

(D) Placement of a Foley catheter

(E) Respiratory isolation of the patient

12-30. A 40-year-old woman with a known seizure disorder presents with an uncomplicated generalized tonic–clonic seizure that lasted about 1 minute. She denies any recent illness or other symptoms. She takes phenytoin. Her physical exam is normal except for a mild tongue laceration. What is the most appropriate diagnostic workup?

(A) Electrolytes, renal function, glucose level, liver function tests, coagulation studies, urine toxicology screen, and phenytoin level

(B) Electrolytes, renal function, glucose level, liver function tests, coagulation studies, urine toxicology screen, phenytoin level, and CT scan of the head

(C) Glucose and phenytoin levels

(D) Glucose and phenytoin levels and CT scan of the head

(E) Glucose and phenytoin levels, urine toxicology screen, and CT scan of the head

12-31. Which of the following is associated with a higher risk of stroke after a transient ischemic attack (TIA)?

(A) Age <60

(B) Anemia

(C) Duration of TIA symptoms >10 minutes

(D) Family history of coronary artery disease

(E) Visual symptoms during TIA

12-32. A 3-year-old boy with a ventriculoperitoneal shunt placed 2 years ago for hydrocephalus presents with headache, vomiting, and listlessness. On exam, he is afebrile, lethargic, and ataxic. There is no meningismus or abdominal tenderness. Plain film shunt series is negative. What is the most likely cause of his symptoms?

(A) Abdominal pseudocyst

(B) Shunt fracture

(C) Shunt infection

(D) Shunt misplacement

(E) Shunt obstruction

12-33. A 55-year-old woman with myasthenia gravis being treated with azathioprine, prednisone, and high-dose pyridostigmine complains of weakness progressing over the past 1 week. She has also had vomiting, diarrhea, and a cough productive of clear sputum associated with shortness of breath. Physical exam reveals bradycardia, diffuse mild-moderate weakness, coarse upper airway rhonchi, and mild wheezing. Her breathing is unlabored and her forced vital capacity is 50 mL/kg. What is the most appropriate intervention?

(A) Hold pyridostigmine, give bronchodilators and atropine

(B) Intravenous edrophonium, full-dose (10 mg)

(C) Intravenous methylprednisolone

(D) Intravenous neostigmine

(E) Intubation

12-34. Which of the following decreases the chance that a headache is due to SAH?

(A) Associated cough and myalgia

(B) Meningismus

(C) Occipital–nuchal location

(D) Older age patient

(E) Onset during exertion

12-35. A 25-year-old man was brought to the ED by paramedics for a seizure. He had been seizing with generalized tonic–clonic jerking for 30 minutes continuously; this stopped after multiple doses of lorazepam and a 20 mg/kg loading dose of fosphenytoin. It has been 40 minutes since the seizure stopped and he was intubated. He remains unresponsive to verbal stimuli. He is afebrile, pupils are equal and reactive, and the neck is supple. Glucose level is 150 mg/dL. Besides CT of the head, LP, and a broad laboratory workup, what needs to be ordered for the patient immediately?

(A) Continuous electroencephalography

(B) Hyperventilation

(C) Hypertonic saline

(D) Mannitol

(E) Thiamine

12-36. A 45-year-old woman complains of dizziness that started suddenly a few hours ago while getting out of bed. If she moves her head toward the right, particularly when lying down, she develops a strong feeling that the room is spinning and becomes nauseated; she has vomited several times. When her head is kept still, the symptoms resolve completely. She denies hearing loss or tinnitus. She has no medical problems and does not smoke or use illicit drugs. Neurologic examination, including coordination, is normal. When the Dix–Hallpike maneuver is performed and the head is tilted to the right, her symptoms as well as rotatory nystagmus ensue after a 3-second delay and resolve after 30 seconds. What is the diagnosis?

(A) Benign paroxysmal positional vertigo (BPPV)

(B) Cerebellar stroke

(C) Méniére disease

(D) Vertebral artery dissection

(E) Vertebrobasilar insufficiency

12-37. A 25-year-old man is brought to the ED by a friend after a seizure that occurred an hour ago. The friend says that the patient has not been himself lately—he has been sleepy with a poor attention span and either does not talk much or spews expletives inappropriately. The patient is awake and complains of severe tooth pain and a headache. On exam, his temperature is 38.1°C. He refuses to answer most questions. He has swelling, redness, and purulent discharge from the left second maxillary molar tooth (no. 15). There is no meningismus. He has a mild right pronator drift. Noncontrast head CT is normal. What diagnostic study should be ordered next?

(A) Complete blood count

(B) Contrast head CT

(C) Erythrocyte sedimentation rate

(D) Lumbar puncture

(E) Panorex film of the teeth

Nervous System Disorders
Answers and Explanations

12-1. **The answer is B** (Chapter 160). Patients with intracranial hemorrhage (ICH) and coagulopathy are critically ill with a high mortality rate, even if the bleed is small and they look well. The coagulopathy, which is usually due to warfarin therapy, must be reversed immediately by the fastest available means—vitamin K and fresh frozen plasma (FFP) are the traditional means and are effective. More expensive but fast and reliable alternatives include prothrombin complex concentrates and recombinant-activated factor VII. Rapid reversal by any means markedly reduces mortality. Aspirin is absolutely contraindicated in ICH. Intubation is not yet indicated in this awake and talking patient. Lowering systolic blood pressure below 180 mm Hg is recommended in ICH—beyond that, there is mixed evidence on the value of further lowering; regardless, reversal of coagulopathy is a higher priority. Therapeutic hypothermia is probably beneficial postcardiac arrest, but has not yet been shown to be helpful in ICH or brain injury.

12-2. **The answer is D** (Chapter 164). The Ramsay Hunt syndrome (herpes zoster oticus) is an acute neuropathy of cranial nerve VII associated with a herpetic rash. It is caused by the varicella zoster virus (VZV). Findings include unilateral lower motor neuron facial weakness (including the periorbital and forehead muscles, indicating peripheral nerve dysfunction), as seen in Figure 12-1, and a rash in the sensory distribution of the facial nerve (anterior tongue, auricle, and/or external auditory canal). Nearby cranial nerve VIII may also be involved, causing hearing loss, vertigo, and/or tinnitus. Bell palsy is *idiopathic* cranial nerve VII neuropathy. It is a diagnosis of exclusion after other causes, such as acute VZV infection or intracranial mass, have been considered. Otitis externa presents with ear pain and an erythematous auditory canal, but neither a vesicular rash nor neurologic abnormalities. Otitis media causes ear pain and hearing loss, and mastoiditis causes postauricular pain and can rarely affect cranial nerve VII in the temporal bone, but these infections are far more common in children and neither explains this patient's rash. A right middle cerebral artery stroke would cause left *lower* facial weakness (sparing the periorbital and forehead muscles) and does not explain the other findings.

12-3. **The answer is D** (Chapters 159 and 160). This presentation is concerning for SAH. Sudden-onset headache (i.e., reaching maximal intensity within minutes) is always concerning for SAH, especially if it starts during exertion. Occipital–nuchal location of pain is common in SAH, and the patient says this headache is unusual for her. Her hypertension and smoking are risk factors for SAH. Finally, 2 weeks ago, she had what sounds like a sentinel headache, which is usually a small leak from an aneurysm that is ready to rupture. The negative head CT decreases the likelihood of SAH, but not enough to obviate LP. Admission without further workup could dangerously delay the diagnosis. Carotid ultrasound might be helpful if carotid dissection were suspected, but not here. Occasionally, patients with frequent ED visits for pain without organic explanations do need to be confronted about secondary gain, but not this patient. Pain control and discharge would be appropriate if the patient did not have high-risk features or if this were a typical headache for her.

12-4. **The answer is C** (Chapter 165). Intravenous lorazepam is the first-line treatment of choice in status epilepticus or impending status epilepticus, the latter being defined as seizure(s) for more than 5 minutes without recovery of consciousness. Lorazepam is effective, can be rapidly administered, and has a short onset of action. Doses of 2–4 mg can be given and repeated. The fact that the patient failed diazepam in the field does not change lorazepam's first-line status. Glucose is not indicated in normoglycemia. Fosphenytoin, a water-soluble prodrug of phenytoin that can be rapidly administered, is a second-line agent and would be useful to abort a seizure that breaks through benzodiazepines or to prevent further seizures after control is established with benzodiazepines. Phenobarbital is a third-line agent in status epilepticus. Rectal diazepam and buccal midazolam are useful when there is no IV access.

12-5. **The answer is A** (Chapter 159). The patient has trigeminal neuralgia (tic douloureux), which presents with paroxysms of severe unilateral electric-like or lancinating pain in one or more of the trigeminal nerve distributions of the face. Episodes last only a few seconds but may occur repeatedly during a flare. Carbamazepine, starting at 100 mg twice daily, is very effective in controlling pain in this disease. It should be started in the ED when the diagnosis is made and should be restarted or increased in patients who are having a flare. Side effects include leukopenia and, rarely, aplastic anemia; thus, patients should have a complete blood count prior to starting therapy and in follow-up. Persons of Asian descent (including Indians) are at risk for Stevens–Johnson syndrome with carbamazepine, so choose an alternative or consult a neurologist for these patients.

12-6. **The answer is E** (Chapter 160). Xanthochromia is yellow discoloration of the CSF due to bilirubin accumulation from the enzymatic breakdown of hemoglobin in RBCs. It is diagnostic of SAH. Xanthochromia develops within 12 hours of SAH and lasts for up to 3 weeks. Unfortunately, most hospital laboratories determine the presence of xanthochromia simply by holding up the specimen against a white background; spectrophotometry is the more sensitive gold standard method. The RBC count in the CSF is important, especially in the first 12 hours after headache onset. The presence of RBCs in a CSF specimen is common due to trauma during the LP, so the presence of RBCs in tube no. 1 is not by itself specific for SAH. However, the RBC count in tube no. 4 should be normal (or in a traumatic tap, it should be substantially decreased from tube no. 1 and nearly normal) to exclude SAH. An elevated opening pressure or a slight elevation in the white blood count in the CSF may be seen in SAH, but is not diagnostic. The glucose level in the CSF should not be altered.

12-7. **The answer is A** (Chapter 168). The patient very likely has herpes simplex virus (HSV) meningoencephalitis. The virus usually infects both the meninges (causing headache, fever, and nuchal rigidity) and the brain parenchyma (encephalitis), in particular the temporal lobe and/or the anterior frontal lobe resulting in cortical signs such as memory deficits and aphasia; seizures are common as well. MRI and sometimes CT show characteristic changes. CSF usually contains a viral pleocytosis (WBC 10–300 with lymphocyte predominance) as well as elevated RBCs due to HSV's destructive nature in this infection. Early initiation of acyclovir is important as it markedly reduces mortality. Ampicillin is indicated when the CSF cell count suggests meningitis and the patient is at risk for Listeria infection (age >50, neonate, or immunocompromised). In bacterial meningitis, dexamethasone should be given just before or concomitant with the first dose of antibiotics, not after the antibiotic has already been given. There is no role for cooling or a neurosurgeon in this case.

12-8. **The answer is A** (Chapter 161). On first glance, this patient may appear to be a good candidate for thrombolysis; *however*, we do not know whether the stroke occurred within the time window (maximum 4.5 hrs) for thrombolysis—therefore, it should be withheld. In patients with stroke, it is critical to ascertain when they were last normal. This patient was last known to be normal the previous night. She awoke with her deficits, so the stroke could have occurred at any point between the onset of sleep and awakening. Aspirin is the appropriate ED treatment for acute nonhemorrhagic stroke, though if thrombolytics are administered aspirin should be withheld for the first 24 hours. Heparin and other anticoagulants have been shown to be either nonbeneficial or harmful in acute stroke, even in the presence of atrial fibrillation. Nimodipine helps prevent vasospasm in SAH, but antihypertensives are contraindicated in acute ischemic stroke unless the blood pressure is above 220/120 mm Hg, and even then treatment should be very gentle, parenteral, and with close monitoring. Vasopressor therapy to induce hypertension is being studied in acute stroke, but is not standard care at this time.

12-9. **The answer is E** (Chapter 255). In acute spinal cord injury, preserved perianal/perineal sensation, which is dependent on the sacral nerve roots, is an important finding that indicates a partial rather than complete cord injury. The other answer choices are useful functions to test, but they do not distinguish partial from complete cord injury. Maximum inspiratory force is important in upper cervical cord injury to determine the need for ventilatory support. Pain and temperature sensation in the upper extremities is affected by most partial and all complete cervical cord injuries. Reflexes may not be abnormal in acute cord injury—hyperreflexia may take hours to manifest. Interestingly, sensation at the angle of the mandible is carried by the C3 nerve root (rather than the trigeminal nerve).

12-10. **The answer is A** (Chapter 162). This patient is delirious. He has waxing and waning disorientation and attention deficit—he was more disoriented at triage than during examination. He cannot focus his attention. He has been worse at night and his sleep–wake cycle is abnormal. Finally, he has concerning vital sign abnormalities that indicate an underlying acute medical condition. With a history of benign prostatic hyperplasia, a complaint of penile burning, and a fever with tachycardia and narrow pulse pressure, perhaps he has urosepsis, a very common cause of delirium in the elderly. Because of his schizophrenia, he is manifesting delirium with more paranoia than is typical, but psychosis alone does not cause disorientation, attention deficit, or vital sign abnormalities, nor does mania or paranoid personality. Dementia makes one more vulnerable to delirium but does not cause acute changes in mental status.

12-11. **The answer is C** (Chapter 159). Migraine headaches are common and manifest in myriad ways, but there are some features that are fairly typical and when present together are suggestive of migraine: pulsatile quality, duration of 4–72 hours, unilateral location, associated nausea/vomiting, and disabling severity. Migraines, however, rarely start suddenly. A patient with headache should always be asked about the onset of pain: if the pain started suddenly and/or is unusual to the patient, then even if there is a history of migraines alternative diagnoses (particularly SAH) should be ruled out.

12-12. **The answer is A** (Chapter 161). Carotid artery dissection is uncommon but is a significant cause of stroke in the young. It usually occurs after major or minor neck trauma. The most common symptom is headache, which is usually frontotemporal, followed by neck pain; pulsatile tinnitus (hearing the heartbeat) occurs occasionally. Neurologic abnormalities, classically a partial ipsilateral Horner syndrome (no anhydrosis), often occur days after the onset of pain and can be quite subtle. In Figure 12-2, the patient's right eye miosis is obvious, but the ptosis is very mild.

Neck strain would be a diagnosis of exclusion and is less likely here given the classic presentation of carotid dissection. Third cranial nerve palsy produces severe ptosis, pupillary dilation, and ophthalmoplegia. Temporal arteritis occurs almost exclusively in those older than 50 years and is not associated with trauma. Vertebral artery dissection also occurs after neck trauma but usually causes occipital and nuchal pain and brainstem deficits such as vertigo and ataxia.

12-13.   The answer is B (Chapter 166). This patient has wound botulism. Historically, most cases of botulism have been due to ingestion of contaminated food (such as home-canned food), but increasingly it is being reported in injection drug users with wounds infected with *Clostridium botulinum*. Botulinum toxin binds to presynaptic nerve terminals and blocks the release of acetylcholine. It presents with a myriad of symptoms, including nonspecific ones such as abdominal cramping, which can lead to a misdiagnosis of a gastrointestinal disorder. But it also causes a descending paralysis, with cranial nerve dysfunction leading to findings such as diplopia, dysarthria, and dysphagia. Anticholinergic signs such as dilated pupils, dry skin, hyperthermia, and urinary retention can be seen as well. The treatment is botulinum antitoxin. Patients need to be admitted to the ICU for close monitoring of respiratory function. Antibiotics may be needed for the wound but are not the highest priority. Edrophonium could temporarily help reverse and diagnose myasthenia gravis, which also causes bulbar weakness, but myasthenia does not cause anticholinergic findings such as pupillary dilation and is less likely in this patient with a suspicious wound. Steroids would be unhelpful. Imaging is not useful in acute peripheral neuropathies.

12-14.   The answer is B (Chapter 167). Myasthenia gravis is caused by autoantibodies directed against the acetylcholine receptor in the neuromuscular junction. Clinically, it involves the muscles of the eye in 90% of cases and presents solely with ocular abnormalities in half of initial presentations of the disease. Both ptosis and ophthalmoplegia are seen; a common exam finding is progressive ptosis during sustained upward gaze. Weakness of other bulbar muscles (mastication, swallowing), neck extensors, and proximal muscles is also typical. Distal muscles would be affected much later in the disease course. Gait, reflexes, and sensation are not affected.

12-15.   The answer is E (Chapter 161). Homonymous hemianopsia is loss of one half of the visual field and is always due to a lesion posterior to the optic chiasm contralateral to the affected visual field. A typical example is occlusion of the posterior cerebral artery, which causes an occipital stroke with loss of the contralateral visual field. The cortex corresponding to the macula is spared; thus, visual acuity is normal. Patients with this deficit sometimes complain of loss of sight in "one eye" if they have not tested each eye separately. Left central retinal artery occlusion causes blindness in the affected eye. Left posterior cerebral artery occlusion causes a right homonymous hemianopsia. Anterior and middle cerebral artery occlusions should not affect vision.

12-16.   The answer is D (Chapter 161). Large cerebellar infarctions, usually due to occlusion of the posterior inferior cerebellar artery, can be life threatening because the cerebellum can become edematous and impinge on the brainstem and may even herniate into the brainstem. Thus, patients can rapidly deteriorate and must be monitored closely in consultation with a neurosurgeon. Obstructing hydrocephalus implies a poorer outcome and the possible need for acute surgical decompression. Carotid ultrasound is not useful in a posterior circulation stroke. Patients with possible elevated intracranial pressure (ICP) should be placed at 30 degrees of head elevation, not Trendelenburg. Heparin is rarely part of the initial treatment of any acute stroke. Thrombolysis is contraindicated in cerebellar stroke because any bleeding can lead to cerebellar herniation. This coupled with the fact that head CT may be normal in cerebellar stroke (due to artifact from bones of the posterior fossa) highlights the importance of the neurologic exam in distinguishing stroke territories.

12-17. The answer is D (Chapter 163). This patient probably has a severe deficit of proprioception (position sense), as evidenced by her incoordination in the absence of visual input. The next step on physical exam would be to formally test proprioception by asking her if she knows which way you move her toes or distal fingers while her eyes are closed. Proprioception is transmitted up the posterior column of the spinal cord, along with vibratory sensation. There are many etiologies of posterior column dysfunction. A classic one is vitamin B_{12} deficiency, which this patient probably has due to inadequate B_{12} intake. It is important for the emergency physician to be familiar with this diagnosis because if it is not treated promptly, it can lead to permanent disability. Basal ganglia dysfunction causes parkinsonism. Cerebellar lesions cause ataxia of the limbs and/or trunk that is present even when there is visual input. Cortical lesions cause abnormalities such as unilateral weakness and numbness, aphasia, and neglect. Thalamic lesions cause unilateral sensory deficits.

12-18. The answer is A (Chapter 160). Modern multidetector CT scanners are very sensitive for SAH and other ICH soon after the onset of bleeding—the earlier, the better. Recent studies find such scanners to be almost 100% sensitive for SAH within 12 hours of the onset of symptoms and more than 90% sensitive between 12 and 24 hours after onset. CT is only about 50% sensitive at 1 week. It is possible that in the near future patients presenting early after the onset of a high-risk headache will not need more than a CT scan to rule out SAH. But at this time, the standard of care is to follow a negative head CT with an LP.

12-19. The answer is B (Chapter 168). This patient has bacterial meningitis until proven otherwise. He needs antibiotics without delay. If an LP could be performed immediately, an-

tibiotics could be ordered to be ready to administer as soon as CSF is obtained. If there is any delay before LP, antibiotics should be given immediately. Ceftriaxone (2 g intravenously) covers the most common meningeal pathogens; other antibiotics can wait until initial CSF studies confirm the diagnosis (unless clinical features strongly suggest a particular uncommon pathogen). If the suspicion for meningitis is high or if CSF is grossly purulent, then dexamethasone should be administered just before or along with ceftriaxone. In one randomized study, this intervention improved outcomes when the pathogen was pneumococcus. Head CT before LP is required if the patient has any of the following risk factors for elevated ICP or brain lesions: age >60, history of central nervous system disease, malignancy, immunocompromised state, altered mental status, an abnormal neurologic exam or papilledema, or a recent seizure. This patient does not have any of the risk factors, and there is nothing about his history that is concerning for a new mass lesion of the brain, so he does not require a head CT. The other choices would delay antibiotics and are therefore incorrect.

12-20. The answer is A (Chapter 159). The patient likely has idiopathic intracranial hypertension (IIH) also known as pseudotumor cerebri. This condition usually occurs in young women, especially those who are obese. It causes typical symptoms of elevated ICP: a headache that is worse in the morning or in the supine position or with activities that raise ICP such as coughing or straining. The headache is often chronic by the time the patient presents for care. Figure 12-3 shows papilledema, a classic fundoscopic finding in IIH that is *not* a cause of vision loss (the worst outcome from IIH) or the transient visual obscurations that are common in this disease. Elevated ICP of any etiology may cause dysfunction of cranial nerves, particularly nerve VI (abducens nerve), which courses through tight canals and can be easily compressed by a downwardly displaced brainstem. Head imaging is normal in IIH, which makes LP safe despite the presence of papilledema. Lumbar puncture shows elevated opening pressure (>20–25 cm H_2O) and otherwise normal CSF.

12-21. **The answer is A** (Chapter 165). Complex partial seizures are focal seizures that affect consciousness or mentation. They usually originate in the temporal lobe and can cause odd symptoms or behaviors, such as olfactory or auditory hallucinations, automatisms, and affective symptoms such as fear or paranoia. LSD causes hallucinations and affective changes but not automatisms with unresponsiveness. Schizophrenia often causes auditory hallucinations and paranoia but is not paroxysmal nor does it affect consciousness. Simple partial seizures could explain all of the findings except the change in consciousness. Tourette syndrome is characterized by recurrent brief motor and verbal tics but not hallucinations or changes in mood or consciousness.

12-22. **The answer is A** (Chapter 166). Guillain–Barré syndrome is an acute demyelinating polyneuropathy that presents with ascending paralysis and loss of deep tendon reflexes. Paresthesias are common, but true sensory deficits are not. It is often preceded by a viral illness or *Campylobacter jejuni* infection. CSF must be analyzed to confirm the diagnosis, and it will show "albuminocytologic dissociation," or elevated protein with a normal cell count. There are several variants of the classic syndrome, including the Miller-Fisher variant, which causes the triad of ophthalmoplegia, ataxia, and areflexia, with minimal or no weakness. It is strongly associated with preceding *C. jejuni*, as this patient likely had in retrospect. Myasthenia gravis might cause ophthalmoplegia but not the other findings. MS typically causes waxing and waning multifocal deficits—diffuse areflexia and symmetric weakness would be unusual. Tick paralysis mimics Guillain–Barré, but it is rare, occurs mostly in children, does not affect CSF, and during symptoms, careful inspection of the skin (including scalp) should reveal a latched tick. Wernicke encephalopathy causes ophthalmoplegia and

ataxia but not areflexia, and the mental status should be abnormal.

12-23. **The answer is C** (Chapter 161). This patient meets all criteria for thrombolysis with rtPA (based on the National Institute for Neurological Disorders [NINDS] trial) except for a blood pressure that is mildly higher than the upper limit (185/110) that is acceptable for thrombolysis. In such a case, the blood pressure should be gently lowered to facilitate thrombolysis. Importantly, we know with certainty that the patient's stroke began within the last 3 hours, a crucial factor in determining eligibility for thrombolysis; of note, though, a recent study European Cooperative Acute Stroke Study (ECASS III) showed a benefit for rtPA in the 3–4.5 hours window, so the acceptable time from symptom onset may be changing soon. Giving aspirin and not lowering blood pressure is a reasonable choice given the mixed evidence and controversies surrounding thrombolysis, but expert guidelines and standard of care would dictate thrombolysis in this case. If thrombolysis is not performed for any reason, then blood pressure should not be lowered unless it is greater than 220 mm Hg systolic or 120 mm Hg diastolic.

12-24. **The answer is D** (Chapter 169). Noncutting pencil-tipped spinal needles (Whitacre or Sprotte) substantially decrease the risk of post-LP headache compared with cutting (Quincke) needles. Smaller spinal needles (i.e., 22 gauge) also decrease the risk. Unfortunately, what comes in the standard LP kit is a 20-gauge Quincke needle; thus, the diligent emergency physician should separately obtain a 22-gauge noncutting needle in most cases. Replacing the stylet before withdrawing the spinal needle prevents arachnoid tissue from being sucked through the hole in the dura and causing a spinal fluid leak, the cause of post-LP headaches. Movement of the legs while the needle is in the subarachnoid space is considered safe. It has traditionally been taught that patients should not sit up for several hours after an LP, but a recent study showed a lower risk of post-LP headache with early mobilization.

12-25. **The answer is E** (Chapter 164). The patient has Wallenberg syndrome, which is infarction of the lateral medulla, usually due to occlusion of the posterior inferior cerebellar artery. Due to the presence of multiple nerve tracts and nuclei in this small section of the brainstem, the syndrome is characterized by seemingly disparate neurologic deficits, including crossed sensory loss (ipsilateral face and contralateral trunk/extremity), vertigo, dysphagia/dysphonia, Horner syndrome, and ataxia (if the cerebellum is affected). Cerebellar stroke causes predominant ataxia and vague, often nonspinning vertigo. Middle cerebral artery stroke causes motor/sensory loss in the contralateral face and upper extremity (less so in the lower extremity) as well as cortical signs such as aphasia or neglect. MS may cause disparate neurologic deficits, but it does so slowly over time. Perilymph fistula is caused by a sudden rise in middle ear pressure resulting in a tear in one of the windows separating the middle ear and vestibular organs; symptoms include peripheral vertigo and hearing loss.

12-26. **The answer is E** (Chapter 165). The most likely cause of this patient's seizure is neurocysticercosis, an infection of the brain by the larvae (cysticerci) of the tapeworm *Taenia solium*. It is the most common parasitic infection of the central nervous system in the world and the most common acquired cause of epilepsy in the developing world, particularly Latin America. The worm is usually acquired via ingestion of undercooked pork or fecally contaminated water. CT or MRI imaging may reveal parenchymal calcifications (scarring) or hypodense or ring-enhancing lesions (active cysts), the latter being seen in the MRI in Figure 12-4. Antiepileptic monotherapy is usually effective in preventing recurrent seizures. Antiparasitics along with or preceded by steroids can be considered in consultation with an infectious diseases specialist if there is evidence of active cysts. A brain tumor could explain this seizure but

is less likely than cysticercosis in this patient from Mexico with no previous symptoms and a normal neurological exam. There is no evidence of cocaine abuse by history or exam. Hyponatremia is unlikely in the absence of a recent illness or medication use. Primary epilepsy is possible, but at the age of 32, this would be late onset, making cysticercosis more likely in a patient from Latin America.

12-27. **The answer is A** (Chapter 163). Ataxia is a common manifestation of many neurologic diseases. Wernicke encephalopathy is due to thiamine deficiency and usually occurs in alcoholics. It is characterized by the triad of altered mental status, ataxia, and ophthalmoplegia. Mortality is up to 20% and the diagnosis is often missed. Thiamine repletion reverses the abnormalities sometimes within hours. Magnesium is a necessary cofactor for thiamine, so it must also be repleted. Normal pressure hydrocephalus occurs in the elderly and presents with the triad of dementia, ataxia, and urinary incontinence. Head imaging shows hydrocephalus with other characteristic findings. Surgical shunting benefits the subgroup of patients who respond well to large-volume CSF drainage. Headache and mydriasis are not typical of either disorder.

12-28. **The answer is D** (Chapter 167). MS is a chronic central demyelinating disease. It is suspected when a patient presents with multiple neurologic abnormalities separated by "space" (occurring in different parts of the brain or spinal cord) and "time" (time of onset of the abnormalities is different). The diagnosis is aided by MRI. Certain neurologic deficits are highly suggestive. This patient has two such deficits: bilateral internuclear ophthalmoplegia and "sensory useless hand." The shooting pain down the spine with neck flexion is called Lhermitte sign and is also characteristic of MS. Optic neuritis causing temporary vision loss is a common initial manifestation. Growing up far from the equator is a risk factor for MS. Amyotrophic lateral sclerosis causes upper and lower motor neuron weakness, not sensory abnormalities. Central cord syndrome presents with upper > lower extremity weakness and numbness usually after traumatic neck extension; it cannot affect the eyes. Conversion disorder is a diagnosis of exclusion and is unlikely in the setting of multiple neurologic deficits. Myasthenia gravis causes ophthalmoplegia, but not of the internuclear variety, and does not cause sensory abnormalities.

12-29. **The answer is C** (Chapters 166 and 167). Respiratory failure is the major life-threatening complication of certain acute neurologic disorders, such as Guillain–Barré, botulism, and cholinergic toxicity, as well as chronic neurologic disorders in exacerbation, especially myasthenia gravis. Respiratory function must be assessed in such cases, ideally with bedside spirometry. Spirometry is usually performed by a respiratory therapist. A forced vital capacity below 25 mL/kg or 50% of predicted is indicative of substantial loss of ventilatory reserve and the likely need for intubation. Other measures such as negative inspiratory force are useful as well. Even patients with milder respiratory compromise may need admission to an intensive care unit for close monitoring. Central venous pressure monitoring is not indicated in these conditions. In the absence of a definite diagnosis, empiric steroids are dangerous in acute weakness as they can cause a myopathy that worsens weakness. A Foley catheter is not the highest priority. Respiratory isolation is not indicated here.

12-30. **The answer is C** (Chapter 165). Patients who have a known seizure disorder and have a single typical seizure do not need an extensive diagnostic workup unless there is reason to suspect that the seizure was provoked by a medically important or treatable factor (e.g., a dehydrated patient may have hyponatremia, which could provoke a seizure and can be treated). A glucose level and an anticonvulsant level suffice in this case. The tests listed in the other answers could all be appropriate in the right clinical circumstance, but not in

this straightforward case. In particular, while imaging of the head is certainly indicated in a first-time seizure, it is rarely needed to work up a typical seizure in a patient with a known seizure disorder.

12-31. **The answer is C** (Chapter 161). TIA is transient neurologic dysfunction like a stroke but usually lasting less than an hour and lacking evidence of cerebral infarction. After a TIA, the 3-month risk of stroke is about 10%. Half of these strokes occur in the first 2 days after the TIA. A validated clinical risk score called ABCD2 stratifies patients' risk of stroke after a TIA. The following features increase the risk of stroke: age >60, hypertension at the time of the TIA, diabetes, duration of symptoms greater than 10 minutes, and weakness or speech disturbance. Adding diffusion-weighted MRI to this score probably improves risk prediction. However, expert guidelines do not yet incorporate this score in decision making about hospital admission; thus in most centers, patients with TIA should be admitted to the hospital for expedited workup and risk modification.

12-32. **The answer is E** (Chapter 169). The patient has typical symptoms of elevated ICP, implying shunt malfunction. Shunt obstruction is the most common mechanism of malfunction. The plain film shunt series (x-rays of skull, chest, and abdomen) helps to identify kinks, malpositioning, and perhaps fracture of the shunt, but does not detect obstruction. CT of the head could be performed, but it exposes the child to ionizing radiation and would likely just confirm the clinical findings of elevated ICP without determining the cause. The valve chamber could be palpated to help diagnose an obstruction—difficulty compressing the chamber indicates a distal obstruction, whereas slow refill of the chamber (more than 3 seconds) indicates a proximal obstruction. Regardless, a neurosurgeon should be consulted. Abdominal pseudocyst is an uncommon cause of shunt malfunction. Shunt fracture is also uncommon and is often evident either on physical exam (e.g., collection of fluid around the clavicle) or the shunt series. There are no signs of shunt infection. Shunt misplacement is a postoperative diagnosis and would usually be identified by the shunt series.

12-33. **The answer is A** (Chapter 167). The patient is having a cholinergic crisis. When patients with myasthenia gravis present with an apparent exacerbation of their disease, you must consider that they could actually be suffering from a cholinergic crisis due to pyridostigmine therapy, which is uncommon and only occurs at high doses. This patient has several characteristic findings: emesis, diarrhea, bronchorrhea, bronchospasm, and bradycardia. Her culprit medication, pyridostigmine, should be held and the muscarinic effects reversed with bronchodilators and atropine. In this case, because her breathing is not labored and her forced vital capacity is normal, intubation is not necessary. Edrophonium or neostigmine would likely precipitate a severe cholinergic crisis and are contraindicated here (edrophonium, starting with a 1–2-mg test dose, is reasonable if the patient does not have clear signs of cholinergic toxicity). Steroids are not indicated in this case, and by causing myopathy might make the patient worse—even in myasthenic crisis, they should only be given after consultation with a neurologist.

12-34. **The answer is A** (Chapters 159 and 160). Diagnosing SAH can be life saving, and taking a good history is the key to suspecting the diagnosis and initiating the workup. Characteristics that increase the risk of SAH include sudden onset; onset during exertion (even coughing or Valsalva); occipital–nuchal location; new, unusual, or particularly severe headache; and family history of SAH or intracranial aneurysm. The risk of SAH increases with age, with a steep rise in the middle ages (45–55 years old). Cough and myalgia suggest a secondary cause of headache, such as influenza, rather than a primary cause such as SAH or migraine.

12-35. **The answer is A** (Chapter 165). This patient has suffered status epilepticus, which is 30

minutes of continuous seizing or multiple seizures without recovery of mental status between seizures. Patients with such long seizures may stop having perceptible muscle activity but may still have ongoing damaging electrical seizures in the brain, so-called nonconvulsive status epilepticus. This should be suspected when a patient is not waking up within 30 minutes of cessation of motor activity. Continuous electroencephalography is essential in these cases. Hyperventilation, hypertonic saline, and mannitol are important short-term treatments in life-threatening elevations of ICP, but there is no evidence of this here. Thiamine deficiency does not cause status epilepticus.

12-36. **The answer is A** (Chapter 164). BPPV is the most common type of peripheral vertigo. Peripheral vertigo is usually described as a strong spinning sensation that is triggered or substantially worsened by head movement. Symptoms often resolve with avoidance of head movement and fatigue after repeated provocation. The finding of vertigo and nystagmus occurring after a few seconds delay during the Dix–Hallpike maneuver and resolving within a minute is almost pathognomonic for BPPV. Cerebellar strokes may cause vertigo but invariably present with ataxia as well. Méniére disease presents with repeated bouts of peripheral vertigo often associated with tinnitus and hearing loss. Vertebral artery dissection may cause central (not peripheral) vertigo, usually occurs after rapid rotation or extreme positioning of the neck, and often the initial symptom is occipital or nuchal pain. Vertebrobasilar insufficiency may cause numerous symptoms referable to the brainstem or cerebellum (including central vertigo) and is a disease of the elderly or those with major atherosclerosis risk factors.

12-37. **The answer is B** (Chapter 168). The patient probably has a brain abscess. His infected tooth is the likely source, via direct spread to the brain (in this case, to the left frontal lobe based on the exam findings). CT scan without contrast may be normal, but with contrast one or multiple ring-enhancing lesions are seen and are diagnostic. Brain abscesses are uncommon now in the developed world, but are critical to diagnose because they are life threatening and the cure usually requires surgery. Direct spread of pathogens in otitis media, sinusitis, and odontogenic infection is responsible for at least a third of cases. The classic clinical triad of headache, fever, and focal neurologic deficits is surprisingly uncommon—therefore, the physician must pick up on subtle risk factors (e.g., signs of sinusitis or a new murmur in a patient with an abnormal heart valve). Complete blood count and erythrocyte sedimentation rate might be abnormal but would not aid in diagnosis. Lumbar puncture is relatively contraindicated if brain abscess is suspected and there are focal findings, but if it were performed, it might show abnormalities similar to bacterial meningitis. Panorex x-rays of the teeth would not be a high priority here.

Orthopedic Emergencies
Questions

13-1. When assessing tendon function in hand injuries, which of the following physical findings is suggestive of a partial extensor tendon laceration?

 (A) Complete inability to extend the digit

 (B) Complete inability to flex the digit

 (C) Inability to flex the digit against resistance

 (D) Inability to visualize the end of the tendon through the overlying laceration

 (E) Pain along the course of the tendon during resistance

13-2. Complete laceration of the extensor tendon over the distal phalanx and distal interphalangeal joint results in the following injury:

 (A) Boutonniere deformity

 (B) Gamekeeper thumb

 (C) Mallet finger

 (D) Trigger finger

 (E) Swan neck deformity

13-3. The following injury is referred to as (Figure 13-1):

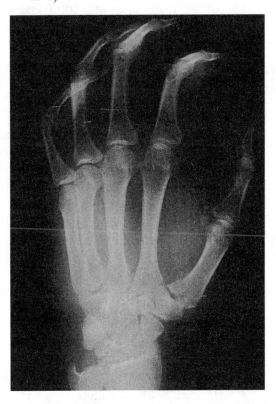

Figure 13-1. Reproduced with permission from Knoop KJ, Stack LB, Storrow AB, Thurman RJ: *The Atlas of Emergency Medicine*, 3rd Edition. Copyright © 2010 The McGraw-Hill Companies, Inc. Photo contributor: Cathleen M. Vossler, MD.

 (A) Bennett fracture

 (B) Destot fracture

 (C) Rolando fracture

 (D) Skier thumb

 (E) Space of Poirier

13-4. A 45-year-old man presents to the emergency department (ED) after sustaining an injury to his left index finger from pressurized spray painter. Examination of the hand reveals a small punctate lesion of the volar aspect of the distal index finger. There is small amount of surrounding pallor, and the entire finger is moderately tender to palpation. The next best steps in the management of this patient include:

(A) Emergent fasciotomy, intravenous antibiotics, administer tetanus prophylaxis.

(B) Immobilize and elevate, intravenous antibiotics, administer tetanus prophylaxis, parenteral analgesia, emergent surgical consultation.

(C) Irrigate, elevate, initiate a 7-day course of cephalexin, administer tetanus prophylaxis, oral pain medications

(D) Irrigate, elevate, initiate a 7-day course of cephalexin, 24-hour follow-up with an orthopedic hand specialist, administer tetanus prophylaxis

(E) Irrigate, x-ray, intravenous antibiotics, administer tetanus prophylaxis, and admit to the orthopedic service for observation and pain control

13-5. Which of the following is the most commonly injured structure in the wrist?

(A) Perilunate ligament
(B) Scapholunate ligament
(C) Space of Poirier
(D) Triangular fibrocartilage complex
(E) Triquetrolunate ligament

13-6. A 30-year-old man fell off a curb onto a dorsiflexed outstretched hand. He complains of wrist pain and has tender generalized pain and swelling in the hand and wrist (Figure 13-2). Which of the following statements best applies to his injury?

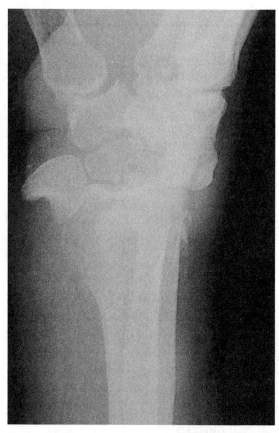

Figure 13-2. Reproduced with permission from Knoop KJ, Stack LB, Storrow AB, Thurman RJ: *The Atlas of Emergency Medicine*, 3rd Edition. Copyright © 2010 The McGraw-Hill Companies, Inc. Photo contributor: Cathleen M. Vossler, MD.

(A) A lunate dislocation is present. The wrist should be immobilized, and a hand specialist should be consulted emergently.

(B) A perilunate dislocation is present. The wrist should be immobilized, and the patient should be referred to a hand specialist urgently.

(C) A perilunate dislocation is present. The wrist should be immobilized, and a hand specialist should be consulted emergently.

(D) A scapholunate dissociation is present. The patient should be immobilized in a volar splint, and a hand specialist consulted emergently.

(E) A triquetrolunate ligament injury is present. The patient should be immobilized and a hand specialist consulted emergently.

13-7. Which of the following is considered gold standard to diagnose a scaphoid fracture in which initial plain films are negative?

(A) Computed tomography of the carpal bones

(B) Bone scan 14 days postinjury

(C) Magnetic resonance imaging

(D) Plain film series of the wrist and hand 14 days postinjury

(E) Plain film series of the wrist and hand with dedicated scaphoid views postinjury

13-8. A 35-year-old man fell while snowboarding and injured his right wrist. He presents to the ED 2 days after the initial injury complaining of pain with movement and swelling over the wrist. He has pain with axial loading of the thumb, and pain with palpation over the anatomic snuffbox. An x-ray of the wrist is obtained (see Figure 13-3). Which of the following is TRUE?

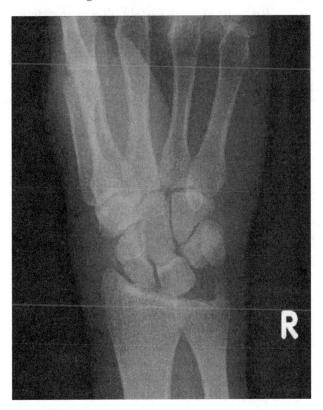

Figure 13-3. Used with permission from C. Hargis.

(A) Left untreated, a scaphoid fracture may develop avascular necrosis of the distal segment that may lead to severe arthritis.

(B) The blood supply to the scaphoid is in the distal segment of bone, and flow from branches of the median and ulnar arteries may be compromised with a fracture and cause avascular necrosis of the proximal segment.

(C) The risk of developing avascular necrosis increases, the more proximal, oblique, or displaced the fracture is.

(D) A scaphoid fracture is considered unstable once there is a minimum of 3 mm of displacement.

(E) Possible complications of untreated scaphoid fractures include avascular necrosis, degenerative arthritis, and carpal tunnel syndrome.

13-9. A radiograph of the wrist that demonstrates volar and proximal displacement of a large fragment of radial articular surface, volar displacement of the carpus, and a radial styloid fracture is most consistent with a:

(A) Barton fracture

(B) Colles fracture

(C) Galeazzi fracture-dislocation

(D) Monteggia fracture-dislocation

(E) Smith fracture

13-10. A 23-year-old man presents after falling while skateboarding. An x-ray is obtained (Figure 13-4). Which of the following is most accurate?

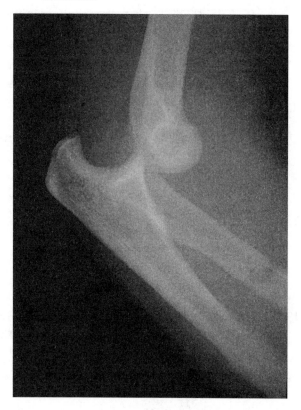

Figure 13-4.

(A) The dislocation is anterior, and possible complications include fractures of the coronoid process, radial head, medial epicondyle, and olecranon.

(B) The dislocation is anterior, and there should be a careful assessment of the brachial artery as well as ulnar, radial, and median nerves.

(C) The dislocation is anterior, and the patient will present with the elbow in 90 degrees of flexion.

(D) The dislocation is posterior. The ulnar nerve and brachial artery are the most frequently injured nerve and vascular structures injured in elbow dislocations.

(E) The dislocation is posterior. Approximately 50% of elbow dislocations are posterolateral.

13-11. Which best describes the injury seen in this radiograph (Figure 13-5)?

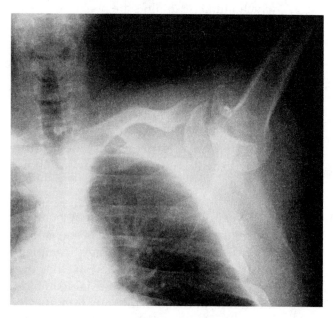

Figure 13-5. Used with permission from Rockford Health System.

(A) Anterior shoulder dislocation

(B) Inferior posterior shoulder dislocation

(C) Luxatio erecta dislocation

(D) Posterior shoulder dislocation

(E) Superior shoulder dislocation

13-12. The patient with the injury seen in the x-ray most likely had which of the following presentations (Figure 13-6)?

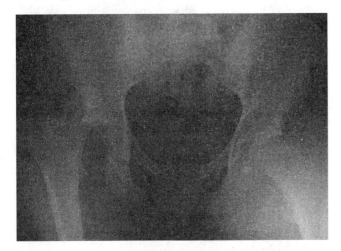

Figure 13-6. Used with permission from Truman Medical Center, Kansas City, MO.

(A) Fell from a 12-ft ladder.

(B) Occurred when the patient's hip was flexed, abducted, and externally rotated.

(C) On physical exam, the affected lower extremity flexed, abducted, and externally rotated.

(D) The front seat passenger was in a high-speed motor vehicle collision.

(E) Was caused by direct force posteriorly to a fully extended hip.

13-13. A 35-year-old woman injured her right ankle when she fell while performing a clown routine. She is unable to walk and in extreme pain. Her ankle appears obviously deformed, and an ankle dislocation is suspected. Which of the following is most accurate?

(A) Anterior is the most common type of ankle dislocation and is caused by force on the dorsiflexed foot.

(B) Anterior is the most common type of ankle dislocation and is associated with fracture of one or both malleoli.

(C) Lateral dislocation causes rupture of the talofibular ligaments or a lateral malleolus fracture.

(D) Posterior is the most common type of ankle dislocation and is caused by backward force on a plantar flexed foot.

(E) Posterior is the most common type of ankle dislocation and is caused by force on a dorsiflexed foot.

13-14. A 32-year-old woman is brought to the ED; her leg is injured by falling debris in an earthquake. The extremity is obviously deformed, and there is a 10-cm laceration overlying the fracture site. The following radiograph is obtained (Figure 13-7). Which of the following is most accurate?

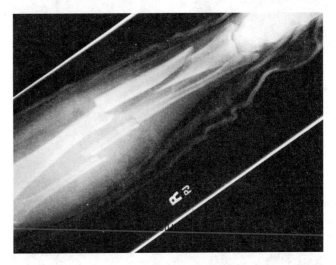

Figure 13-7.

(A) Compartment syndrome is not a concern because the fracture is open.

(B) The fracture pattern and laceration size make this injury a Gustilo Grade 1 injury.

(C) This injury is at increased risk of malunion/nonunion.

(D) This injury may be treated with copious irrigation in the ED and prompt casting.

(E) This injury is likely the result of large rotational forces.

13-15. A 6-year-old boy presents to the ED after falling from the play structure at school. He complains of right arm and elbow pain. The elbow is tender and edematous, and there is a depression proximal to the elbow. A radiograph is obtained (see Figure 13-8). Which of the following is true regarding this injury?

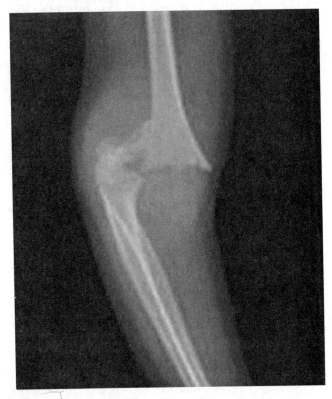

Figure 13-8. Reproduced with permission from Tintinalli JE, Stapczynski JS, Ma OJ, Cline DM, Cydulka RK, Meckler GD: *Tintinalli's Emergency Medicine: A Comprehensive Study Guide*, 7th Edition. Copyright © 2011 The McGraw-Hill Companies, Inc.

(A) Anterior interosseous nerve function should be tested in this injury by assessing sensation over the dorsolateral forearm.

(B) Compartment syndrome of the forearm from a supracondylar fracture should be suspected in the child who will not open their hand, has tenderness with passive finger extension, and has tenderness in the forearm.

(C) The incidence of anterior interosseous injuries is much lower than ulnar nerve injuries in association with supracondylar fractures.

(D) The incidence of neurologic complications approaches 40% in supracondylar fractures.

(E) The most serious complication is Volkmann ischemic contracture, which may be diagnosed by the absence of the radial pulse.

13-16. A 28-year-old man is involved in a moderate speed motorcycle accident. His radiographs reveal a fracture of the proximal third of the ulna with radial head dislocation. This injury is called a:

(A) Essex-Lopresti lesion

(B) Galeazzi-Fracture dislocation

(C) Monteggia fracture dislocation

(D) Nightstick fracture

(E) Reverse Monteggia fracture

13-17. A 60-year-old man is involved in a high-speed motor vehicle collision. He complains of severe pain at the right sternoclavicular joint. The pain is worsened with movement of the right arm as well as lying on his back. On physical examination of this patient, the medial end of the right clavicle is difficult to palpate and appears asymmetric compared with the left. Which of the following is most accurate?

(A) Anterior sternoclavicular dislocation is highly likely, and the patient should be imaged with computed tomography and intravenous contrast.

(B) Anterior sternoclavicular dislocation is highly likely, and the patient may be discharged without attempted reduction.

(C) Posterior sternoclavicular dislocation should be suspected, and complications may include severe injuries to mediastinal injuries and pneumothorax.

(D) Posterior sternoclavicular dislocation should be suspected, and immediate reduction attempted in the ED.

(E) Routine radiographs are the imaging modality of choice and considered gold standard for both anterior and posterior sternoclavicular dislocations.

13-18. Which of the following is true regarding complications of shoulder dislocations?

(A) Associated bony lesions include the Bankart lesion, which is a fracture of the anterior glenoid lip.

(B) Associated bony lesions include the Bankart lesion, which is a fracture of the coracoid.

(C) Associated bony lesions include the Bankart lesion, which is a compression fracture of the humeral head.

(D) Associated bony lesions include the Hill-Sachs deformity, which is a fracture of the anterior lip of the glenoid labrum.

(E) Associated bony lesions include the Hill-Sachs deformity, which is a compression fracture of the acromion.

13-19. A 35-year-old woman twisted her knee while playing soccer. She complains that her "knee cap feels out of joint." Which of the following is most accurate?

(A) Accompanying soft-tissue injury rarely occurs in patella dislocations.

(B) Recurrent dislocation may be expected in 40% of patients with patella dislocation, and all patients should be referred to an orthopedic specialist within 10 days.

(C) Reduction should be accomplished with procedural sedation followed by extending the hip, flexing the knee, and sliding the patella back in place.

(D) The dislocation is most likely to be lateral, and may be reduced with flexion of the hip, hyperextension of the knee, and sliding the patella back in place.

(E) The dislocation is most likely to be medial, and can easily be reduced with almost immediate relief of pain.

13-20. A 20-year-old motorcycle rider is brought to the ED after a crash. He complains of severe pain in his left knee. On physical examination, the knee is grossly swollen, exquisitely tender with range of motion, and a moderate knee effusion is palpable. On plain film, a tibial plateau fracture is present. Which of the following is most accurate?

(A) Anterior cruciate and medial collateral ligament injuries are associated with lateral plateau fractures.

(B) Anterior cruciate and medical collateral ligament injuries are associated with medial plateau fractures.

(C) Ligamentous instability is present in the majority of patients with a tibial plateau fracture.

(D) Posterior cruciate and lateral collateral ligament injuries are associated with lateral plateau fractures.

(E) Posterior cruciate and medial collateral ligament injuries are associated with lateral plateau fractures.

13-21. A 45-year-old man presents to the ED complaining of sudden pain in his right calf and ankle while playing basketball yesterday. He is now unable to run, and has trouble climbing the stairs in his house. Physical examination reveals some calf swelling and a palpable gap in the Achilles tendon 4 cm from the calcaneus. Which of the following is true?

(A) Risk factors for Achilles tendon rupture include prior macrolide antibiotic use, younger age, and prior steroid use.

(B) The diagnosis of Achilles tendon rupture cannot be made without radiographs.

(C) The Thompson test is diagnostic of Achilles tendon rupture when squeezing the patient's calf results in plantar flexion of the foot.

(D) The vascular supply of the Achilles tendon is close to the insertion on the calcaneus, and this is the weakest portion of the tendon.

(E) Ultrasound and magnetic resonance imaging maybe useful in cases where the diagnosis is not clear.

13-22. In the ankle, the lateral ligament complex consists of the lateral malleolus, which attaches to the anterior and posterior aspects of the talus and calcaneus by several ligaments. Which ligament is the weakest and most prone to injury?

    (A) Anterior talofibular ligament

    (B) Calcaneofibular ligament

    (C) Medial collateral ligament

    (D) Medial deltoid ligament

    (E) Posterior talofibular ligament

13-23. A 25-year-old man is involved in a high-speed motor vehicle collision. He sustains a left mid-shaft displaced femur fracture. The left leg appears foreshortened, and the man is in extreme pain from his injury. Which of the following is a contraindication to placing this patient's leg in traction?

    (A) Evidence of sciatic nerve damage

    (B) Evidence of vascular injury

    (C) Fracture is highly comminuted

    (D) Fracture occurred more than 6 hours ago

    (E) Severe pain not controlled with parenteral analgesia

13-24. Which of the following is recommended in the hemodynamically unstable patient with pelvic fracture in whom intra-abdominal causes of bleeding were excluded?

    (A) Computed tomography without intravenous contrast

    (B) Magnetic resonance imaging with gadolinium

    (C) Pelvic angiography

    (D) Pelvic ultrasound

    (E) Tagged red blood cell scan

13-25. A 22-year-old man fell during a volleyball game. He presented to the ED complaining of left fifth digit pain, deformity, and decreased range of motion. The following radiograph was obtained (Figure 13-9). Which of the following is most accurate regarding this injury?

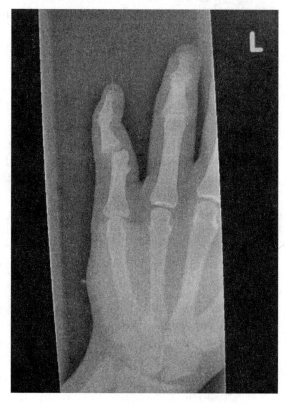

Figure 13-9.

    (A) Complete ligamentous disruption should be treated with immobilization at 30 degrees for 6–8 weeks.

    (B) The finger is most frequently ulnar deviated because the radial collateral ligament is much more likely to rupture than the ulnar collateral ligament.

    (C) This is a common hand injury and is usually the result of axial loading and hyperflexion.

    (D) Palmar dislocation occurs when the volar plate ruptures.

    (E) Volar dislocations are common.

13-26. A 26-year-old jockey is thrown from his horse during a race and presents to the ED as a trauma activation. Physical examination of the patient reveals soft-tissue swelling and bruising around the right arm and shoulder. He has diminished pulses in the distal right arm, as well as decreased motor and sensory function in the extremity. A portable chest x-ray is obtained, and lateral displacement of the right scapula is noted. Which of the following injuries is most likely?

(A) Anterior shoulder dislocation
(B) Distal clavicle fracture
(C) Humeral head fracture
(D) Luxatio erecta
(E) Scapulothoracic dislocation

Orthopedic Emergencies
Answers and Explanations

13-1. **The answer is E** (Chapters 47 and 265). Tendon injuries, both partial and complete, can be difficult to diagnose. The extensors of the hand are connected by junctura. Consequently, a complete tendon laceration proximal to the junctura may occur, but extensor function seems intact. Further, as much as 90% of a tendon may be lacerated before there is a decrease in range of motion without resistance. For this reason, it is crucial to test the extensors against resistance. Pain along the course of the tendon is also indicative of tendon injury, and can also be elicited with strength testing against resistance. Direct visualization of the tendon injury is ideal but not always possible. If the tendon is lacerated while the fingers are flexed, the cut end of the end of the tendon will retract once the hand is extended, thereby making it difficult to identify. Inability to visualize one end of the tendon indicates that the tendon laceration is most likely complete.

13-2. **The answer is C** (Chapters 47 and 265). Mallet finger is the injury resulting from laceration or rupture of the extensor tendon over Zone I, the distal phalanx, or distal interphalangeal joint. This injury causes the distal interphalangeal joint to be flexed at 40 degrees. It is the most common tendon injury in athletes. Swan neck deformity may result from chronic untreated Mallet finger. Boutonniere deformity results from an injury in Zone III over the proximal interphalangeal joint. Injury of the central tendon and disruption of the lateral bands allow flexion as well as the flexor digitorum profundus to function unopposed. There is retraction of the extensor hood and resultant extension of the metacarpophalangeal and distal interphalangeal joints. Gamekeeper's thumb is the rupture of the ulnar collateral ligament. This occurs as the result of radial deviation of the metacarpophalangeal joint.

13-3. **The answer is A** (Chapter 265). The x-ray demonstrates a Bennett fracture, an intra-articular fracture of the thumb metacarpal with associated subluxation or dislocation of the carpometacarpal joint. Rolando fractures occur through a similar mechanism to Bennett fractures—impaction from striking an object, but are less common. A Rolando fracture refers to a comminuted intra-articular fracture at the base of the metacarpal. Skier thumb is also known as Gamekeeper's thumb, rupture of the ulnar collateral ligament. The Space of Poirier is the area between the two palmar arches at the junction of the capitate and lunate. Destot sign is a hematoma over the inguinal ligament that may be seen in the setting of pelvic fracture.

13-4. **The answer is B** (Chapter 265). High-pressure injection injuries are a surgical emergency. The injection site itself may soon after the injury be quite unimpressive. However, these injuries can be devastating, leading to compartment syndrome, necrosis, and widespread infection. Material injected through a fingertip may be found up in the forearm. Amputation rates as high as 30% are reported with injection injuries. The materials injected are usually highly irritating, and this worsens the inflammatory response.

Treatment of injection injuries must be early and aggressive. In the ED, it is crucial to recognize these injuries, immobilize and elevate the affected limb, initiate broad-spectrum antibiotics, administer tetanus prophylaxis, and facilitate the patient going to the operating room for wide debridement.

13-5. **The answer is B** (Chapter 266). The scapholunate ligament is the most commonly injured ligament in the wrist, usually the result of a fall on an outstretched hand. The scapholunate ligament is an intrinsic ligament binding the scaphoid and lunate together between the proximal and distal rows of carpal bones. Scapholunate dissociation is diagnosed radiographically with a widening of the scapholunate space greater than 3 mm. This is also known as the Terry Thomas sign. Injuries to the triquetrolunate ligament are less common, and usually result from a fall onto an outstretched and dorsiflexed hand. This injury may produce pain on the ulnar aspect of the wrist and can be confused with injury to the triangular fibrocartilage complex. The Space of Poirier refers to the area between the two palmar arches at the junction of the capitate and lunate, and is vulnerable to ligamentous disruption.

13-6. **The answer is A** (Chapter 266). This x-ray demonstrates a lunate dislocation. Best seen on the lateral x-ray, the lunate has lost its relationship with the distal radius and is displaced toward the palm of the hand. This is the "spilled tea cup" or "piece of pie" appearance. Drawing a line from the second metacarpal through to the distal radius, the lunate appears offset. In contrast, in a perilunate dislocation, the lunate will maintain its relationship with the distal radius. The capitate and other carpals will appear dorsal to the lunate. Both injuries are true orthopedic emergencies and require immediate consultation. A scapholunate dislocation is best seen on the AP view and does not require immediate attention. Triquetrolunate ligament injuries may be difficult to diagnose and may appear normal on x-ray.

13-7. **The answer is C** (Chapter 266). Initial radiographs of scaphoid injuries may be negative in up to 10% of instances. Therefore, clinical exam and a high degree of suspicion are both crucial. Initial imaging with plain films is standard. Specialized scaphoid views provide visualization of the scaphoid bone in a lengthwise orientation, and may increase the ability to see subtle fractures. Delayed repeat films are not considered gold standard but rather MRI. Computed tomography is not commonly utilized with this particular injury.

13-8. **The answer is C** (Chapter 266). Two-thirds of the surface of the scaphoid is articular, and any compromise in blood flow can result in avascular necrosis and subsequent degenerative arthritis. The vascular supply to the scaphoid consists of small perforators from the radial artery, palmar, and superficial arteries. The blood supply enters through the distal segment of the scaphoid, and if it is disrupted by fracture, the proximal segment loses its blood supply and can develop avascular necrosis. Fractures are considered unstable with as little as 1 mm of displacement. Comminuted fractures and fractures with any component of rotational deformity are also considered unstable. Unstable fractures are much more likely to cause disruption to the blood flow. Therefore, early immobilization and operative intervention for unstable fractures are crucial.

13-9. **The answer is A** (Chapter 266). This description best describes a Barton fracture. A Colles fracture involves dorsal angulation of the distal radius; the distal radius fragment is displaced proximally and dorsally. Colles fractures have radial displacement of the carpus, and the ulnar styloid may be fractured. Unlike the Colles, the Smith fracture has volar angulation of the distal radius, and the fragment is displaced proximally and volar. The fracture typically extends in an oblique fashion from the dorsal surface 1–2 cm proximal to the articular surface. Galeazzi and Monteggia injuries are fracture dislocations of both of the forearm bones.

13-10. **The answer is D** (Chapter 267). This x-ray demonstrates a posterior elbow dislocation. Elbow dislocations may present as posterior, anterior, medial, lateral and divergent, or a combination. Of these types, posterolateral dislocation is the most common (approximately 90%). Fractures of the coronoid, radial head, medial epicondyle, and olecranon may occur with the dislocation. However, accompanying neurovascular injuries are the most devastating complication of elbow dislocation. The ulnar nerve is the most frequently injured nerve, and the brachial artery is the most frequently injured vessel. Fall on an outstretched hand is the most common mechanism, and patients usually present with their arm held flexed at 45 degrees.

13-11. **The answer is C** (Chapter 268). This x-ray demonstrates a posterior shoulder dislocation also called a luxatio erecta. Inferior dislocation results from forced hyperabduction, and is frequently associated with soft-tissue damage and fractures. Anterior shoulder dislocations are most common. Posterior and superior dislocations are very rare.

13-12. **The answer is D** (Chapter 270). The patient in this film has sustained a posterior hip dislocation. This is a high-energy mechanism where force is directed posteriorly to a flexed hip. High-speed motor vehicle accidents are the most common cause of posterior hip dislocations. Patients typically present with the hip shortened and internally rotated. Patients with anterior hip dislocation present with the hip flexed, abducted, and externally rotated.

13-13. **The answer is D** (Chapter 273). Posterior ankle dislocations are caused by backward force on a plantar flexed foot and are the most common type of ankle dislocation. Posterior ankle dislocations usually rupture the talofibular ligaments and are also commonly seen with a lateral malleolus fracture. Anterior dislocations are less common, and the result of force on a dorsiflexed foot. There is frequently an associated anterior tibial fracture.

13-14. **The answer is C** (Chapter 272). The x-ray demonstrates a comminuted tibia and fibula fracture. There is almost 50 degrees of translational displacement of the tibial shaft, and the fibula is in multiple segments. There is a large overlying tissue defect, making this injury, a Gustilo Grade 3 injury, the most severe in this scoring system. There are four compartments in the leg—all are vulnerable to such a high-energy mechanism. A break in soft tissue does not prevent development of a compartment syndrome. This injury is best managed with analgesia, gross decontamination, broad-spectrum intravenous antibiotics, and transfer to the operating room for definitive irrigation and open reduction internal fixation.

13-15. **The answer is B** (Chapter 267). Supracondylar fractures are the most common pediatric elbow fracture and have numerous serious complications. Displaced fractures require emergent reduction and orthopedic care, as well as careful neurovascular assessment and observation. The rate of neurovascular complications is reported as 7%. While the ulnar nerve is rarely injured, the anterior interosseous nerve (which arises from the median nerve) has a high incidence of injury. The anterior interosseous nerve does not have a sensory component and should be tested by flexion of the thumb interphalangeal joint and the index finger distal interphalangeal joint. Volkmann ischemic contracture refers to the associated compartment syndrome of the forearm. Radial pulse is unreliable in children in assessing this injury, as the artery frequently spasms. Other clinical signs including pain with palpation of the forearm and hand and pain with hand opening should also be assessed.

13-16. **The answer is C** (Chapter 267). Fracture of the proximal third of the ulna with a radial head dislocation is a Monteggia fracture dislocation. Fracture of the distal third of the radius with dislocation of the distal radioulnar joint is a Galeazzi fracture dislocation, or reverse Monteggia fracture. A nightstick fracture is an isolated ulna fracture usually the result of a singular direct blow. The Essex-Lopresti lesion refers to the disruption of the triangular fibrocartilage of the wrist and interosseous membrane in association with radial head fractures.

13-17. **The answer is C** (Chapter 268). This patient sustained a high-energy injury to the chest, and clinically appears to have a posterior sternoclavicular dislocation as the medial end of his clavicle is difficult to visualize and palpate. Computed tomography with intravenous contrast is the next best step to detect associated mediastinal and chest injuries including compression or laceration of the great vessels, trachea, and esophagus, as well as associated pneumothorax. Plain films are frequently inadequate to diagnose this injury. Posterior dislocations are difficult to reduce, and this procedure is performed in the operating room in consultation with a vascular surgeon. Anterior sternoclavicular dislocations are more common and have far fewer complications. These injuries can be safely discharged without reduction, as the injury has little impact on long-term function.

13-18. **The answer is A** (Chapter 268). Bony injuries are common complications of shoulder dislocations and may occur in up to 30% of shoulder dislocations. A Hill-Sachs deformity is a compression fracture of the humeral head. Fracture of the anterior glenoid lip is called a Bankart lesion. Other bony injuries include fractures to the greater tuberosity, coracoid, and acromion.

13-19. **The answer is D** (Chapter 271). Patella dislocation results from twisting an extended knee. The patella dislocates laterally in the majority of cases, and can be reduced by flexing the hip, extending the knee, and gently manipulating the patella back in place. Frequently, there is associated soft-tissue injury, and the patient should be placed in a knee immobilizer. Patients with dislocations other than lateral dislocation may be more difficult

to reduce in the ED and require orthopedic consultation and operative intervention. The rate of recurrent dislocation is approximately 15%.

13-20. **The answer is D** (Chapter 271). Tibial plateau fractures result from direct trauma to the knee, and there is ligamentous instability and injury in about one-third of patient. Fracture of the lateral tibial plateau is more common and is associated with injuries to the anterior cruciate and medial collateral ligaments. Medial plateau fractures are associated with posterior cruciate and lateral collateral ligaments.

13-21. **The answer is E** (Chapter 272). The Achilles tendon is the largest and strongest tendon in the human body. The insertion of the vascular supply is 2–6 cm proximal to the calcaneus, and this is where the majority of injuries occur. Risk factors include older age, infrequent or periodic strenuous exercise, prior fluoroquinolone antibiotic use, and prior steroid use. Achilles tendon ruptures can often be diagnosed clinically without x-rays by palpating the defect in the tendon 2–6 cm above the calcaneus in the setting of a suspicious mechanism. Patients usually complain of pain with walking and running, and inability to climb stairs. The Thompson test is performed by having the patient lie prone with the affected leg flexed to 90 degrees. The calf is then squeezed. An intact Achilles tendon will transmit the force and plantarflex the foot. If the tendon is ruptured, the foot will not move. Ultrasound and magnetic resonance imaging are indicated in cases where the diagnosis is not obvious.

13-22. **The answer is A** (Chapter 273). The ankle is stabilized by three groups of ligaments: the medial deltoid ligament, the lateral ligament complex, and the syndesmosis. The medial deltoid ligament is also called the medial collateral ligament and is the strongest of all the ligaments. The lateral ligament complex is made up of the anterior talofibular ligament, the posterior talofibular ligament, and the calcaneofibular ligament. The anterior talofibular ligament is the weakest.

13-23. **The answer is A** (Chapter 270) Traction splints should be applied to most femur fractures at the time of injury. Traction can relieve pain as well as stabilize the fracture and reduce blood loss into the thigh compartment. However, traction is contraindicated if the fracture is open with the ends of the bone grossly contamination, or if there is evidence of sciatic nerve involvement. Traction may worsen the nerve injury. In this case, it is recommend to splint the extremity without applying traction.

13-24. **The answer is C** (Chapter 269). The pelvis is a highly vascular structure, and any injury where there are two breaks in the pelvic ring is considered unstable with the potential for displacement. Plain films are acceptable for initial survey in the hemodynamically stable patient, although computed tomography is more sensitive and considered gold standard for evaluating pelvic injuries. Contrast extravasation seen on computed tomography and the hemodynamically unstable patient with pelvic fracture are both indications for pelvic angiography.

13-25. **The answer is B** (Chapter 265). The injury in this x-ray shows a fracture dislocation of the proximal interphalangeal joint, a common injury resulting from axial loading and hyperextension. Lateral dislocations occur when there is rupture of the collateral ligaments and partial avulsion from the volar plate. Complete volar plate rupture occurs with dorsal not palmar dislocation. Digits will frequently be ulnar deviated because the radial collateral ligament ruptures six times more often than the ulnar collateral ligament.

13-26. **The answer is E** (Chapter 268). The physical exam and x-ray findings are most consistent with scapulothoracic dislocation. This injury occurs in the setting of severe trauma, and is the result of sudden traction to the upper extremity and shoulder girdle. Clinical signs include extensive swelling and bruising, and 90% of patients will have associated nerve and vessel damage, including axillary and subclavian artery injuries and brachial plexus injuries. The classic chest x-ray finding is lateral displacement of the scapula.

CHAPTER 14

Pediatrics
Questions

14-1. A 10-day-old, full-term boy presents with concern for blood in the diaper. Past medical history reveals a normal pregnancy and delivery, group B streptococcus negative, and jaundice noted on third day of life. Bilirubin level has decreased as well as yellow color of skin per mother. Infant is exclusively breast-fed and has been otherwise well, no fevers. Physical exam is normal. Upon inspection of the diaper in question, a red brick color is present. What is the most appropriate next step?

(A) Apt test
(B) Complete blood count (CBC) with pro-thrombin time (PT) and partial thrombo-plastin time (PTT)
(C) Full sepsis evaluation
(D) Reassurance
(E) Urinalysis and culture

14-2. A 3-day-old presents with respiratory rates in the 40s followed by periods of pauses in breathing lasting up to 5 seconds. Which additional exam finding would most likely be present?

(A) Bradycardia
(B) Change in muscle tone
(C) Cyanosis
(D) Fever
(E) No other findings

14-3. An infant is brought in for poor feeding and constipation. The child is afebrile with hoarse cry. Two noticeable findings on exam are a large anterior fontanelle and decreased body tone for age. What test is warranted?

(A) Barium enema
(B) Botulism toxin assay
(C) Rectal biopsy
(D) Sweat chloride test
(E) Thyroid studies

14-4. Which of the following is true regarding apnea in infants?

(A) Associated with periodic breathing
(B) Can occur with pertussis
(C) Defined as stoppage of breathing for >10 seconds
(D) More common in term versus premature infants
(E) Occurs in the later stages with respiratory syncytial virus (RSV) bronchiolitis

14-5. A 2-year-old boy with 1 week of upper respiratory infection presents with fever of 38.7°C. His left eye area has redness and swelling. The eyelids are edematous, but he can still open them and able to look around without difficulty. Aside from nasal discharge, the rest of the physical exam is normal. What is the next appropriate step?

(A) Admit for parental antibiotics
(B) Computed tomography (CT) of the orbit
(C) Prescribe 10-day course of amoxicillin–clavulanate
(D) Ophthalmology referral
(E) Recommend warm compresses along with topic antibiotic ointment

14-6. A 5-year-old boy brought in by his father after he dislodged one of his front teeth. Child was on a school field trip when he fell. At the time, the avulsed tooth could not be found, but a school official with the tooth in milk is on the way to the emergency department. Your exam is normal except for the missing left central incisor and a 5-mm nongapping tongue laceration. Your plan includes:

(A) CT scan of the face

(B) In-hospital dental consultation

(C) Follow-up with the dentist as an outpatient and no need for tooth reimplantation

(D) No intervention required for the tooth but you will repair the tongue laceration

(E) Reimplantation of the tooth once it arrives

14-7. A 9-month-old boy is brought in by his mother due to fever and decreased oral intake, although he has good urine production. The child has a mild upper respiratory infection over the past few days. On exam, he is playful, and breathing normally. Child has oral ulcers and the following extremity lesions. The rest of the exam is normal. Temperature is 39.2°C, heart rate 130, respiratory rate 27, and room air oxygen saturation is 99% (Figure 14-1). What is the most appropriate management?

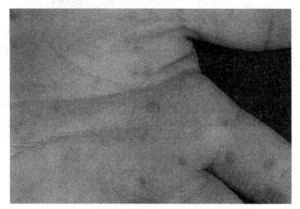

Figure 14-1. Reproduced with permission from Shah BR, Lucchesi M: *Atlas of Pediatric Emergency Medicine.* Copyright © 2006 The McGraw-Hill Companies, Inc.

(A) Antipyretics and supportive care measures

(B) CBC with differential and blood culture

(C) Intravenous normal saline fluids

(D) Oral acyclovir

(E) Undergo evaluation for Rocky Mountain spotted fever (RMSF) (*Rickettsia rickettsii*)

14-8. An 18-month-old girl brought in by mother due to neck mass. The area has increased in size over the past couple of days. The child has had no fever and does not appear to be bothered by the mass. Only finding is a painless, midline, 1-cm neck mass that moves with swallowing. There is fluctuance but no redness. Mother is frantic about possibility of cancer. What is the most likely diagnosis?

(A) Brachial cleft cyst

(B) Cystic hygroma

(C) Dermoid cyst

(D) Lymphadenitis

(E) Thyroglossal duct cyst

14-9. An 18-month-old boy presents with 2 days of runny nose and cough. Tonight he awoke with fever and difficulty breathing. Mother reports child has improved a little since leaving home. Temperature is 39.5°C, heart rate 180, respiratory rate 42, and room air oxygen saturations 95%. The child is awake, flushed, and breathing labored. He has inspiratory stridor and suprasternal retractions. Your initial management should be:

(A) Albuterol sulfate nebulized treatment

(B) CBC and blood culture

(C) Minimize patient agitation

(D) Racemic epinephrine nebulized treatment

(E) Soft-tissue neck radiograph

14-10. What is the most common cause of congenital stridor in children?

(A) Hemangioma

(B) Laryngomalacia

(C) Subglottic stenosis

(D) Vascular ring

(E) Vocal cord paralysis

14-11. What is the most common difference between a peritonsillar and retropharyngeal abscess?

(A) Presence of respiratory distress

(B) Age of child

(C) Dysphagia

(D) Presence of drooling

(E) Type of antibiotics for proper coverage

14-12. A 16-month-old boy referred by their physician after he ingested something 2 hours ago. Child has been acting well per father but keeps gagging when he takes a drink from his bottle. You evaluate the child and his exam is completely normal. A chest radiograph reveals abnormality (Figure 14-2). What is the appropriate management?

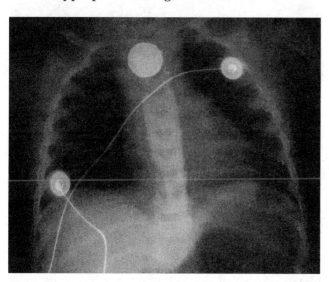

Figure 14-2. Reproduced with permission from Shah BR, Lucchesi M: *Atlas of Pediatric Emergency Medicine.* Copyright © 2006 The McGraw-Hill Companies, Inc.

(A) Admit for observation and repeat radiographs

(B) Consult surgery emergently

(C) Discharge with instructions to have follow-up radiograph in 1 day

(D) Pass feeding tube in an attempt to move object to stomach

(E) Repeat radiograph in 4–6 hours to see if the object passes to the stomach

14-13. An infant with unrepaired congenital heart disease is brought in by mother for cyanosis. Mother states she cannot recall the name of her child's condition but knows it starts with a "T." Child is usually pink but on occasion turns blue. Mother says oxygen sometimes helps but sometimes they have to put in an IV and give him medicine. What is this child's diagnosis?

(A) Tetralogy of Fallot (TOF)

(B) Total anomalous pulmonary venous return

(C) Transposition of the great arteries

(D) Tricuspid atresia

(E) Truncus arteriosus

14-14. A 10-day-old boy is brought in by his mother due to poor feeding and not looking right. The child is mottled, tachypneic, has a weak cry, and his body temperature is 35.8°C. You auscultate a harsh systolic murmur and have trouble finding femoral pulses. Which of the interventions can lead to further clinical deterioration?

(A) Broad-spectrum antibiotics

(B) Intravenous fluid (IVF) bolus with normal saline

(C) Prostaglandin E_1 intravenously

(D) Sodium bicarbonate intravenously

(E) Supplement oxygen therapy

14-15. You are evaluating a child for fever and rash. The 4-year-old has had 6 days of fever along with a rash involving the trunk and extremities. Also present are bilateral conjunctival injection without discharge and a 2-cm cervical lymphadenopathy. Which of the following would help confirm your suspicion?

(A) C-reactive protein (CRP), erythrocyte sedimentation rate (ESR), CBC, urinalysis

(B) CRP, ESR, antistreptolysin titer (ASO)

(C) CBC with differential

(D) Chest radiograph

(E) Ebstein–Barr virus titers

14-16. A 1-month-old boy is brought in by his teenage mother due to vomiting. Emesis has been nonbloody and nonbilious, but it has progressively increased over past week. Mother has attempted three different formulas without improvement. No reported fever or other pertinent finds on review of systems. On your exam, the child appears mildly dehydrated. Bedside glucose reads 72. IVF therapy is begun and the basic metabolic panel (BMP) reveals sodium 130, potassium 2.8, chloride 92, and bicarbonate 32. What test will confirm your suspicion for this etiology of this child's problems?

(A) Abdominal radiograph

(B) Abdominal ultrasound

(C) Cerebrospinal fluid (CSF) studies

(D) Milk protein allergy panel

(E) Upper gastrointestinal (GI) radiograph

14-17. Which of the following is least likely to be present in a 5-year-old child with the diagnosis of Henoch–Schönlein purpura (HSP)?

(A) Abdominal pain

(B) Hematuria

(C) Rash

(D) Refusal to bear weight

(E) Testicular torsion

14-18. A 14-month-old boy arrives to the emergency department with 1 day of nonbilious, nonbloody emesis. There is no fever, diarrhea, or rash. Parents report child will occasionally cry out in discomfort and that he is just not acting right. Child does attend daycare and there have been contacts with stomach flu. The child is tired appearing, nontoxic, and his abdomen has diminished bowel sounds, nondistended, no masses, but cries with palpation. Stool examination reveals no gross blood but is positive for occult blood. You obtain an abdominal radiograph (Figure 14-3). What is the most likely diagnosis?

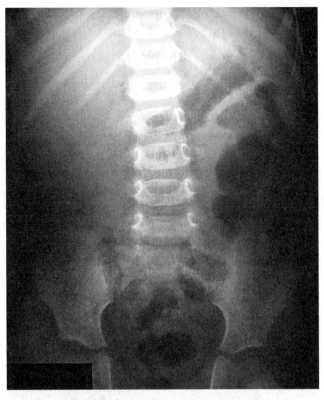

Figure 14-3. Reproduced with permission from Schwartz DT: *Emergency Radiology: Case Studies.* Copyright © 2008 The McGraw-Hill Companies, Inc.

(A) Constipation

(B) Gastroenteritis

(C) Intussusception

(D) Malrotation with volvulus

(E) Pneumatosis intestinalis

14-19. Which of the following would be the most common presentation for a urologic emergency in a 6-month-old boy?

(A) High-flow priapism

(B) Hydrocele

(C) Testicular torsion

(D) Tourniquet syndrome

(E) Varicocele

14-20. A 9-year-old girl is brought in by her grandmother while on Spring break for eyelid swelling. No complaints of eye drainage or pruritus. The child is well appearing with bilateral eyelid swelling and no conjunctival injection. You decide the most appropriate action is:

(A) Antimicrobial eye drops

(B) BMP

(C) Recommend over-the-counter antihistamine preparation

(D) Recommend cool compresses

(E) Urinalysis

14-21. An 11-year-old boy presents to the emergency department for vomiting and diarrhea with parental concern for dehydration. Stool was described as watery at onset but now is grossly bloody. Child appears moderately dehydrated, fecal occult blood positive, and rest of the physical exam unremarkable. You start an IVF bolus and send off stool studies. Her appearance improves with the IV fluids but her BMP reveals the following: sodium 131, potassium 4, bicarbonate 14, BUN 45, creatinine 1.5. Next appropriate step is:

(A) Check a CBC and urinalysis.

(B) Consult gastroenterologist for the hematochezia.

(C) Continue further IV fluid bolus.

(D) Discharge home with primary physician follow-up tomorrow.

(E) Empirically treat with antibiotics for infectious enteritis.

14-22. A 2-year-old girl brought in by emergency medical services (EMS) because of a seizure. Upon EMS arrival at the child's home, the seizure had stopped and the child was slowly returning to baseline. Mother states the child was shaking with her eyes rolled back for 2–3 minutes. Past few days, the child has been coughing with runny nose. In the emergency department, you evaluate an interactive child who is clinging to her mother's side. Her right tympanic membrane is red and bulging with yellow effusion. Vital signs reveal fever oth-

erwise normal. You determine the child had a simple febrile seizure and proceed to:

(A) Consult a pediatric neurologist

(B) Obtain a CBC, urinalysis, and cultures

(C) Order a head CT

(D) Prescribe course of amoxicillin and discharge home

(E) Refer child for an electroencephalogram (EEG)

14-23. An infant with DiGeorge syndrome presents with seizure activity. Which of the following would most likely help in stopping seizure?

(A) 3% sodium chloride

(B) 10% dextrose

(C) Calcium gluconate

(D) Fosphenytoin

(E) Magnesium sulfate

14-24. Which is the least likely finding in a child with intussusception?

(A) Abdominal pain

(B) Abdominal mass

(C) Altered mental status

(D) Currant jelly stool

(E) Vomiting

14-25. Refusal to bear weight in a 3-year-old boy can be due to various etiologies. Which of the following would not be a cause?

(A) HSP

(B) Legg–Calvé–Perthes disease

(C) Slipped capital femoral epiphysis (SCFE)

(D) Toddler's fracture

(E) Toxic synovitis

14-26. A 16-month-old boy who has been walking since 11 months of age presents with refusal to bear weight on his left leg. There has been no witnessed trauma. Child is cared for by parents, no other caregivers. You elicit pain with palpation over the mid-shaft of his tibia. Radiograph is shown in Figure 14-4. What is your next action?

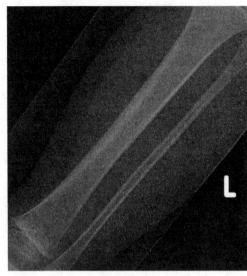

Figure 14-4. Used with permission from Wake Medical Center, Raleigh, NC.

(A) Contact the appropriate authorities due to concern of nonaccidental trauma

(B) Interview parents separately about nature of injury

(C) Skeletal survey

(D) Social worker consult

(E) Splint and refer to orthopedics as an outpatient

14-27. A 3-year-old boy presents with refusing to bear weight on his left leg. Parents state that the child awoke in this condition. No known trauma or recent activity to cause abnormality. Child has been well since getting over a cold last week. On exam, the child is afebrile, well appearing sitting in his mother's lap. The child guards with range of motion with the left hip and lifts his left leg when placed in standing position. The rest of the physical exam is normal. Radiographs of the hip is read as normal per radiologist; therefore, you obtain laboratory studies: white blood cell (WBC) count 8900, CRP <0.2, ESR 18 mm/hr. Next course of action is:

(A) Aspiration of the hip by interventional radiologist

(B) Bone scan pelvis

(C) Magnetic resonance imaging (MRI) of the hip

(D) Scheduled ibuprofen with primary medical doctor (PMD) follow-up

(E) Ultrasound of the hip

14-28. A child presents with abdominal and leg pain. Aside from the rash depicted below, he is well appearing (Figure 14-5).
Which laboratory study is most likely to aid in the management this patient?

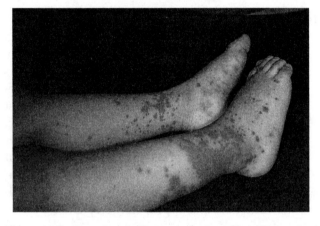

Figure 14-5. Reproduced with permission from Shah BR, Lucchesi M: *Atlas of Pediatric Emergency Medicine.* Copyright © 2006 The McGraw-Hill Companies, Inc.

(A) Blood culture

(B) Hemoglobin

(C) PT and PTT

(D) Platelet count

(E) Urinalysis

14-29. A 10-month-old African American girl brought in by her mother for hand abnormality. She became progressively fussy when mother noted bilateral hand swelling. No fevers or known trauma. Which of the following would be most useful in confirming the diagnosis?

(A) CBC with differential

(B) ESR

(C) Radiograph of the hands

(D) Renal function panel

(E) Serum albumin

14-30. A 5-year-old boy with hemophilia A fell from counter top in kitchen 2 hours prior to arrival. He has vomited once since the event. Mother reports the child is acting normal. The child has a small hematoma to the right forehead region and the physical exam is otherwise normal. Your next action is to:

(A) Admit for observation and factor IX infusion

(B) Intravenous factor replacement

(C) Obtain factor levels; if normal discharge home

(D) Obtain PT, PTT, platelet counts; if normal discharge home

(E) Send child for head CT

14-31. Rapid multidirectional eye movements along with involuntary extremity movements can be associated with which of the following oncologic condition?

(A) Brainstem glioma

(B) Hodgkin lymphoma

(C) Medulloblastoma

(D) Nephroblastoma

(E) Neuroblastoma

14-32. What is the most common presentation of retinoblastoma?

(A) Eye pain

(B) Leukocoria

(C) Strabismus

(D) Unilateral fixed pupil

(E) Visual loss

14-33. An 8-week-old, full-term infant is undergoing workup for a fever. Other than mild respiratory symptoms, the child appears well. You review all the result and the only thing that catches your eye is the hemoglobin of 9.2 g/dL. The child's parent asks why the hemoglobin is low. What is your explanation?

(A) Autoimmune hemolytic disorder

(B) Iron-deficient anemia

(C) Normal development

(D) Parvovirus B-19 infection

(E) Possible oncologic process

14-34. A 3-week-old boy presents with vomiting and lethargy. The infant is tachypneic and moderately dehydrated, remaining listless throughout the evaluation. The infant is intubated. A full sepsis workup is initiated. Laboratory analyses reveal elevated ammonia level. Of the following, which will be detrimental to the patient outcome?

(A) Arginine HCL 10% intravenously

(B) Continued IVF hydration with normal saline

(C) Mannitol for suspected cerebral edema

(D) Sodium benzoate intravenously

(E) Steroids intravenously for suspected cerebral edema

14-35. A child presenting with an acute crisis of their congenital adrenal hyperplasia (CAH) will likely have the following abnormality?

(A) Hypoglycemia with absence of urinary ketones

(B) Hypoglycemia with ketonuria

(C) Metabolic acidosis with hyperammonemia

(D) Metabolic acidosis with hypernatremia and hypokalemia

(E) Metabolic acidosis with hyponatremia and hyperkalemia

14-36. A 12-year-old boy arrives by EMS due to lethargy and dehydration. Parents report that he has been tired the past few days with increase thirst and going to the bathroom a lot. You appreciate a fruity odor to his breath along with tachypnea and dehydration. Diabetic ketoacidosis (DKA) is suspected. Bedside glucose reads as high. Venous blood gas has pH of 7.12 and HCO_3 of 8. You instruct the nurse that the priority is:

(A) Administer insulin subcutaneously

(B) Administer sodium bicarbonate

(C) IVF therapy

(D) Obtain serum ketone level

(E) Portable chest radiograph

14-37. Which of the following is NOT a risk factor for severity of illness in a dehydrated diabetic child?

(A) Acidosis in a type I diabetic

(B) Acidosis in a type II diabetic

(C) Age less than 5 years

(D) Hypernatremia

(E) Hyperosmolality

14-38. A 1½-year-old boy is brought in by EMS for seizure. The child is healthy with no chronic problems. Mother states child was playing when she took away a top in preparation for nap time. The child was sitting on the floor, cried, and then became cyanotic. This was followed by loss of body tone with brief shaking of extremities. The boy was back to baseline upon EMS arrival to house. After you determine the 18-month-old child has a normal exam, the next appropriate action is:

(A) EEG

(B) Head CT

(C) MRI of the brain

(D) Neurology consultation

(E) Reassurance

14-39. What is the most reliable indicator for severity of dehydration in an infant?

(A) Capillary refill time

(B) Mucous membrane appearance

(C) Sunken fontanelle

(D) Urine output

(E) Weight loss

14-40. An 8-month-old boy presents to the emergency department with 2 days of not feeding well. No fevers or other associated symptoms. Child's past medical history is unremarkable and no recent medications. Infant is alert, pink, and breathing unlabored but noticeable tachycardia. His temperature is 37.8°C and does not appear dehydrated. An ECG is obtained (Figure 14-6).

Which of the following interventions should be avoided?

(A) Adenosine

(B) Amiodarone

(C) Digoxin

(D) Synchronized cardioversion

(E) Vagal maneuvers

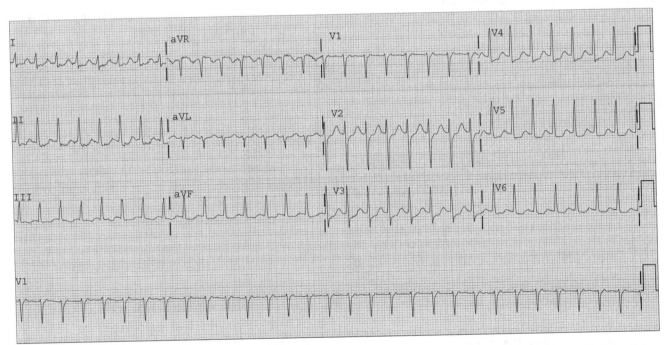

Figure 14-6. Reproduced with permission from Knoop KJ, Stack LB, Storrow AB, Thurman RJ: *The Atlas of Emergency Medicine*, 3rd Edition. Copyright © 2010 The McGraw-Hill Companies, Inc. ECG contributor: R. Jason Thurman, MD.

Pediatrics
Answers and Explanations

14-1. The answer is D (Chapters 111 and 125). A common cause for infants with red or orange appearance in their diapers is amorphous crystals. As breast milk supply increases, infant hydration improves and discoloration to the diaper resolves. Apt-Downey test can be performed if there is suspicion of swallowed maternal blood. Laboratory tests such as CBC, PT, PTT, urinalysis, and culture and sepsis evaluation are unnecessary in this well-appearing child with diaper findings.

14-2. The answer is E (Chapter 111). Periodic breathing of newborn is more common in premature infants but also seen in term infants. The infant will have periods of normal fast breathing followed by slowing of breathing and at times pauses of breathing for 3–10 seconds. This is due to immature regulatory centers of the infant. Normal respiratory rates range from 30 to 60 breaths/min. Bradycardia, cyanosis, fever, and change in muscle tone are concerning and not normal. These require further investigation.

14-3. The answer is E (Chapter 111). This child has classic findings of hypothyroidism, which could also include coarse facial features, hypothermia, and peripheral edema. Thyroid studies will help confirm diagnosis. Barium enema and rectal biopsy are studies indicated when undergoing evaluation for Hirschsprung disease. Diagnostic study will reveal absence of ganglion cell on biopsy. Sweat chloride test is useful with a workup in a child with suspected cystic fibrosis. A history of meconium ileus, poor weight gain, and constipation may be presenting findings. Infantile botulism can present with poor feeding, abnormal cry, decreased tone, constipation, and potential respiratory insufficiency.

14-4. The answer is B (Chapter 111). Apnea can occur early in infants with pertussis even without cough or nasal congestion. The definition of apnea is pauses in breathing greater than 20 seconds or apnea associated with pallor/cyanosis, decreased tone, or bradycardia. Periodic breathing of newborn is normal and described as rapid breathing followed by slowing of respirations and pauses lasting 3–10 seconds. Apnea of prematurity occurs in up to 25% of premature infants and usually outgrown by 37 weeks postconceptual age. Apnea can occur without symptoms in RSV as in pertussis. RSV can also be the result of obstructive apnea due to thick mucus production.

14-5. The answer is C (Chapter 115). Outpatient management with oral antibiotics is indicated with your diagnosis of periorbital cellulitis. Well-appearing children with no evidence of proptosis or pain with eye movement do not require a CT scan of the orbits. Failure of outpatient management with oral antibiotics or development of orbital cellulitis warrants parental antibiotics as well as an ophthalmology consult. Topical antibiotic would be helpful for a conjunctivitis but not in periorbital cellulitis.

14-6. The answer is C (Chapter 117). Since it is a primary tooth, you could cause damage to the future permanent tooth if reimplanted. No need for emergent dental consultation, since this can be followed up in the dental office. CT scan is unnecessary due to mechanism of injury and absence of clinical findings. Ionizing radiation exposure outweighs benefit. Oral lacerations heal remarkably well and tongue lacerations generally do not require primary closure.

14-7. **The answer is A** (Chapter 117). Antipyretics and supportive care measures are the usual management strategies for hand–foot–mouth disease. Coxsackie virus has been found to be the main pathogen and the illness is typically self-limited. Laboratory studies are not necessary in the majority of cases unless dehydration is present. IVFs are required only if signs of dehydration were present: ill appearance, sticky mucus membranes, poor urine output, or delayed capillary refill. RMSF is unlikely due to the presence of classic oral lesions, the absence of petechial rash, and appearance of child. Acyclovir not indicated for treating coxsackie and for most cases of herpes virus infections in the immune-competent individuals.

14-8. **The answer is E** (Chapter 118). Thyroglossal duct cyst is the most common midline neck mass in children. They are usually surgically excised but at times do require antibiotics for acute infections. These are distinguished from dermoid cyst by movement with swallowing or tongue protrusion. Branchial cleft cysts are not midline and usually nontender, round, and mobile masses if not infected. Cystic hygromas of the neck arise along the jugular chain of the lymphatics and are large, painless, compressible masses. Lymphadenitis can vary in size but is generally tender and nonmidline.

14-9. **The answer is D** (Chapter 119). Croup is the most common cause for stridor in children older than 6 months. Most common pathogen is the parainfluenza virus but others such as RSV and human bocavirus can be infectious etiologies. Initial management of stridor at rest causing distress is racemic epinephrine nebulization. This can aide in airway edema reduction from its vasoconstrictor effects. Albuterol nebulization is not indicated and may worsen situation by vasodilatation of vascular beta-receptors. Laboratory studies are unnecessary as these are viral process with clinical diagnosis. Soft-tissue radiography is not indicated for initial management but may be useful if patient has atypical response to routine croup treatments. Minimizing agitation may be of some benefit but will not reduce respiratory distress significantly in children with moderate-to-severe croup.

14-10. **The answer is B** (Chapter 119). Laryngomalacia accounts for 60% of congenital stridor and is due to developmentally immature cartilaginous structures of the epiglottis, aryepiglottic folds, and arytenoids. The condition usually self-resolves as the child grows. Vocal cord paralysis can be congenital or acquired and unilateral or bilateral. Subglottic stenosis may also be congenital or acquired and will usually resolve by a few years of age. Hemangiomas cause congenital stridor when involved in the airway. It becomes noticeable as it grows during the first year of life. Suspicion of hemangioma arises with finding of other hemangiomas on the surface of the skin. A rare but concerning cause of congenital stridor is vascular rings, which require comprehensive imaging for diagnosis.

14-11. **The answer is B** (Chapter 119). Retropharyngeal abscess occurs in young children, whereas peritonsillar abscess is more common in adolescence. The lymph nodes that cause suppurative infections in the retropharyngeal space usually resolve by the age of 4 years. Both types of infections can be polymicrobial and include staphylococcal, streptococcal species, as well as oral anaerobes. Coverage of antibiotics for the treatment of the two types of illness includes clindamycin and/or ampicillin–sulbactam (amoxicillin–clavulanate). Both illnesses can present with fever, dysphagia, drooling. Peritonsillar abscess usually has a bulging tonsil with uvular deviation, whereas retropharyngeal abscess may have a bulging posterior oropharynx.

14-12. **The answer is B** (Chapter 119). The radiograph reveals a metallic circular object that can be easily confused with a coin (Figure 14-7). The outer ring is found in button batteries and requires surgical consultation for urgent removal. This can lead to erosion into local tissue structures and liquefaction necrosis. Prompt removal is necessary. Passing a feeding tube blindly is contraindicated due to potential for damaged structures. Choosing to wait and observe can increase morbidity and mortality.

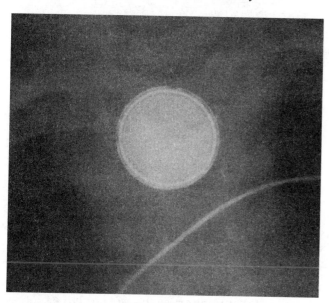

Figure 14-7. Reproduced with permission from Shah BR, Lucchesi M: *Atlas of Pediatric Emergency Medicine*. Copyright © 2006 The McGraw-Hill Companies, Inc.

14-13. **The answer is A** (Chapter 122 A). TOF is one of the cyanotic heart lesions that can also present "pink" without cyanosis. Structural abnormalities lead to mixing of deoxygenated and oxygenated blood that is circulated throughout the body. TOF has a large ventricular septal defect, right ventricular outflow tract obstruction, over-riding aorta, and right ventricular hypertrophy. The degree of right ventricular outflow obstruction dictates if the child will be cyanotic versus acyanotic. The infant described above has baseline left-to-right ventricular shunting of blood, but during a "Tet" spell, the shunting is reversed, right to left. This leads to cyanotic state. Maneuvers to increase preload, pro-

mote pulmonary vasodilatation, and increase afterload are recommended to terminate a Tet spell. Management options include 100% oxygen via non-rebreather mask, calming the child, flexing knees to chest, IVFs, and morphine sulfate. The other congenital heart conditions are all cyanotic.

14-14. **The answer is E** (Chapter 122 A). The child's presentation of shock, combined with the physical examination finding of a murmur, is highly suspicious for a congenital heart defect. The age of the child and presentation strongly suggest a ductal-dependent lesion. Although placement of 100% oxygen in a very sick infant is routine, in this case oxygen may actually lead to significant deterioration. Oxygen has vasoconstrictor effects on the ductus arteriosus and is a potent pulmonary vasodilator, which can inadvertently lead to decreased systemic perfusion. Maintaining patency of the ductus arteriosus is accomplished with prostaglandin E_1 intravenously. IVF administration needs to be closely monitored due to potential exacerbation of congestive heart failure. Sodium bicarbonate may help in cases of severe metabolic acidosis. Sepsis is always at the top of the differential diagnosis and coverage with broad-spectrum antibiotics can be potentially life saving.

14-15. **The answer is A** (Chapter 122 B). You suspect incomplete Kawasaki disease, which requires fever for 5 days and two to three of classic Kawasaki disease criteria (see Table 14-1). Laboratory criteria include CRP ≥3, ESR ≥40 mm/hr along with three or more laboratory findings: albumin <3 g/dL, anemia, elevated alanine transaminase, thrombocytosis, WBC count >12,000, or sterile pyuria. Chest radiograph would not add any additional information for diagnosis. Etiology of Kawasaki disease is unknown, so EBV titers are not useful in diagnosis.

14-16. **The answer is B** (Chapters 111, 123, and 125). The infant presents with the classic abnormalities associated with hypertrophic pyloric stenosis: hyponatremic, hypokalemic, and

TABLE 14-1. DIAGNOSTIC CRITERIA FOR KAWASAKI DISEASE

Classic Kawasaki Disease	Incomplete Kawasaki Disease
Fever for 5 days or more plus four of the following symptoms	Fever for 5 days and two to three clinical criteria of classic Kawasaki disease *plus*
	CRP $\geq$3.0 and/or ESR $\geq$40 mm/hr plus three or more of the following supplemental labs *or* positive echo
1. Bilateral nonexudative conjunctivitis	1. Albumin <3 g/dL
2. Mucus membrane changes (erythema, peeling, cracking of lips, "strawberry tongue," or diffuse oropharyngeal mucosae)	2. Anemia for age
3. Changes of the extremities (erythema or swelling of hands/feet, peeling of finger tips/toes in the convalescent stage)	3. Elevated ALT
4. Rash (see text)	4. Platelets >450,000 after 7 days of fever onset
5. Cervical adenopathy (>1 node >1.5 cm unusually unilateral anterior cervical)	5. WBC >12,000
	6. Presence of pyuria

ALT, alanine transaminase; CRP, C-reactive protein; ESR, erythrocyte sedimentation rate; WBC, white blood cell.
Notes: Kawasaki disease: Irritability in an infant with Kawasaki disease. Note also the conjunctivitis and red, cracked lips. (Courtesy of Tomisaku Kawasaki, MD.)

hypochloremic metabolic alkalosis (HPS). HPS usually presents in the first month of life with progressive nonbilious emesis that is often reported as being projectile. Laboratory studies are not always abnormal due to earlier diagnosis with ultrasound. An olive-shaped mass below the liver may be felt on physical examination, but ultrasound is the diagnostic gold standard. CSF studies are not indicated due to history of present illness, absence of fever, and other physical exam findings. Abdominal radiograph would most likely reveal a nonspecific gas pattern and is not diagnostic standard for pyloric stenosis. Upper GI may be indicated if there is concern for other obstructive processes such as malrotation. In malrotation, the emesis is more likely to be bilious. The emesis with HPS is always nonbilious. Milk protein allergy typically presents with vomiting and diarrhea and blood in stool.

14-17.   **The answer is E** (Chapter 124). HSP is a vasculitic process with unclear etiology. Children typically present with abdominal pain with or without rash. As disease progresses, rash evolves and can be ecchymotic, purpuric, petechial, or erythema multiforme. Lower extremity pain can be initial complaint from arthralgia or arthritis. Renal findings of HSP include microscopic hematuria, proteinuria, and hypertension. Testicular torsion is not a common finding in a patient with HSP, although testicular pain, scrotal pain, or edema may prompt an emergency department visit.

14-18.   **The answer is C** (Chapter 124). Intussusception can occur between 3 months and 6 years of age when there is telescoping of the intestine into itself. Location is classically ileocolic. Children develop intermittent colicky abdominal pain and appear well between episodes. As intervals increase, the child can appear very ill and sometimes lethargic. Vomiting presents as obstructive process persists. Currant jelly stool is a rare and late finding but commonly reported in textbooks. The radiograph reveals a filling defect on the right upper quadrant. Ultrasound is a useful imaging modality for diagnosis. Air contrast enema is diagnostic and can be therapeutic. Malrotation usually presents in a younger child, and abdominal distention, ill appearance, and bilious vomiting persist until obstruction corrected. Pneumatosis intestinalis is also more common in infants with necrotizing enterocolitis. Radiographic findings of air bubbles within the intestinal wall are seen with pneumatosis intestinalis. Gastroenteritis will have nonspecific findings but usually scattered air fluid levels. Constipation will have varying degrees of fecal retention.

14-19.   **The answer is D** (Chapter 127). Tourniquet syndrome of the penis usually is caused by hair and will lead to diminished tissue perfusion secondary to venous congestion. Removal of hair or thread by means of a depilatory agent or cutting is required. Testicular torsion is a urologic emergency but more common in the immediate neonatal period or early adolescence. High-flow priapism usually is a result of direct trauma and not a true urologic emergency due to nonischemic nature. Low-flow priapism (ischemic type) is a urologic emergency, usually seen with sickle cell anemia. Hydrocele and varicocele are nonemergent and may require elective surgical intervention.

14-20. **The answer is E** (Chapter 128). Urinalysis is an easy, noninvasive study for this child. Findings of proteinuria would indicate further testing to evaluate for nephrotic syndrome. Obtaining a CBC, complete metabolic panel, complement-3 level, complement-4 level, and antinuclear antibody will help the pediatric nephrologists manage the child as an outpatient. Conjunctival injection with or without drainage would require topical antimicrobial coverage but absent in this patient. BMP is not a first-line test; if the urinalysis is normal, then supportive care measures recommended such as cool compresses and over-the-counter antihistamine preparation for possible allergic component.

14-21. **The answer is A** (Chapter 128). These laboratory abnormalities could be the result of dehydration from infectious gastroenteritis, but further investigation is necessary to evaluate for hemolytic uremic syndrome (HUS). HUS is the most common cause for acute renal failure in children. Laboratory abnormalities will show anemia, thrombocytopenia, microscopic hematuria, hyponatremia, and hyperkalemia. Stool cultures need to be obtained with specific request for *Escherichia coli* O157:H7. Additional IVF resuscitation not indicated once hypovolemia corrected due to potential iatrogenic fluid overload. Antibiotics could increase risk of HUS and are not recommended empirically in a child with diarrheal illness. All children

with a diagnosis of HUS will require inpatient management.

14-22. **The answer is D** (Chapter 129). Findings consistent with simple febrile seizure require reassurance with supportive care measures and antibiotic for the child's otitis media. If a focal seizure, abnormal neurologic exam, and prolonged seizure, then neuroimaging may be part of the patient's evaluation. American Academy of Pediatrics does not recommend blood studies, neuroimaging, or EEG for simple febrile seizures. The primary care provider can follow up the child without the involvement of a neurologist for simple febrile seizures.

14-23. **The answer is C** (Chapters 122A and 129). DiGeorge syndrome is the result of chromosomal abnormality. These children have truncus arteriosus, midline facial abnormalities, hypoplastic thymus, and hypoparathyroidism. The infant would benefit most from intravenous calcium replacement to stop the seizure. Calcium gluconate is preferred over calcium chloride due to less irritating effects on the vein. Benzodiazepines can be attempted but usually not effective. Fosphenytoin would not stop the seizure and considered a second-line agent for infants and children with seizures. Hypoglycemia, hyponatremia, and hypomagnesemia are not likely causes for seizure activity in this child.

14-24. **The answer is D** (Chapters 124 and 131). Currant jelly stool is due to bowel ischemia and is a late finding with intussusception. Altered mental status can be the only presenting finding in up to 10% of cases. Other nonspecific symptoms such as vomiting and colicky abdominal pain along with a palpable mass are seen in children with intussusception.

14-25. **The answer is C** (Chapter 133). HSP classic presentation includes rash, abdominal pain, and arthralgias, which lead to pain with ambulation. This can occur between ages 2 and 11 years. Toxic (transient) synovitis is an inflammatory process of the hip with peak incidence between 3 and 6 years. Toddler fracture is an oblique nondisplaced fracture of the distal tibia seen in the toddler years. Legg–Calvé–Perthes disease is due to avascular necrosis of the femoral head and presents between 2 and 13 years of age. SCFE would not be a cause of weight bearing refusal in this child, because this condition is seen in adolescence.

14-26. **The answer is E** (Chapter 133). Toddler fracture is a unique injury in children. They are caused by rotational forces while the foot is planted and the knee flexed. Radiographs may be normal on initial presentation, but if repeated in a week, the abnormality is apparent. This spiral fracture of the tibia does not warrant suspicion of abuse unless other physical findings or fractures are present. Long leg posterior splint with orthopedic follow-up is the appropriate action.

14-27. **The answer is D** (Chapter 133). Nonsteroidal anti-inflammatory drugs with PMD follow-up is all that is needed for transient synovitis. A child with septic arthritis would likely appear ill, likely febrile, and have significant guarding with the hip exam. The CRP and WBC would be elevated in a septic joint. Ultrasound can show effusion in 50–95% of children with transient synovitis and is unnecessary in a well-appearing child with reassuring laboratory studies. Arthrocentesis is not indicated unless suspicion of septic joint. Bone scan and MRI may be useful if other diagnostic modalities and exam still question strong possibility of infectious etiology.

14-28. **The answer is E** (Chapter 134). The child is presenting with the most common vasculitic process in children, HSP. Reasons for emergency department visits are usually rash, abdominal pain, and joint discomfort. Other nonspecific complaints of nausea, vomiting, and diarrhea can be present but fever not typical. Urinalysis can reveal renal involvement with microscopic hematuria or proteinuria, which would prompt renal function studies. The classic appearance and lack of other exam findings make other conditions such as idiopathic thrombocytopenia, meningococcemia,

and sepsis unlikely. Therefore, hemoglobin, PT/PTT, and platelets would be normal and no additional management implications. Abnormal urine would require close follow-up with potential oral steroids and nephrology involvement.

14-29. **The answer is A** (Chapter 135). Dactylitis is a clinical presentation of a vaso-occlusive crisis in a child with sickle cell anemia. If febrile, they are typically low grade. CBC would reveal some degree of anemia depending on the type of sickle cell disease. There may be mild leukocytosis as well as sickling reported on peripheral smear. Hemoglobin electrophoresis would be gold standard for diagnosis, but would not alter management in the emergency department. ESR is nonspecific and unreliable in patients with sickle cell disease. If this was related to protein losing condition, other areas of swelling would be present and not just isolated hand edema. Hypoalbuminemia would cause edema but hand pain. Renal function panel would not have abnormalities specific to the vaso-occlusive crisis. The symmetry of hand swelling makes infection and trauma less likely.

14-30. **The answer is B** (Chapter 136). Intracranial bleed is the most common cause of death in a child with hemophilia. This child requires immediate factor VIII replacement at 100% correction. A head CT is to be obtained after factor infusion. Children with hemophilia A and B will have elevated PTT and normal PT and platelets. This information as well as factor level would provide no benefit in a hemophiliac after closed head injury. Waiting could delay possible life-saving intervention with factor replacement. Admission with scheduled factor VIII replacement may be necessary in a child with a small intracranial bleed and no current surgical intervention determined by neurosurgeon. Factor XI replacement is for a patient with hemophilia B (Christmas disease).

14-31. **The answer is E** (Chapter 136). Opsoclonus-myoclonus (dancing eyes–dancing feet) is highly suggestive of neuroblastoma due to effects of autoantibodies on the neural tissues. Neuroblastoma is the most common neoplasm in the first year of life. Hodgkin lymphoma presents with painless enlarging lymph node and/or identifying mediastinal mass on chest radiograph. Medulloblastoma and brainstem glioma are poster fossa tumors and usually present with signs of increased intracranial pressure (e.g., headache, vomiting) with or without ataxia. Nephroblastoma (Wilms tumor) presents with abdominal mass.

14-32. **The answer is B** (Chapter 136). Leukocoria, loss of the red reflex, is the most common presentation in retinoblastoma. The other complaints/findings can occur in retinoblastoma but not as common in the initial presentation. This intraocular malignancy is at times picked up by a caregiver when an absence of red eye on photography (Figure 14-8).

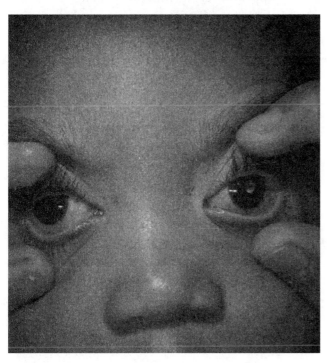

Figure 14-8. Reproduced with permission from Shah BR, Lucchesi M: *Atlas of Pediatric Emergency Medicine.* Copyright © 2006 The McGraw-Hill Companies, Inc.

14-33. **The answer is C** (Chapter 136). Physiologic nadir occurs around 6–9 weeks of age as fetal hemoglobin levels decrease and the adult form takes over. Normal hemoglobin ranges around 9–11 g/dL. No intervention is needed other than normal scheduled visits with the PMD. Iron-deficient anemia is not seen until 4–6 months of age when iron stores depleted. Iron deficiency is most commonly due to excessive whole milk intake. Parvovirus B-19 is classically described as fifths disease with slapped cheek rash appearance. If red cell aplasia were involved, the infant's hemoglobin would likely be lower and the child ill appearing. An infant with autoimmune hemolytic anemia would appear ill and anemia would be clinically evident before hemoglobin measured. The peripheral blood would have spherocytes and schistocytes. Oncologic process is unlikely with isolated cell line involvement and expected hemoglobin for age.

14-34. **The answer is E** (Chapter 137). With significantly elevated ammonia levels, a metabolic disorder is the likely cause of infant's encephalopathy. Continue aggressive hydration with normal saline after initial IVF boluses will help clear some of the toxic metabolites into the urine. Hypotonic fluid could exacerbate cerebral edema. Arginine HCL 10%, sodium benzoate, and sodium phenylacetate intravenous preparations help to reduce ammonia levels. Mannitol and steroids can be treatment options for cerebral edema, but steroids in this case are contraindicated. Steroids can potentially elevate ammonia levels.

14-35. **The answer is E** (Chapter 137). Classic findings from salt wasting CAH crisis include metabolic acidosis with hyponatremia and hyperkalemia. Hypoglycemia can be present but not always. This condition is due to a cortisol deficiency leading to hyperaldosteronism and resultant electrolyte abnormalities. Urea cycle, mitochondrial, respiratory chain, and fatty acid oxidation defects lead to metabolic acidosis with elevated ammonia levels. Hypoglycemia with absence of urinary ketones suggests fatty acid oxidation defect and hypoglycemia with ketonuria can be due to organic acidemias.

14-36. **The answer is C** (Chapter 139). If presenting in shock, 20 mL/kg IVF bolus with normal saline is indicated, but once patient and vital signs stabilize, correction of dehydration over 24–48 hours provides best outcomes. Sodium bicarbonate infusion is not recommended and can increase chances of cerebral edema in children with DKA. Insulin therapy is key to halting ketone production and acidosis after IVFs begun. Controlled correction is best achieved by regular insulin infusion at 0.1 units/kg per hour. Subcutaneous regular insulin can complicate management in children due to risk of decreasing glucose levels too quickly and hypokalemia. Serum ketone levels are not helpful for initial management of DKA. Severity of acidosis and hyperosmolar state would be more useful in assessing risk factors for cerebral edema. Portable chest radiograph is not indicated, since patient's tachypnea (Kussmaul breathing) is a response to his metabolic derangement.

14-37. **The answer is D** (Chapter 139). Sodium is depleted in the DKA state and hypernatremia is not a risk factor in determining potential severity of illness. In children presenting with DKA, about 1% will develop significant cerebral edema. Factors that place the child at increased risk for cerebral edema include age less than 5 years, severe acidosis, severe hyperosmolality, and persistent hyponatremia. An uncommon but worrisome condition is hyperglycemic, hyperosmolar nonketotic syndrome. This occurs in type II diabetic patients with severe electrolyte abnormalities and dehydration.

14-38. **The answer is E** (Chapter 140). Breath holding spells are very frightening but only require reassurance. They can occur as early as 6 months through toddler age. It is a neurally mediated event typically triggered by anger or frustration. When children cry, they hold their breath causing pallor or cyanosis followed by brief loss of body tone. Myoclonic jerks or seizure-like activity is sometimes seen. These are self-limited events. MRI brain and head CT would likely be normal and not give any additional information. Since this is related to syncopal event and not seizure, an EEG and neurology consult are not necessary.

14-39. **The answer is E** (Chapter 142). Preillness weight is the best way to determine degree of dehydration. This information is usually not available to the emergency physician. Using a variety of indicators together can help quantify degree of dehydration such as capillary refill time, urine output, mucous membrane appearance, and anterior fontanelle.

14-40. **The answer is C** (Chapter 143D). The ECG illustrates the classic delta wave associated with Wolff–Parkinson–White (WPW) syndrome. This patient is currently in supraventricular tachycardia. With the exception of digoxin, all of the options listed are considered safe and effective in the management of SVT in patients with WPW. Digoxin is contraindicated as it could lead to a lethal arrhythmia. In a stable child, vagal maneuvers are the first option followed by intravenous adenosine if unsuccessful. If no evidence of prolonged QTc, then amiodarone is another choice for SVT. Synchronized cardioversion (0.5 J/kg) is reserved for children with unstable SVT or those not responsive to medications.

CHAPTER 15

Prehospital Care and Disaster Preparedness
Questions

15-1. What is generally considered to be the weakest link of most disaster responses?

(A) Access to care
(B) Communications
(C) Documentation
(D) Personnel
(E) Transportation

15-2. Which piece of equipment is most important for survival from cardiac arrest?

(A) Cervical collar
(B) Defibrillator
(C) Intravenous catheter
(D) Laryngoscope
(E) Splint

15-3. Which part of a typical child needs the most padding to help maintain neutral neck position during cervical spine immobilization?

(A) Head
(B) Lumbar spine
(C) Neck
(D) Pelvis
(E) Shoulders

15-4. Which of the following factors, if present, would likely suggest the use of a ground emergency medical services (EMS) unit in preference to an air EMS unit?

(A) Bad weather
(B) Long transport distance

(C) Need for advanced airway procedure
(D) Obstetric patient
(E) Urban environment

15-5. In the United States, who is responsible for arranging an appropriate mode of transport for interfacility transfers?

(A) Charge nurse
(B) Hospital administrator
(C) Primary care provider
(D) Receiving physician
(E) Referring physician

15-6. What is the first therapy for infant respiratory distress syndrome?

(A) Albuterol
(B) Continuous positive airway pressure
(C) Epinephrine
(D) Intubation
(E) Surfactant

15-7. What is the preferred therapy for hyponatremia in athletes during prolonged events?

(A) Hypertonic saline intravenously
(B) Magnesium orally
(C) Normal saline intravenously
(D) Oral rehydration
(E) Salt tablets

15-8. What is the key defining characteristic of a disaster?

(A) Location

(B) Mismatch between available and required resources

(C) Number of patients

(D) Types of injuries involved

(E) Use of chemical, biological, or radiological agents

15-9. What is the main goal of triage during a disaster?

(A) Determine who needs comfort care rather than resuscitation

(B) Identify the sickest patients first

(C) Obtain primary insurance authorization for treatment

(D) Optimize individual patient outcome

(E) To do the most good for the most people

15-10. What deficit is uniformly present in postdisaster communities?

(A) Inability to access health care facilities

(B) Lack of clean water

(C) Limited law enforcement capability

(D) Loss of resources

(E) Poor access to prescription medications

15-11. Which of the following is frequently a major health threat in disaster-affected populations?

(A) Cadaver-transmitted infections

(B) Exacerbation of chronic diseases

(C) Malaria

(D) Tuberculosis

(E) Yellow fever

15-12. What constitutes the vast majority of blast injuries?

(A) Aircraft incidents

(B) Fireworks-related incidents

(C) Industrial incidents

(D) Motor vehicle collisions

(E) Terrorist bombings

15-13. What is the most common fatal primary blast injury?

(A) Compartment syndrome

(B) Intestinal perforation

(C) Pulmonary barotrauma

(D) Shrapnel injuries

(E) Tympanic membrane perforation

15-14. What is the most common and consistent feature of compartment syndrome?

(A) Acidosis

(B) Electrolyte abnormality

(C) Pain

(D) Pulselessness

(E) Renal failure

15-15. What is the primary role of hazardous materials (HAZMAT) personnel in a chemical hot zone?

(A) Decontaminating victims

(B) Extinguishing fires

(C) Identifying the involved agent

(D) Rescuing the victims

(E) Resuscitation of victims

15-16. What is the "universal" decontamination agent?

(A) Bleach

(B) Decontamination foam

(C) Fuller's earth

(D) Neutralizing alkali

(E) Water

15-17. A patient presents with urinary and fecal incontinence, drooling, vomiting, and irritated eyes after exposure to an unknown vapor. Which of the following antidotes should be empirically given?

(A) Atropine

(B) Diazepam

(C) Hydroxocobalamin

(D) N-acetylcysteine

(E) Sodium thiosulfate

15-18. A patient presents with fever, myalgias, and vesicular skin lesions all in the same stage. The lesions are most abundant on the face and distal extremities. Name the most likely biological agent this patient was exposed to.

(A) Anthrax

(B) Chicken pox

(C) Ebola

(D) Smallpox

(E) Tularemia

15-19. Which of the following protective methods is appropriate for most infectious agents of concern for bioterrorism?

(A) Airborne precautions

(B) Contact precautions

(C) Droplet precautions

(D) Patient isolation

(E) Standard precautions

15-20. Which of the following organ systems is most sensitive to the effects of ionizing radiation?

(A) Cardiovascular

(B) Hematopoietic

(C) Musculoskeletal

(D) Nervous

(E) Respiratory

15-21. What is the most important treatment priority for victims of a radiologic dispersion device (RDD; dirty bomb)?

(A) Decontaminate with soap and water

(B) Administer an antidote

(C) Notify law enforcement

(D) Remove the victim's clothing

(E) Treat major traumatic injuries

15-22. Which of the following should be monitored as an indicator of the extent of radiation injury?

(A) Erythrocytes

(B) Lymphocytes

(C) Neutrophils

(D) Platelets

(E) Schistocytes

15-23. Which symptoms are most likely to be the first encountered with acute radiation syndrome?

(A) Altered mental status

(B) Fever and fatigue

(C) Hypotension

(D) Nausea and vomiting

(E) Seizures

Prehospital Care and Disaster Preparedness
Answers and Explanations

15-1. **The answer is B** (Chapter 1). Communication has historically been the weakest component of disaster responses, which has led to a focus on communication redundancy as a key to effective response. Transportation and manpower are generally sufficient or able to be augmented rapidly through national mutual aid compacts and other national resources such as (in the United States) the National Disaster Medical System. Access to care, while often a problem in routine provision of health care, can be paradoxically less problematic during disasters due to an increased availability of charity care; in fact, some experts have noted concerns in returning communities to their predisaster level of care, which may be lower than that provided after a disaster. Documentation needs during disasters are often streamlined, although careful documentation is still needed to track patient outcomes and maintain the ability to receive reimbursement for care.

15-2. **The answer is B** (Chapter 2). The defibrillator provides what some studies suggest is the only significant factor in survival from cardiac arrest—early defibrillation. Intravenous catheters provide a route for administration of advanced cardiac life support (ACLS) medications, but the evidence supporting the benefit of these medications is weak. Laryngoscopes (and thus intubation) were historically given precedence in resuscitation, but recent studies have supported the provision of defibrillation prior to intubation (in contravention to the previously

taught "ABC" [airway-breathing-circulation] mantra of resuscitation further noting that over-ventilation during cardiac arrest can decrease survival). Cervical collars and splints are used for immobilizing injured or possibly injured skeletal structures and do not have a direct role in cardiac arrest therapy.

15-3. **The answer is E** (Chapter 2). Children's occiputs are large compared with the rest of their bodies, causing forward flexion of the neck if laid directly down upon a flat, rigid spine board. Accordingly, placing padding under the shoulders will allow the child to be placed in a more spine-neutral position. Alternatively, some pediatric spine boards have a hole cut out for the occiput, allowing the head to fall slightly through the board and maintain a neutral position. Placing padding under the head would exacerbate the forward flexion of the neck, while placing padding under the lumbar spine or pelvis would not have any significant impact upon neck position. Placing more padding under the neck would also be unlikely to have a significant impact upon neck position, but might cause pressure to be applied directly to an injured area, making this maneuver contraindicated.

15-4. **The answer is A** (Chapter 3). Bad weather is a major limitation to the use of aeromedical EMS; even instrument flight rules (IFR) capable aircraft may need to abort or decline a mission due to bad weather. Weather issues can present a serious threat to safety.

This is a concern of such significance that pilots are generally asked to make flight safety decisions related to weather and other factors before they are told what the mission is, to avoid any bias in this critical decision process. A long distance between the scene and the receiving facility generally favors the use of aeromedical EMS, due to the higher speeds attainable. Providers on both ground and aeromedical units can perform advanced airway procedures, although some aeromedical unit personnel have access to providers with a broader range of skills and training for more difficult airway procedures. Outcomes for obstetric patients are rarely dependent on mode of transportation. Responses in an urban environment often are just as prompt with ground units as aeromedical units due to the absence of a need for creating landing zones and verifying a safe location for landing zones, but traffic congestion can make aeromedical transportation favorable. The use of aeromedical units in an urban environment is highly situational.

15-5. **The answer is E** (Chapter 4). The referring physician must arrange for appropriate transportation capable of providing the needed services and stabilizing the patient to the best of his or her ability. Although responsibilities of the other listed occupations are not specifically delineated in law, it is generally expected that the referring physician, in concert with the charge nurse and perhaps the primary physician, will assist in having a current copy of the medical record, old records, recent laboratory and radiography results, documentation of physician-to-physician contact, and consent for transfer arranged prior to transport. The receiving physician's responsibilities begin when the patient arrives at his or her facility, but receiving physicians will often provide advice and general assistance related to the safe transport of the patient. Hospital administrators are responsible for ensuring that protocols for safe transport, transfer agreements, and appropriate memoranda of understanding are in place to facilitate emergent interfacility transfers.

15-6. **The answer is B** (Chapter 4). Continuous positive airway pressure at 4–6 cm H_2O is the initial therapy to stent open airways and reduce further lung damage. Intubation and surfactant therapy may follow closely behind, but require more expertise in the management of respiratory distress syndrome. Intravenous epinephrine has no role in the treatment of this syndrome unless the child progresses to cardiac arrest. Nebulized albuterol also has no role in this therapeutic pathway.

15-7. **The answer is D** (Chapter 5). Oral rehydration, in combination with fluid balance maintenance at less than 500 mL/hr of oral fluids, is the best preventative management of hyponatremia in these circumstances. Patients not responding to oral rehydration may be treated with intravenous normal saline. Intravenous hypertonic saline should be used very cautiously, if at all, due to the risk of central pontine myelinolysis with rapid correction of serum sodium. Magnesium is used to treat muscle cramps. Oral salt tablets do not have a generally recognized role in the treatment of hyponatremia in athletes.

15-8. **The answer is B** (Chapter 6). A disaster by definition is an event that overwhelms the available resources to immediately manage the event; although a ten-car crash on the interstate may not be a disaster in a large urban EMS system, a single car rollover might overwhelm local resources in a rural area. The number of patients, location, and types of injuries involved may contribute to this resource mismatch but are not the defining characteristics. Chemical, biological, and radiological events will likely be disasters due to the extensive decontamination, law enforcement, and other resource-intensive components required, but other events such as transportation incidents, building collapses, and explosion events are just as capable of becoming disasters.

15-9. **The answer is E** (Chapter 6). The main goal of disaster triage is to do the most good for the most people. This is in contrast to the main goal of routine emergency department triage, which is to identify the sickest patients first; in a disaster, the sickest patients may not be salvageable with the available resources, requiring a change in how priorities for patient care are assigned. Determining who needs comfort care rather than resuscitation is a function of some disaster triage systems, but is not the main goal; further, while the comfort care designation does exist in some systems, resuscitation is generally not performed during disasters due to the intensive use of resources and often-poor outcomes of resuscitation. Consequently, optimizing individual patient outcome (an individual goal) becomes secondary to the community goal of optimizing the overall outcome. Obtaining primary insurance authorization for treatment is a registration function, not a triage function.

15-10. **The answer is D** (Chapter 7). Although many specific problems can occur in postdisaster communities, such as inability to access health care facilities, lack of clean water, limited law enforcement capability, and poor access to prescription medications, the underlying and constant theme is loss of resources. Communities may be faced with a variety of economic, social, and health deficits that can often be lessened by appropriate preparation.

15-11. **The answer is B** (Chapter 7). Inability to access regular sources of health care frequently leads to exacerbations of chronic diseases, such as hypertension and diabetes. Tuberculosis, yellow fever, and malaria are not expected in a postdisaster population at any significantly different rate than in the predisaster population. Cadaver-transmitted infections are very rare, with psychological illnesses being the most likely result of prolonged exposure to cadavers.

15-12. **The answer is E** (Chapter 8). Terrorism-related bombings using conventional explosives comprise the vast majority of blast injuries. Aircraft incidents, fireworks-related incidents, and motor vehicle collisions are much less likely to result in blast injury, resulting instead in burns and other trauma. Industrial incidents may lead to blast injury, but generally do so in small numbers of patients at any given incident.

15-13. **The answer is C** (Chapter 8). Pulmonary barotrauma including parenchymal disruption, hemorrhage, hemopneumothorax, and eventual acute respiratory distress syndrome is the most common fatal primary injury associated with blast injuries. Intestinal perforation, while having a high potential for morbidity, is less common. Tympanic membrane perforation is fairly common but does not correlate well with injury severity and does not generally result in mortality. Shrapnel injuries may result in severe vascular injuries, possibly leading to compartment syndrome, but this would be considered a form of secondary blast injury (not primary).

15-14. **The answer is C** (Chapter 8). Pain is the most consistent feature of compartment syndrome. Pulselessness, while a critical finding suggestive of poor outcomes, is almost always delayed and often absent even in significant compartment syndrome, as the syndrome is a disease of the microvasculature. Acidosis and electrolyte abnormalities may be found in crush syndrome, the systemic manifestation of crush injury (of which compartment syndrome is a subset). Renal failure is the most serious complication of crush syndrome, not compartment syndrome.

15-15. **The answer is D** (Chapter 9). Rescuing the victims by removing them from further exposure is the primary role of hot zone HAZMAT personnel. Resuscitation of victims, although intuitively desirable, puts other victims at risk due to further exposure to the agent; longer exposures cause more severe results. Further, victims who are already pulseless or apneic, and thus requiring ACLS interventions, are much less likely to be salvageable then the possibly large number of victims not yet in cardiopulmonary arrest. Decontaminating victims does not occur in the hot zone—this occurs in the warm zone. Extinguishing fires is an important role, but not the primary role for HAZMAT personnel. Identifying the involved agent is also important, but again is secondary to victim rescue. Also, it is more important to identify the toxidrome than the specific agent so that providers can institute a general course of therapy. Specific identification can generally be delayed.

15-16. **The answer is E** (Chapter 10). Tepid water, often used with a mild soap and a brush, is the preferred decontamination agent for almost all chemicals (the major exceptions being reactive metals) due to easy availability in large volumes. Even for reactive metals, removing clothing and rapidly washing with large volumes of warm water may minimize exothermic reactions that are likely already occurring due to moisture on the victims' skin. Decontamination foam is a newer technology which is still being tested and validated and may have a future role in decontamination. Fuller's earth, a dry agent, may be useful for reactive metals and dusts. Bleach is generally not recommended due to the possibility of tissue injury and the lack of availability in large volumes, but might be of some use for specific exposures. Neutralizing acids and alkalis are not recommended due to the danger of heat released from exothermic neutralizing reactions.

15-17. **The answer is A** (Chapter 9). This patient is suffering from exposure to an organic phosphorus (or organophosphate) agent, and is demonstrating key features of the "SLUD" (salivation, lacrimation, urination, and defecation) or "SLUDGE" syndrome (salivation, lacrimation, urination, defecation, gastrointestinal upset, and emesis). Atropine and pralidoxime are indicated to help relieve these symptoms; atropine is given for hypersalivation, bronchorrhea, and bradycardia, and is titrated to clearing of respiratory secretions (with doses possibly as large as 20 mg that are not withheld for tachycardia or pupillary response), while pralidoxime helps reactivate acetylcholinesterase if given promptly before chemical aging has

occurred. Diazepam may be used if the patient is seizing, but is not the primary antidote for this toxidrome. *N*-acetylcysteine is indicated in acetaminophen toxicity to help prevent the formation of the toxic metabolite *N*-acetylparabenzoquinoneimine, while sodium thiosulfate is used to treat cyanide toxicity.

15-18. **The answer is D** (Chapter 10). Vesicular lesions all in the same stage of development in a centrifugal distribution are a hallmark of smallpox. While chicken pox can also present with fever, myalgias, and vesicular lesions, these occur in a centripetal (central) presentation and are found in varying stages. Ebola is marked by fever, but the skin lesions are generally nonvesicular (often petechial or purpuric). The most common presentations of tularemia include fever and possibly ulcerative skin lesions, while anthrax has several forms that may include fever but not vesicular lesions.

15-19. **The answer is E** (Chapter 10). Standard precautions are sufficient for the majority of biological agents. Agents that are contagious through airborne or droplet transmission are a troublesome minority of these agents and include pneumonic plague (requiring droplet precautions and patient isolation), viral hemorrhagic fevers (requiring droplet precautions), and smallpox (requiring airborne precautions, contact precautions, and patient isolation).

15-20. **The answer is B** (Chapter 11). The hematopoietic system, along with other systems containing rapidly proliferating cells with high turnover rates such as the gastrointestinal and reproductive systems, is highly sensitive to the effects of ionizing radiation. Systems with more slowly dividing cells, such as the cardiovascular, musculoskeletal, nervous, and respiratory systems are less immediately affected.

15-21. **The answer is E** (Chapter 11). Treating traumatic injuries is the first treatment priority, as patients are more likely to die of major trauma from blast effects than from radiation exposure from an RDD. An RDD, or "dirty bomb," is a weapon that has combined explosive effects and radiation exposure. While decontamination by removing the victims' clothing and washing with water is important, the amount of radiation exposure is generally minimal so this takes second priority after treating traumatic injuries. Detonation of an RDD is a terrorist event and law enforcement authorities must be notified early. In addition, if the radionuclide can be identified and this information communicated to receiving health care facilities, time-sensitive antidotes can be prepared if appropriate.

15-22.   **The answer is B** (Chapter 11). Lymphocytes are rapidly destroyed and slowly replenished after acute radiation injury, causing a rapid decline, which is a hallmark of the hematopoietic syndrome and an excellent indicator of the extent of radiation injury. Neutrophils, and platelets to a lesser extent, initially increase in number then show a steady decline, with a nadir at about 30 days after exposure. Erythrocyte counts decline to a lesser extent. Schistocytes are not typically seen in acute radiation syndrome, but are instead found in other disease processes such as hemolytic anemia.

15-23.   **The answer is D** (Chapter 11). Nausea and vomiting, along with other gastrointestinal symptoms, are part of the prodromal phase that occurs first in the progression of acute radiation syndrome. These symptoms are sufficiently reliable to allow some experts to suggest using vomiting within 2 hours of exposure as a useful sign to help triage patients who are more likely to have received a clinically significant radiation dose. Fever and fatigue, as well as hypotension, may occur as well, but less commonly than nausea and vomiting. Severe hypotension, altered mental status, and seizures are indicative of cardiovascular and central nervous syndrome, the most severe manifestation of acute radiation syndrome, but these symptoms are preceded by nausea and vomiting.

Psychobehavioral Disorders
Questions

16-1. Which feature is MOST suggestive of an organic etiology in a patient with acute psychosis?

(A) Auditory hallucinations
(B) Family history of psychosis
(C) Normal mental status
(D) Onset before 40 years of age
(E) Visual hallucinations

16-2. The "Mini Mental State Examination" is MOST useful in determining which of the following?

(A) Cognitive impairment
(B) Disorientation due to drugs or alcohol
(C) Occult depression
(D) Prognosis posthead injury
(E) Psychosis

16-3. A 25-year-old male patient is brought to the emergency department (ED) for violent, agitated behavior. The patient was handcuffed by law enforcement who suspect drug intoxication or psychiatric disease. The patient is yelling, spitting, and uncooperative with emergency personnel. What is the MOST compelling justification for placing this patient in four-point restraints?

(A) Allow the placement of an intravenous line and blood draw for diagnostic testing.
(B) Ensure safety of patient and ED personnel.
(C) Facilitate transfer for psychiatric evaluation.

(D) Minimize impact of behavior on other sick patients nearby.
(E) Permit a medical screening exam to be performed.

16-4. Which of the following best describes the use of laboratory testing and neuroimaging in the evaluation of the patient with new behavioral changes?

(A) A positive screen for alcohol or drugs of abuse obviates the need for further testing.
(B) Computerized tomography of the brain should be routinely performed in the setting of a new psychotic break.
(C) Diagnostic investigation tends to be more intensive in the younger patient.
(D) Routine metabolic and electrolyte testing can be omitted since these are unusual causes of behavioral abnormalities.
(E) Testing should be directed by a careful history, physical examination, and consideration of probable organic etiologies.

16-5. A young patient with a history of psychiatric disease is brought to your ED after creating a public disturbance. In the course of his evaluation, you witness the patient verbalizing physical threats against a specific member of his family. When later asked again about the threats, the patient denies ever having made them. Which of the following best describes the limit of your responsibility in this matter?

(A) Avoid documenting the specifics of the threat in order to protect patient–physician confidentiality.

(B) Contact police in order to warn target individual.

(C) Enlist social worker to assist in assessing risk of violence toward the family member.

(D) Fully document the affirmation and denial in the medical record.

(E) Medically sedate the patient to mitigate the risk of physical violence.

16-6. Which of the following describes a patient group at comparatively high risk of death by suicide?

(A) Chronically ill

(B) Females

(C) Married with children in the home

(D) Non-Caucasians

(E) Teenagers

16-7. Which of the following statements best describes the role of the *DSM-IV* (diagnostic and statistical manual of mental disorders)?

(A) Allows patients to be placed into fixed diagnostic categories in order to standardize management.

(B) Clearly distinguishes between psychiatric and medical illnesses.

(C) Excludes behavior disorders due to substance abuse.

(D) Prioritizes the making of precise psychiatric diagnoses in the ED.

(E) Provides a diagnostic framework and method of organizing complex clinical information for communicating between medical providers.

16-8. An elderly male presents to the ED after being found wandering in a nearby neighborhood. You learn that he has mild Alzheimer disease and resides in an assisted living facility. The staff are surprised by this behavior since he normally cares for himself and has never wandered off before. Which of the following would be the most appropriate ED course of action?

(A) Admit patient for placement in a skilled nursing facility.

(B) Contact social services to investigate the assisted living facility for failure to adequately supervise patient.

(C) Immediately return patient to assisted living facility with instructions for a higher level of surveillance.

(D) Perform a careful clinical evaluation to rule out underlying organic disease explaining the change in mental status.

(E) Perform a medical screening examination, prescribe a medication for behavior control and return to assisted living facility.

16-9. Which of the following would suggest that a patient's cognitive impairment is due to dementia rather than delirium?

(A) Absence of underlying medical condition

(B) Clouding of consciousness

(C) Rapid onset

(D) Visual hallucinations

(E) Waxing and waning course

16-10. Why was a "black box" Food and Drug Administration (FDA) warning issued for haloperidol and droperidol?

(A) Adverse hemodynamic effects

(B) Excessive sedation

(C) Extrapyramidal syndromes

(D) Hepatic toxicity

(E) Prolongation of the Q-T interval and ventricular arrhythmias

16-11. A 25-year-old male with a history of schizophrenia presents to the ED with 30 minutes of neck and jaw stiffness and difficulty breathing. A friend confirms that the patient was started on a new antipsychotic regimen 2 days earlier by his psychiatrist. Vital signs are unremarkable, but the physical examination reveals neck and jaw rigidity, and audible stridor to the upper airway. There is no rash, tongue swelling, or wheezing. What would be the most appropriate initial management?

(A) Diazepam 5 mg intravenously

(B) Diphenhydramine 50 mg intravenously

(C) Fiberoptic intubation after direct airway visualization

(D) Methylprednisolone 125 mg intravenously

(E) Oral-tracheal intubation using rapid sequence induction

16-12. Which of the following statements about panic attacks is NOT accurate?

(A) Attacks usually last less than 1 hour and are often associated with somatic complaints and agoraphobia.

(B) Cross-cultural studies have documented that features of panic attacks are very similar throughout varying societies.

(C) Increased use of the ED in patients with panic disorder can precede the ultimate diagnosis by up to 10 years.

(D) Occurrence of panic disorders is bimodal with the largest peak during adolescence and another peak in the third decade of life.

(E) Typical somatic complaints of attacks include tachycardia, tachypnea, dyspnea, chest tightness, weakness, nausea, dizziness, and paresthesias.

16-13. With respect to making a diagnosis of panic attack or panic disorder, which of the following statements is most accurate?

(A) By definition, panic attacks are spontaneous without situational or other obvious triggers.

(B) Common triggers include caffeine use, street drugs, and smoking.

(C) Domestic violence should be considered as victims commonly present with panic attacks.

(D) Laboratory tests that may be helpful in making the diagnosis include a mild leukocytosis without a left shift and elevated bicarbonate levels.

(E) The course of this illness is chronic with attacks occurring at fairly consistent intervals.

16-14. Which of the following treatments is NOT considered an option for panic disorder patients?

(A) Antidepressants

(B) Antipsychotics

(C) Benzodiazepines

(D) Cognitive behavioral therapy

(E) Social services intervention

16-15. Which of the following is NOT considered a core feature of conversion disorder?

(A) At least one prior similar event has occurred.

(B) Symptom expressed is a change or loss of physical function suggesting a physical disorder.

(C) Recent psychological stressor or conflict.

(D) Symptom produced unconsciously.

(E) Symptom cannot be explained by a known organic etiology or culturally sanctioned response pattern.

16-16. Which of the following most accurately describes typical characteristics of alcohol withdrawal seizures?

(A) Focal seizures are common.

(B) Most patients only have a single seizure.

(C) Majority of patients who experience alcohol withdrawal seizures later develop delirium.

(D) Onset 6–48 hours after the last drink.

(E) Time frame from the first to the last seizure is generally 12 hours.

16-17. According to DSM-IV-TR guidelines, a substance abuse diagnosis requires one of four symptoms in the preceding 12 months. Which of the following is NOT one of those qualifying symptoms?

(A) Failure to fulfill major obligations

(B) Assault

(C) Recurrent substance use in physically hazardous situations

(D) Recurrent substance-related legal problems

(E) Continued substance use despite persistent social or interpersonal problems

16-18. All of the following can be used to treat alcohol withdrawal EXCEPT:

(A) Chlordiazepoxide

(B) Diazepam

(C) Haloperidol

(D) Lorazepam

(E) Phenytoin

Psychobehavioral Disorders
Answers and Explanations

16-1. **The answer is E** (Chapter 284). While visual hallucinations can occur in functional psychotic illness (schizophrenia or affective disorder), they are much more common and indicative of organic disease. The opposite is true for auditory hallucinations. Functional psychiatric illness typically presents in young adulthood—well before age 40. There are strong inheritance patterns for a number of psychiatric disorders, particularly schizophrenia and depression, so family history of behavior disorders can be an important clue. Patients with organic psychosis often manifest some degree of cognitive impairment, delirium, or altered mental status related to their underlying disease process.

16-2. **The answer is A** (Chapter 283). The Mini Mental Status Examination consists of a series of tasks that assess orientation, memory, attention, calculation, language, and visual construction. A below normal score on this cognitive test is highly predictive of delirium or some form of dementia such as Alzheimer disease and vascular cerebral pathology. Drugs and alcohol impact mental status and affect cognition primarily through sedation and intoxication. Occult depression may mimic dementia and the physician should look for clues in the patient's mood, effect, as well as other "organic" signs of depression. Prognosis after head injury is best assessed using the Glasgow Coma Scale.

16-3. **The answer is B** (Chapter 283). The patient described represents a clear danger to himself and others. The rule of "safety first" must take precedence. Physical restraints, when placed carefully and humanely, assure patient and provider safety as well as facilitate further workup. Alternatives include the use of sedation drugs: the so-called medical restraint. The patient's undifferentiated behavior abnormality will likely require laboratory testing, a careful physical examination, and possible psychiatric consultation. The impact on other patients can best be managed by relocating to a more secluded area of the department.

16-4. **The answer is E** (Chapter 283). There is no such thing as a routine workup for new onset behavioral changes. Each patient deserves a careful history, physical examination, and consideration of a reasonable list of differential diagnoses. In older patients as well as those with important comorbidities such as diabetes, cerebral vascular disease, and HIV, a broader investigation will be necessary. Although most patients undergo drug and alcohol testing, a positive result does not exclude important concomitant disease such as occult head trauma, metabolic and electrolyte derangements, and stroke.

16-5. **The answer is B** (Chapter 283). When evaluating a patient with a behavioral disorder, the physician must make a judgment regarding the patient's likelihood of violence toward self or others. In the latter case, candidate victims may need to be warned despite clear concerns for patient confidentiality. This question was codified in law by *Tarasoff v. Regents of University of California, 1976*. The physician's responsibility includes the option of notifying a psychiatrist involved in the case, police, or the targeted individual.

16-6.   The answer is A (Chapter 283). The risk of suicide is increasing across all demographic groups. The rate of fatal suicide continues to be highest among older, white males, living alone, with chronic medical illnesses. In contrast, the rate of nonfatal suicide attempts is greatest in females, between the ages of 15 and 19. Other features that increase the probability of fatal suicide include poor prognosis/degenerative diseases such as HIV, cancer, stroke and spinal cord injuries, coexisting psychiatric disease, or a history of violent attempts in the past, for example, jumping, hanging, or firearms.

16-7.   The answer is E (Chapter 284). The *DSM-IV* provides a standardized nomenclature for describing mental and behavioral disorders. The diagnostic criteria are provided for each disorder as well as information on demographics, associated symptoms, and differential diagnoses. The system is divided into five general axes that in turn provide an algorithmic "tree" leading to a more precise disorder. The diagnostic axes include primary psychiatric disease as well as medical diseases that may have behavioral manifestations. Any given patient may possess features of several axes at the same time, presenting a mosaic of different psychiatric disorders requiring highly individualized approaches to care. For the emergency physician, the DSM-IV classification should not take priority over good medical care and a fastidious search for medical disease underlying the patient's behavioral problem.

16-8.   The answer is D (Chapter 284). Cognitive disorders such as Alzheimer's typically followed a slow and progressive clinical course. In the early stages, a perceived high functional status can belie the fact that patients have minimal cognitive or physiologic reserve. Abrupt changes in behavior can be brought on by relatively innocent physical or emotional stressors, such as, change in living status, minor infections, dehydration, new

medications, etc. A careful history, physical examination, and basic metabolic and infection screen are essential. In the absence of an obvious organic etiology, social workers, patient caregivers, and family may be enlisted in evaluating the potential psychosocial underpinnings of the patient's behavioral change.

16-9.   The answer is A (Chapter 284). Dementia tends to be a slow and progressive disorder with a consistent pattern and the notable absence of any clouding of consciousness. In contrast, the hallmark feature of delirium is decreased alertness and/or awareness of the external environment. The impairment may range from simple inattention to drowsiness, even stupor. Dementia and delirium may coexist in the same patient with the latter typically a response to some underlying medical condition: infection, metabolic derangement, intoxication, trauma, medication intolerance, etc. Visual hallucinations are common as is a rapid onset of symptoms and variable pattern often matching the underlying medical condition.

16-10.   The answer is E (Chapter 285). The FDA issued a "black box" warning against the use of droperidol and haloperidol in patients with a history of cardiac arrhythmia and/or prolongation of the Q-T interval. Particularly in the setting of rapid intravenous administration, this class of drugs can cause Q-T prolongation risking the polymorphic ventricular tachycardia, torsades de pointes. While expressed recommendations do not exist, it has been suggested that a screening electrocardiography (EKG) and electrolyte panel be obtained prior to using this class of drugs. Extrapyramidal syndromes, excess sedation, and hypotension are side effects that have been described with virtually all neuroleptic medications, including droperidol and haloperidol. The FDA has also placed a "black box" warning on the use of olanzapine, an atypical antipsychotic, in elderly patients with dementia due to an increased risk of stroke.

16-11.   The answer is B (Chapter 285). Acute dystonias are the most common side effect of antipsychotic medication. Typically, these include muscle spasms of the neck and back but may manifest as oculogyric crises (fixed or sustained rotational deviation of the eyes) or even laryngospasm. It is common for these side effects to be misdiagnosed as a primary neurologic disorder, muscle strain, angioedema, etc. A careful and complete medication history is essential. Symptoms resolve quickly after the administration of anticholinergic agents such as diphenhydramine or benztropine and airway management is rarely, if ever, required. The offending psychotropic agent must be discontinued and anticholinergic therapy should be continued for 3 days after discharge. Since this is not an allergic reaction, steroids are not beneficial.

16-12. **The answer is B** (Chapter 287). Given the growing diversity of our patient populations, it is critical to recognize significant cultural differences. Sleep paralysis is a common symptom of panic disorder in the African American population and orthostatic-induced dizziness is a common trigger for panic attacks in Vietnamese refugees. Somatic complaints are very common but must be taken seriously. Panic disorder is a diagnosis of exclusion in the ED.

16-13. **The answer is C** (Chapter 287). It is always critical to consider domestic violence when a patient presents with a panic attack. Many victims present with a panic attack. Triggers may include caffeine or street drugs, but there is no association with smoking. Although patients may not immediately recognize the cause for their attack, exposure to a situation or specific trigger is common. Laboratory studies are usually within normal limits but changes consistent with hyperventilation such as a low bicarbonate level may be noted. The illness is chronic by nature, but attacks are most often random.

16-14. **The answer is B** (Chapter 287). Antipsychotic medications are not considered a viable option to treat panic disorder patients. Antidepressant medication is the mainstay of treatment for panic disorders because the potential complications of abuse, dependence, and withdrawal are not associated with their use. In addition, antidepressants may be beneficial in treating comorbid mood and anxiety disorders, including posttraumatic stress disorder and premenstrual dysphoric disorder. However, behavioral therapy and benzodiazepines are used in selected cases and situations. Occasionally family counselling or social service may be of benefit.

16-15. **The answer is A** (Chapter 288). In order to diagnose a conversion disorder, a patient must meet the following five criteria: symptoms is expressed where there is a loss or change of physical function; there has been a recent stressor; symptom is produced unconsciously; the symptom cannot be explained by an organic or cultural means; and the symptom is not limited to pain or sexual dysfunction.

16-16. **The answer is D** (Chapter 289). About 40% of patients will have a single seizure. Most patients have multiple seizures when they are withdrawing from alcohol. Up to one-third of patients may go on to develop a state of delirium. Focal seizures are uncommon and demand further evaluation. The time frame from first to last seizure is 6 hours in the vast majority (85%) of patients.

16-17. **The answer is B** (Chapter 289). A patient who has any one of the following four symptoms meets DSM criteria for substance abuse: failure to fulfill major obligations; recurrent use of substance in situations that are physically hazardous; legal problems related to substance use; and continued use despite interpersonal and social problems.

16-18. **The answer is C** (Chapter 289). Benzodiazepines are the first-line treatment for alcohol withdrawal symptoms. Haldol may also be used to treat alcohol withdrawal especially if hallucinosis is a primary symptom. Phenytoin is not recommended for the treatment of alcohol withdrawal seizures, as it may actually lower the seizure threshold.

Pulmonary Emergencies
Questions

17-1. The most common infectious cause of acute exacerbation of bronchitis is:

(A) *Bordetella pertussis*

(B) *Haemophilus influenzae*

(C) Legionella

(D) Respiratory viruses

(E) *Streptococcus pneumoniae*

17-2. Which of the following best describes chronic bronchitis?

(A) Change in the characteristic of a productive cough that has lasted for more than 3 months for 2 consecutive years.

(B) Nonproductive cough for 2 months each year for 3 consecutive years, often with dyspnea and partially reversible airway obstruction.

(C) Nonproductive cough for 3 months each year for 2 consecutive years, often with dyspnea and partially reversible airway obstruction.

(D) Productive cough for 2 months each year for 3 consecutive years, often with dyspnea.

(E) Productive cough for 3 months each year for 2 consecutive years, often with dyspnea and partially reversible airway obstruction.

17-3. Which of the following statements about respiratory illnesses is correct?

(A) Acute bronchitis is usually associated with a cough for at least more than 3 days.

(B) Common cold is associated with persistent cough, low-grade fever that is followed by sore throat, and rhinorrhea.

(C) Fever is less common in pertussis than in viral bronchitis.

(D) Influenza is associated with malaise, myalgias, and low-grade fever.

(E) Rhinorrhea and repetitive throat clearing is associated with gastroesophageal reflux disease (GERD).

17-4. Which of the following is considered a risk factor for penicillin resistance?

(A) Asplenia

(B) History of unsuccessful treatment with macrolide

(C) Immunosuppression from alcoholism or cancer

(D) Penicillin allergy

(E) Premature infants

17-5. An 80-year-old male with several comorbidities presents with a productive cough, malaise, confusion, and fever of 38.4°C for 7 days. Which of the following is the most appropriate treatment plan?

    (A) Obtain blood cultures, chest radiograph, and consider admission.

    (B) Possible lymphoma, obtain complete blood count, and recommend follow-up with primary care physician.

    (C) Prescribe a cough suppressant, fever control instructions, and discharge home.

    (D) Recheck temperature and if below 38°C, discharge home with fever instructions.

    (E) Treat his viral illness with acetaminophen and discharge home.

17-6. A 40-year-old male with mental illness and chronic alcoholism left the hospital a week ago after a diagnosis of pneumonia. He now presents with fever, cough, and right-sided chest pain. Chest x-ray is shown. Which of the following is the most likely etiologic agent (Figure 17-1)?

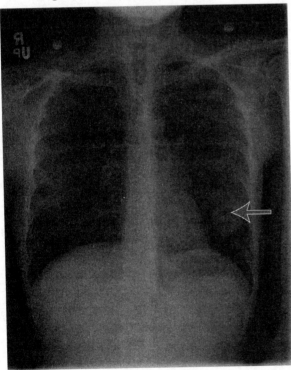

Figure 17-1. Reproduced with permission from Tintinalli JE, Stapczynski JS, Ma OJ, Cline DM, Cydulka RK, Meckler GD: *Tintinalli's Emergency Medicine: A Comprehensive Study Guide*, 7th Edition. Copyright © 2011 The McGraw-Hill Companies, Inc.

    (A) *H. influenzae*

    (B) Legionella

    (C) *Staphylococcus aureus*

    (D) Tuberculosis

    (E) Viral pneumonia

17-7. The patient from the question above develops acute respiratory distress while in the emergency department (ED). After administering supplemental oxygen and establishing intravenous (IV) access and IV bolus of crystalloids, what is the next most appropriate step?

    (A) Obtain arterial blood gas

    (B) Check coagulation studies

    (C) IV antibiotics

    (D) Needle decompression

    (E) Thoracentesis/thoracostomy

17-8. A patient arrives with respiratory distress. You obtain an arterial blood gas and discover an elevated alveolar–arterial (A–a) gradient. Which of the following conditions can explain the discrepancy?

    (A) Anemia with a hemoglobin concentration of less than 10 g/dL

    (B) Aortic stenosis

    (C) Heroin overdose with respiratory depression

    (D) Interstitial lung disease

    (E) Severe upper airway compromise due to laryngeal edema

17-9. Which of the following statement is correct with regard to how the following situations affect PAO_2 or A–a gradient?

    (A) Higher altitude will decrease PAO_2.

    (B) Increasing a person's hemoglobin will increase PAO_2.

    (C) Increasing respiratory rate will increase PAO_2.

    (D) Lower altitude will decrease PAO_2.

    (E) Supplying supplemental oxygen always significantly increases the PaO_2.

17-10. All of the following conditions have an elevated A–a gradient. Which one will NOT be corrected by supplemental oxygen administration?

(A) Age-related decrease A–a gradient due to decreased PaO_2

(B) Arteriovenous (AV) shunt

(C) Congestive heart failure

(D) Lobar pneumonia

(E) Pleural effusion

17-11. Which of the following represent increased dead space ventilation?

(A) Acute respiratory distress syndrome (ARDS)

(B) Cyanide toxicity

(C) Pulmonary embolus

(D) Pulmonary hemorrhage

(E) Pneumonia

17-12. In distinguishing a chronic obstructive pulmonary disease (COPD) exacerbation from congestive heart failure (CHF), which of the following clinical or laboratory features is helpful?

(A) B-type natriuretic peptide level

(B) Body habitus

(C) Distended neck veins

(D) History of COPD

(E) Peripheral edema

17-13. A 30-year-old female is intubated and placed on mechanical ventilator due to respiratory failure. The patient's initial ventilator settings include an assist control mode with a ventilator rate of 16 breaths/min, tidal volume of 650, FiO_2 of 60%, inspiratory flow rate of 70 L/min, and no positive end-expiratory pressure (PEEP). Approximately 20 minutes later, the respiratory therapist calls you because the patient's blood pressure has dropped from 120/60 to 70/50 mm Hg. On physical examination, the patient displays bilaterally diminished breath sounds. What is the next intervention?

(A) Add PEEP

(B) Bolus 1 L normal saline

(C) Decrease inspiratory flow rate

(D) Perform bilateral needle decompressions

(E) Reduce respiratory rate

17-14. A 38-year-old female with a history of type 2 diabetes mellitus presents with a complaint of 6 days of cough and body aches. Patient states that her right chest is tender with deep breathing. Upon initial assessment, the patient's vital signs are the following: temperature (T), 37.1; blood pressure (BP), 150/97; heart rate (HR), 100; respiratory rate (RR), 18; and pulse oximetry, 93%. On physical examination, she has diminished breath sounds and appears comfortable at rest (Figure 17-2). What are diagnostic considerations?

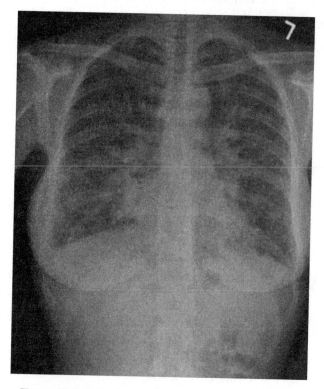

Figure 17-2. Reproduced with permission from Tintinalli JE, Stapczynski JS, Ma OJ, Cline DM, Cydulka RK, Meckler GD: *Tintinalli's Emergency Medicine: A Comprehensive Study Guide,* 7th Edition. Copyright © 2011 The McGraw-Hill Companies, Inc.

(A) Atypical pneumonia

(B) Congestive heart failure

(C) Empyema

(D) Pleural effusion

(E) Pulmonary embolism

17-15. Which of the following is NOT a cause of chronic cough of more than 8 weeks?

(A) Asthma

(B) Bronchiectasis

(C) GERD

(D) Pulmonary embolism

(E) Upper airway cough syndrome

17-16. A patient with history of coronary artery disease, hypertension, and respiratory distress presents to the ED with shortness of breath. He has no history of fever and his symptoms are worsened by the recumbent position. On physical examination, his vital signs are BP, 180/100; HR, 98; RR, 20; and T, 37.8. You notice that in the seated position he has jugular venous distention. His breath sounds are significant for course expiratory rales and diminished sounds at the bases. His chest x-ray demonstrates bilateral pleural effusions seen at the bases obscuring approximately 15% of his lung. Which of the following is an appropriate management strategy?

(A) Administer broad-spectrum antibiotic.

(B) Administer bronchodilators via nebulizer.

(C) Initiate afterload reduction and antidiuretic therapy.

(D) Obtain a high resolution CT of the chest.

(E) Perform a thoracentesis.

17-17. A patient presents with massive hemoptysis. Which of the following is most likely the source of the bleeding?

(A) Alveolar vessel

(B) Bronchial vessel

(C) Intercostal artery

(D) Intercostal vein

(E) Internal mammary artery

17-18. What is the primary reason that patients with brisk hemoptysis require emergent airway management?

(A) Asphyxiation

(B) Aspiration

(C) Exsanguination

(D) Infection

(E) Nausea and subsequent vomiting

17-19. A 50-year-old male patient presents with massive hemoptysis and hypotension. Clinically, the bleeding is continuous, patient is in respiratory distress, and oxygenation has become compromised. The patient has normal coagulation studies and a hematocrit of 12. In addition to IV access, which of the following is the most appropriate management?

(A) Bolus infusion of normal saline, supplemental oxygen, arrange for platelet and fresh frozen plasma (FFP) infusion.

(B) Bolus infusion of normal saline, supplemental oxygen, type and cross red blood cells, arrange for emergent bronchoscopy or selective arterial embolization, selective intubation.

(C) Bolus infusion of normal saline, supplemental oxygen, and IV antibiotics.

(D) Supplemental oxygen, CT angiogram, and sedation.

(E) Supplemental oxygen, transfuse O positive red blood cells, consider intubation, and arrange for emergent bronchoscopy or selective arterial embolization.

17-20. A patient taking warfarin arrives to the ED with severe hemoptysis. Which of the following would be best initial management?

(A) Administer FFP

(B) Check complete blood cell count

(C) Cryoprecipitate

(D) Transfusion of uncrossmatched red blood cells

(E) Withhold warfarin for 1 day

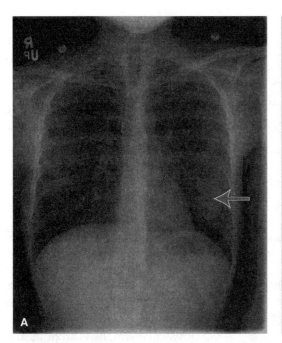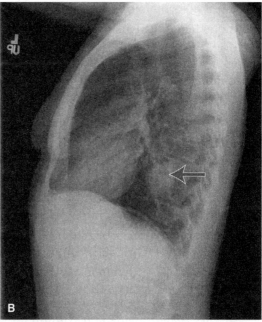

Figure 17-3. Reproduced with permission from Tintinalli JE, Stapczynski JS, Ma OJ, Cline DM, Cydulka RK, Meckler GD: *Tintinalli's Emergency Medicine: A Comprehensive Study Guide*, 7th Edition. Copyright © 2011 The McGraw-Hill Companies, Inc.

17-21. A patient with a 6-day history of productive cough, fever, and malaise presents with increasing chest pain. The patient has tried cough suppressants and "borrowed" some green antibiotic pills from his relative and presents today appearing very ill with significant respiratory distress. On physical examination, you find diminished breath sounds, dullness on percussion, and the chest x-ray is displayed (Figure 17-3). What is the diagnosis?

(A) Abscess

(B) Congestive heart failure

(C) Hospital acquired pneumonia

(D) Mycoplasma pneumonia

(E) Tuberculosis

17-22. A recently immigrated 4-year-old boy is brought in by his mother because of poor feeding, weight loss, and swellings in his neck consistent with lymphadenopathy. The child is diagnosed with likely tuberculosis on chest x-ray. Which of the following statements is true?

(A) Child is highly contagious.

(B) Children rarely present with primary stage tuberculosis.

(C) Drug therapy for children is similar for adult tuberculosis.

(D) Extra pulmonary manifestations are common.

(E) Severe respiratory distress is common.

17-23. A 44-year-old male with a history of AIDS and a CD4 count of 100 was recently started on oral antiretroviral therapy and antituberculosis medications during a recent hospital admission. He presents with a fever, worsening cough, and difficulty breathing. The patient affirms that he has been compliant with all medications prescribed and a "pill count" confirms the patient's assertion. This apparent worsening of symptoms could be attributed to:

(A) Anxiety

(B) Drug interaction

(C) Immune reconstitution syndrome

(D) Misdiagnosis of pneumonia

(E) Reaction to antituberculosis medications

17-24. A patient with acute respiratory failure secondary to a severe acute asthma exacerbation was intubated. The respiratory therapist speaks to you to ask for recommendations regarding initial ventilator settings. Which of the following approaches is recommended?

(A) Maintain a higher respiratory rate (16–20) to decrease CO_2, which may have been retained during exacerbation.

(B) Maintain a higher respiratory rate (16–20) because patient had rapid shallow breaths before requiring intubation.

(C) Use a tidal volume of 6–8 cc/kg of ideal body weight even if there is mild respiratory acidosis.

(D) Use a tidal volume of 10–15 cc/kg of ideal body weight.

(E) Use a pH of 7.40 as your goal to guide future ventilator settings.

17-25. A 24-year-old pregnant female with a 20-week gestation presents in acute respiratory distress. Past medical history is significant for asthma normally controlled with a metered dose inhaler on an as needed basis. She states that she used her inhaler at least eight times before arrival and feels no better. On arrival to the ED, she was in acute distress, bilateral wheezes on physical examination. Pulse oximetry 92% on room air. An arterial blood gas has the following values: pH, 7.34; PCO_2, 40; HCO_3^-, 30; PAO_2, 68; SAO_2, 91%. What is your assessment and plan?

(A) The patient has a moderate asthma exacerbation and should receive supplemental oxygen, albuterol by metered dose inhaler.

(B) The patient has a moderate asthma exacerbation and should receive supplemental oxygen, albuterol by metered dose inhaler, and oral steroids.

(C) The patient has a moderate exacerbation of asthma and should receive supplemental oxygen, nebulized albuterol, and ipratropium, as well as begin steroids.

(D) The patient has a severe exacerbation of asthma with evidence of respiratory failure. Administer supplemental oxygen, initiate nebulized albuterol, and begin steroids as soon as possible.

(E) The patient has a severe exacerbation of asthma with evidence of respiratory failure. Administer supplemental oxygen, initiate nebulized albuterol and ipratropium, begin steroids, and initiate fetal monitoring.

17-26. A 70-year-old male with a 40-pack-year smoking history presents with a complaint of progressively worsening shortness of breath over the last 2 days. He has tried using his "orange" inhaler and increasing the flow on his home oxygen which has not worked for him. On physical exam, he is anxious and demonstrates significant retractions with the following vitals: T, 37.4; RR, 16; HR, 110; BP, 110/60; pulse oximetry, 92% on 2 L nasal cannula. Which of the following interventions will most improve his work of breathing acutely?

(A) Albuterol 2.5 mg nebulized treatment

(B) Ipratropium 0.5 mg nebulized treatment

(C) Noninvasive positive pressure ventilation

(D) Oxygen by 100% non-rebreather mask

(E) Solumedrol 125 mg IV bolus

17-27. Which of the following is LEAST efficacious in the treatment of an acute exacerbation of COPD?

(A) Albuterol

(B) Ipratropium

(C) Magnesium

(D) Steroids

(E) Supplemental oxygen

17-28. A patient with a longstanding history of COPD on home O_2 supplementation was admitted to the ED for an exacerbation. The patient improved significantly with treatment. The patient is currently comfortable and is no longer requiring frequent breathing treatments and is back to his baseline requirement of 2 L/min of supplemental oxygen. Upon discharge, which of the following is warranted?

(A) Increased home oxygen flow to 3 L/min per nasal cannula
(B) Magnesium supplementation
(C) Physical rehabilitation
(D) Steroid taper
(E) Switching from metered dose inhaler to nebulizer for albuterol administration

17-29. When entertaining the diagnosis of COPD, which of the following historical findings would be least helpful?

(A) Occupational/environmental exposures
(B) Presence of ankle swelling
(C) Presence of hemoptysis
(D) Presence of pets
(E) Severity of shortness of breath with activity

17-30. Which of the following is the most likely clinical history for the patient whose plain film and CT scan are shown (Figure 17-4)?

(A) Acute onset fever, chills, and night sweats
(B) Lung cancer history now with increasing shortness of breath
(C) Productive cough and fever
(D) Recent coronary bypass surgery
(E) Smoker with a change in the character in his sputum

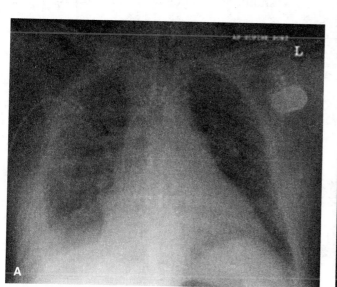

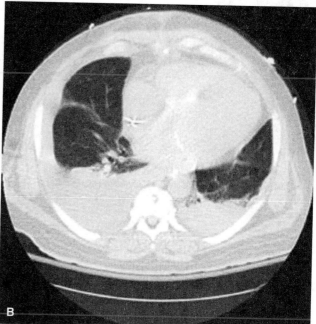

Figure 17-4. Reproduced with permission from Tintinalli JE, Stapczynski JS, Ma OJ, Cline DM, Cydulka RK, Meckler GD: *Tintinalli's Emergency Medicine: A Comprehensive Study Guide,* 7th Edition. Copyright © 2011 The McGraw-Hill Companies, Inc.

17-31. A 72-year-old male with a 60-pack-year history of smoking cigarettes presents with increasing shortness of breath. The patient has a history of myocardial infarction 5 years ago and an echocardiogram that reveals an ejection fraction of 35–40%. The patient states that he has been coughing but can't really say if there has been a change in color or amount. In addition, the patient states he has been sweating but does not recall having a fever. You obtain a 12-lead ECG that reveals no new abnormality and a pulse oximetry reading of 95% on room air. Chest x-ray is shown (Figure 17-5). Which of the following would be helpful in determining the etiology of this patient's shortness of breath?

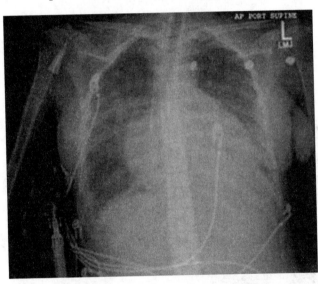

Figure 17-5. Reproduced with permission from Tintinalli JE, Stapczynski JS, Ma OJ, Cline DM, Cydulka RK, Meckler GD: *Tintinalli's Emergency Medicine: A Comprehensive Study Guide,* 7th Edition. Copyright © 2011 The McGraw-Hill Companies, Inc.

(A) Arterial blood gas

(B) Chest CT with contrast to rule out pulmonary embolism

(C) Decubitus chest films

(D) Repeat pulse oximetry after patient has ambulated

(E) Serum B-type natriuretic peptide

17-32. A patient with a history of longstanding COPD and home oxygen therapy presents with sudden worsening shortness of breath after a coughing spell. The patient ambulates on a regular basis. When you examine him, you notice his vitals are the following: BP, 130/90; HR, 100; RR, 24 with some splinting. His pulse oximetry reading is 89% on room air. His breath sounds are distant in both lung fields but particularly on the right. After administering supplemental O_2, his pulse oximetry reading is now 98% and he feels somewhat better. Which of the following should you consider diagnostically?

(A) Arterial blood gas

(B) Chest x-ray (PA and lateral)

(C) Chest pulmonary toilet

(D) Decubitus chest films

(E) Peak flow

17-33. A thoracostomy tube was inserted into a 30-year-old male with a large pneumothorax. There was a gush of air noted with the insertion. Which of the following complications should you watch for in this patient?

(A) Hemothorax from injury to intercostals vessels

(B) Infection of thoracostomy site

(C) Mucous plugging of thoracostomy tube

(D) Persistent air leak and reexpansion pulmonary edema

(E) Tension pneumothorax

17-34. A 50-year-old female with history of cirrhosis secondary to hepatitis C complains of shortness of breath for 2 weeks with no other symptoms. Her vital signs are within normal limits and her physical examination is unremarkable. Her chest x-ray is shown (Figure 17-6). What is the most likely diagnosis?

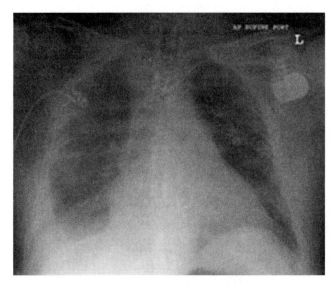

Figure 17-6. Reproduced with permission from Tintinalli JE, Stapczynski JS, Ma OJ, Cline DM, Cydulka RK, Meckler GD: *Tintinalli's Emergency Medicine: A Comprehensive Study Guide,* 7th Edition. Copyright © 2011 The McGraw-Hill Companies, Inc.

(A) Abscess
(B) Diaphragmatic hernia
(C) Hydrothorax
(D) Pneumonia
(E) Pulmonary embolism

17-35. A 19-year-old male presents with a rapid onset of shortness of breath. There is no history of trauma or chronic medical disease. The patient has no risk factors for thromboembolic disease. The following x-ray is consistent with which of the following conditions (Figure 17-7)?

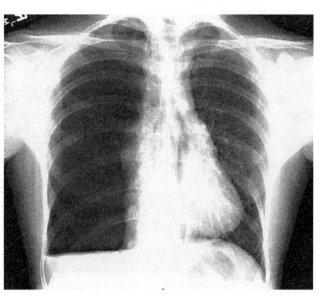

Figure 17-7. Reproduced with permission from Tintinalli JE, Stapczynski JS, Ma OJ, Cline DM, Cydulka RK, Meckler GD: *Tintinalli's Emergency Medicine: A Comprehensive Study Guide,* 7th Edition. Copyright © 2011 The McGraw-Hill Companies, Inc.

(A) Atypical pneumonia
(B) Hampton hump
(C) Metabolic bone disease
(D) Rib fracture
(E) Spontaneous pneumothorax

17-36. A 35-year-old male presents to the ED with sudden onset chest pain. The patient has a history of substance abuse. On examination, the patient's chest wall is tender to palpation. An ECG is obtained that is normal. An ultrasound of the patient's chest is performed and shown here (Figure 71-8). What is the patient's diagnosis?

(A) Abscess
(B) Contusion
(C) Hemothorax
(D) Pneumothorax
(E) Rib fracture

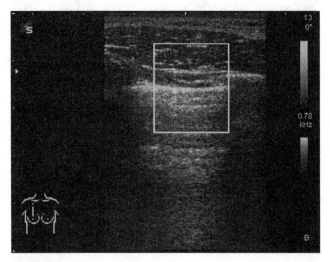

Figure 17-8. Reproduced with permission from Tintinalli JE, Stapczynski JS, Ma OJ, Cline DM, Cydulka RK, Meckler GD: *Tintinalli's Emergency Medicine: A Comprehensive Study Guide,* 7th Edition. Copyright © 2011 The McGraw-Hill Companies, Inc.

Pulmonary Emergencies
Answers and Explanations

17-1. **The answer is D** (Chapter 67). Respiratory viruses such as influenza A and B, parainfluenza, respiratory syncytial virus, and coronavirus have all been attributed to acute bronchitis. *S. pneumoniae* and *H. influenzae* are common causes of bacterial pneumonia. Legionella is an atypical bacteria associated with outbreaks of Legionella pneumonia. *B. pertussis* causes a subacute cough and is becoming more prevalent due to waning immunity.

17-2. **The answer is E** (Chapter 67). Chronic bronchitis is defined as a productive cough for 3 months of the year for 2 consecutive years often with dyspnea along with partially reversible airway obstruction. Patients usually present to the ED due to acute exacerbation of chronic bronchitis. These episodes may manifest cough with up to 50% of patients with acute bronchitis reporting production of purulent sputum. An acute exacerbation of chronic bronchitis is defined as a change in the characteristic of a productive cough that has lasted for more than 3 months for 2 consecutive years.

17-3. **The answer is C** (Chapter 67). Rhinorrhea and repetitive throat clearing are hallmarks of upper respiratory cough syndrome previously termed "postnasal drip." GERD can produce a cough but not postnasal drip. Fever is common in patients with viral respiratory illnesses and is less common with pertussis infections. The common cold is most commonly associated with sore throat, low-grade fever followed by cough and rhinorrhea. Influenza is associated with malaise, myalgias, and high-grade fever. Acute bronchitis is usually associated with a cough of at least 5 days duration and can persist up to 20 days.

17-4. **The answer is C** (Chapter 68). Immunosuppression from alcoholism and cancer has been associated with penicillin resistance. A history of penicillin allergy may predispose an individual to a serious allergic reaction upon rechallenge with a penicillin but is not associated with penicillin resistance. Prematurity is not a predisposing factor for penicillin resistance. There is no structural similarity between macrolides and penicillin so there is no known cross-resistance. A history of asplenia may predispose an individual to streptococcal infection but not to penicillin resistance.

17-5. **The answer is A** (Chapter 68). The severity of the patient's symptoms warrants admission. In the case of an elderly patient with productive cough and fever, it is better to err on the side of caution as the mortality for an elderly patient with pneumonia is close to 40%. When an elderly patient mounts a febrile reaction, a search for its etiology is warranted. Fever is evanescent and a lower temperature on recheck does not rule out serious respiratory illness. Poor prognostic factors in elderly are fever greater than 38.3°C, leucopenia, immunosuppression, gram-negative or staphylococcal infection, cardiac disease, and bilateral infiltrates. In addition, the Pneumonia Patient Outcomes Research Team (PORT) score was devised to identify low-risk patients who could be discharged. The PORT score includes factors such as age, certain comorbidities, and mental confusion among other factors to derive a score and identify mortality risk. Elderly patients with pneumonia frequently require hospitalization and in this case, in which the patient has multiple comorbidities if the chest radiograph confirms clinical suspicion admission, should be strongly considered. A cough suppression and fever control may only mask symptoms in this case and the duration of fever warrants further diagnostic evaluation. The clinical history and physical exam point toward a respiratory cause of fever rather lymphoma.

17-6. **The answer is C** (Chapter 69). This x-ray demonstrates a pneumonia complicated by an empyema. These are seen in patients with necrotizing infections of local parenchyma or due to bacteremia from a nonpulmonary source. Patients with chronic alcoholism are predisposed to aspiration. *S. aureus*, *S. pneumoniae*, *Klebsiella pneumoniae*, and *Pseudomonas aeruginosa* are possible etiologic agents. Viral pneumonias are less likely to produce an abscess. Tuberculosis is a distinct possibility but is incorrect. In the right clinical and sociodemographic setting, or if in doubt, as is often the case, then ruling out tuberculosis would be prudent. In this case, there is no information such as a history of homelessness, living in a shelter or coming from a place where tuberculosis is endemic. Legionellosis is an atypical cause of pneumonia and can cause an abscess, but this patient's history of alcoholism is more consistent with staphylococcus. Haemophilus pneumonia is also another possibility, but the patient's historical information points more toward a pulmonary abscess from aspiration.

17-7. **The answer is E** (Chapter 69). No doubt this patient deserves antibiotics, but given the patient's change in respiratory status, the most important next step is to remove some of the fluid either via thoracentesis or thoracostomy. The patient's respiratory status could benefit from drainage and reexpansion of the affected lung. Needle decompression is used for temporary relief of a tension pneumothorax and in the case of an empyema in which significant inflammatory fluid must be drained a needle will not be sufficient. Antibiotics should then be attended to. The choice of antibiotic is based upon the most likely organisms and Piperacillin–Tazobactam will provide adequate coverage. Obtaining an arterial blood gas is incorrect, although it would give additional information regarding oxygenation but can wait until the patient is more stable. Coagulation studies can be performed in patients with a high risk of bleeding, but in this setting, attention should be directed to supporting respiration.

17-8. **The answer is D** (Chapter 65). A patient with anemia has decreased arterial oxygen content due to the low concentration of oxygen-carrying hemoglobin, but the partial pressure of oxygen is not decreased. Anemia will therefore not affect the value of the A–a gradient. The same is true with a patient who is exposed to carbon monoxide. They will have decreased oxygen content as carbon monoxide displaces oxygen on the hemoglobin molecule, but the partial pressure of oxygen will remain the same. A patient with aortic stenosis has a partial mechanical obstruction to forward flow of blood from the left ventricle, and although this decreases the overall delivery of oxygenated blood, it should not affect the A–a gradient. A patient with upper airway obstruction will continue to absorb oxygen as much as possible and in the initial setting will have a normal partial pressure of oxygen. As less oxygen is absorbed, they will essentially have hypoventilation that can be corrected by supplemental oxygen and ventilation. A patient with significant interstitial lung disease will have an impediment to oxygen diffusion across alveolar membrane and thus leading to a decrease in the partial pressure of oxygen. There will be oxygen arriving to the alveolus, but due to the interstitial disease, oxygen will not readily diffuse across alveolar membrane. This discrepancy will be more notable during exertion when red blood cell transport cannot keep up with the increased demand and manifest as an elevated A–a gradient. A patient who overdoses on heroin will have significant respiratory depression due to stimulation μ-opiates receptors, which leads to decreased breathing frequency and tidal volume, but this will not affect partial pressure of oxygen.

17-9. **The answer is A** (Chapter 65). Being at higher altitude affects oxygen availability due to the decreased oxygen tension at a particular level. The partial pressure of inspired oxygen PiO_2 and the barometric pressure will have a decremental change as you ascend. For example, at sea level, the barometric pressure P_B will be 760 mm Hg with a fraction of inspired oxygen of 21% (FiO_2). The partial pressure of inspired oxygen PiO_2 will be 150 mm Hg, alveolar partial pressure PAO_2 is approximately 102, and partial pressure of oxygen in arterial blood PaO_2 is 95. When a person ascends to a higher altitude such as Pikes Peak in Colorado Springs at an altitude of 14,000 feet, the barometric pressure drops to 450 mm Hg. At this altitude with a fraction of inspired oxygen of 21%, the PiO_2 drops to 85 mm Hg, PAO_2 is 62 and PaO_2 is 55. Increasing a person's hemoglobin may increase their oxygen carrying capacity but does affect the partial pressure of oxygen in blood. Increasing respiratory rate will increase ventilation and thus decrease partial pressure of CO_2 but should not increase the partial pressure of oxygen in the alveoli. Supplemental oxygen will not significantly increase PaO_2 in cases of anemia or carbon monoxide poisoning with the caveat that hyperbaric oxygen therapy in the latter case can augment PaO_2 by displacing CO at a faster rate than with conventional supplemental oxygen.

17-10. **The answer is B** (Chapter 65). An arterial venous shunt will not have an appreciable difference in PaO_2 by providing supplemental oxygen. With a pleural effusion, there is a ventilation perfusion mismatch. Increasing oxygen supply will allow for greater delivery of oxygen to well-ventilated areas. Pulmonary edema from CHF can be thought of

as a problem occupying the alveolar space and supplemental oxygen should improve the A–a gradient. Lobar pneumonia is incorrect due to a similar scenario when the airspace is occluded with inflammatory fluid due to infection. Age-related changes cause an increase in the A–a gradient that ultimately lower the partial pressure of oxygen in arterial blood (PaO_2). Again, supplemental oxygen will be helpful.

17-11. **The answer is C** (Chapter 65). With a pulmonary embolism, there is increased dead space ventilation with a relatively higher proportion of ventilation to perfusion (i.e., high V/Q ratio). An area of the lung is receiving oxygen, but due to thrombotic obstruction of pulmonary vessel, there is an area of under perfusion. Pneumonia represents a situation where inflammatory fluid due to infection impairs ventilation while maintaining adequate perfusion (low V/Q). Pulmonary hemorrhage is similar in that blood is present in airspace while maintaining adequate perfusion (low V/Q). ARDS is an extreme case of airway inflammation that compromises oxygenation and sometimes ventilation while maintaining perfusion. Cyanide toxicity represents a cellular inability to upload oxygen due to cyanide.

17-12. **The answer is A** (Chapter 73). Given the overlapping epidemiology of patients with COPD and CHF, distinguishing between patients with both comorbidities can be challenging for the emergency physician. Patients may have coexisting COPD and CHF. Patients with COPD may have latent CHF that has previously not been diagnosed or masked by their more prevalent bronchitic symptoms. Distended neck veins are a helpful clinical feature for identifying patients with CHF but unfortunately may also be present in patient with elevated right-sided heart pressures due to right-sided heart failure seen in patients with advance lung disease including COPD and emphysema. Body habitus such as the classic "blue bloater" and "pink puffer" are associations with emphysema more so than

COPD. Moreover, patients with advanced CHF develop "cardiac cachexia" that may bear resemblance to a "pink puffer." Patients with significant fluid retention in CHF may resemble a "blue bloater." Peripheral edema is often seen in acutely decompensated CHF; however, the cause of peripheral edema can be due to decreased oncotic pressure from decreased protein levels present in patients with significant wasting due to advance lung disease. B-type natriuretic peptide is a useful noninvasive adjunct to differentiate between COPD and CHF due to its release by the left ventricle in response to cardiac stress. When the levels are decreased, it makes CHF very unlikely.

17-13.   The answer is E (Chapter 72). This asthmatic patient has an underlying expiratory flow limitation due to inflammation and thus is susceptible to air trapping that manifests as auto-PEEP. This auto-PEEP can compromise venous return and lead to hypotension. In asthmatic patients, inspiratory flow rate can be adjusted up and devise a low inspiratory–expiratory ratio, which will increase expiratory phase. To avoid breath stacking, the ventilation rate can be decreased as part of a permissive hypoventilation strategy. Choice C is incorrect because you actually want to maintain a vigorous inspiratory flow rate. Choice B is incorrect because the hypotension is due to physiologic obstruction of preload rather than strict volume depletion. Choice A is incorrect because with an elevated auto-PEEP, you want to avoid extrinsic PEEP. Choice D is incorrect because with relief of auto-PEEP, the ventilation and breath sounds should return to normal. Needle decompression is tenuous intervention because if executed, it must be followed by thoracostomy tubes, which is very complicated in a patient receiving positive pressure mechanical ventilation and thus should be avoided.

17-14.   The answer is A (Chapter 68). Choice B is incorrect because evaluation of the chest x-ray does not demonstrate significant cardiomegaly, although there appears to be bilateral interstitial pattern. There is no suggestion of cephalization. In addition, history does not mention orthopnea, paroxysmal nocturnal dyspnea, or history of cardiac disease. Choice E is incorrect, as pulmonary embolism is difficult to diagnose on chest x-ray. Classic findings of Hampton hump and wedge sign are absent and in fact the lack of a clear x-ray makes pulmonary embolism less likely to explain difficulty with respiration. Choice A is correct, an atypical pneumonia is favored given the indolent course. The patient does have a low oxygenation and the systemic symptoms are consistent with atypical pneumonia. Initiate empiric antibiotics to cover atypical organisms. Choices D and C are very unlikely given the lack of fluid layering for either of these diagnoses and additionally the patient does not appear ill enough to expect an empyema.

17-15.   The answer is D (Chapter 65). A chronic cough by definition is a cough that lasts more than 8 weeks. Choices A, C, and E are incorrect because asthma, GERD, and upper airway cough syndrome (previously called "postnasal drip syndrome") can cause a chronic cough. Choice B is incorrect because bronchiectasis is a condition that results from a process, mass, or infection that permanently disrupts conducting bronchi and infrequently leads to a disabling cough. Choice D is correct as pulmonary embolism usually manifests with rapid onset, chest pain, and acute respiratory distress. The cough seen with pulmonary embolism may manifest as hemoptysis and usually signifies pulmonary infarct.

17-16.   The answer is C (Chapter 65). This case represents a case of pulmonary edema from systolic dysfunction. Patients with this condition are responsible for a large number of admissions to the hospital. Choice A is incorrect and would be a reasonable choice if there were more historical or physical examination findings pointing toward an infectious etiology, but this patient is afebrile. In addition, the patient has a significant coronary disease. Choice E is incorrect because an urgent thoracentesis would only be indicated if patient was hypoxic or having significant respiratory distress. A diagnostic thoracentesis would not be helpful, since bilateral pleural effusions are frequently seen with CHF and the risk does not outweigh any benefit. Choice C is correct, as this is the appropriate management of CHF with pulmonary edema. Choice B, initiating bronchodilator therapy, is incorrect and would not serve to treat the underlying cause. Obtaining a CT, choice D, is incorrect and is indicated for diagnosis of parenchymal processes but would not add much to the management of this patient.

17-17. **The answer is B** (Chapter 66). The answer "bronchial vessel" is correct, as they are under systemic pressure and thus are more likely to bleed briskly as opposed to choice A, an alveolar vessel, which is under relatively lower pressure. Choices C and D are incorrect, as these vessels do not communicate with the conducting airways and would be an unlikely source of hemoptysis. Choice E, internal mammary artery, is a frequently used vessel for coronary bypass but does not communicate with conducting airway and an unlikely source for brisk hemoptysis.

17-18. **The answer is A** (Chapter 66). Massive hemoptysis can lead to asphyxiation from obliteration of airspaces due to blood. Aspiration, choice B, is plausible and may occur to varying degrees depending on the patient's level of consciousness and position but is not the primary reason airway management is needed. Choice C is incorrect, although significant blood loss can occur and exsanguination would be possible if not for the obliteration of airway patency and a patient succumbing to asphyxiation first. Infection is a likely cause of hemoptysis as well as a possible complication of hemoptysis especially if a patient is unable to clear their secretions, but it is not the immediate concern during the acute episode of massive hemoptysis.

Choice E is incorrect even though blood can induce nausea when swallowed. It is for this reason that patient should be placed in either upright position or with the bleeding lung (if known) in dependent position. It is important to have suction available and possibly treat patient for nausea expectantly, but the nausea is not the immediate concern during the acute event.

17-19. **The answer is E** (Chapter 66). In situations where there is respiratory embarrassment, a more aggressive approach is necessary to control bleeding. Supportive care for hypotension due to blood loss and oxygen for hypoxia is indicated. Choice A is incorrect because it includes mention of the blood products, platelets, and FFP. There is nothing in the history to suggest that the patient requires supplemental platelets or coagulation factors to control the current bleeding. This might be a consideration if the patient has an underlying hematologic disorder needing platelets or is being treated with anticoagulation therapy. Choice B is a reasonable approach but incorrect given the patient's considerable anemia awaiting full type and cross-match may be too great a delay. Choice C is incorrect: antibiotics do not a play a role at this point in the management of this patient. Choice D is incorrect but would be reasonable if the patient was more stable. Sedating a patient who is prone to aspiration is ill advised. Choice E is the most appropriate choice, as it addresses the need for supportive care, addresses the ongoing blood loss as well as a reasonable diagnostic plan. If the patient was more stable, they could be transferred to a facility or department with expertise in selective intubation, rigid bronchoscopy, and/or cardiothoracic intervention to alleviate hemorrhage if selective embolization or rigid bronchoscopy cannot control bleeding. The next option would be to perform surgical resection of the affected area of lung.

17-20. **The answer is A** (Chapter 66). Warfarin depletes vitamin K dependent coagulation factors II, VII, IX, X, and proteins C and S.

FFP contains all of these plus several other coagulation factors. Cryoprecipitate that is derived from FFP only contains factors VIII, XIII, fibrinogen, fibronectin, and von Willebrand factor. Choice B is incorrect as checking the patient's complete blood count (CBC) may not fully quantify blood loss but can serve as a baseline. Choice B is correct for this case of a patient who is known to be on warfarin and develops sudden hemoptysis. It is prudent to request FFP, as this will take several minutes to thaw units of FFP. FFP will effectively replace the coagulation factors that are most likely inactivated by warfarin. Vitamin K administration could be used in less severe bleeding as it would allow time for vitamin K to reactivate the warfarin inactivated factors. Cryoprecipitate does not contain the factors necessary to reverse the effects of warfarin. Transfusion of uncrossmatched red blood cells is an important step in the management of patients with massive bleeding but will not address the underlying medication-induced coagulopathy. With holding his medication (warfarin) will not make a significant impact on his current state and may need to be reinforced when patient is more stable and is ready for discharge.

17-21.   **The answer is A** (Chapter 69). The patient has a history of an indolent course with worsening respiratory status. The patient has an infection that is apparently resistant to an incomplete course of antibiotics. The dullness on examination is probably due to focal consolidation of the affected lobe. Choice A is the correct answer due to the history and x-ray findings. Note the air fluid level at the left base on PA view. Thoracic CT makes the necrotic area more apparent. Choice C is not correct, as there is no indication in the clinical history about the patient being hospitalized recently. Mycoplasma pneumonia usually presents with more subtle clinical and radiographic findings. Tuberculosis is a serious consideration but once again based upon the history provided; there are no obvious risk factors for exposure and contraction of tuberculosis. Choice B, CHF, can cause significant dyspnea and would also not re-

spond to oral antibiotics but would not have the chest x-ray findings displayed. Congestive heart failure may present with a myriad of x-ray finding including bilateral pleural effusions.

17-22.   **The answer is D** (Chapter 70). Choice D is correct as TB progresses rapidly from primary disease and seeds other organs by the time children present for medical assistance. Choice A is not the right choice because children with tuberculosis are often very ill and have a weak cough and have a smaller tuberculosis burden than a larger adult. Nonetheless, all patients with tuberculosis should be appropriately isolated. Choice B is incorrect as this is the opposite of what occurs in children who contract tuberculosis. Choice C is incorrect as the prevailing recommendation is to treat all children with a positive purified protein derivative (PPD) and an abnormal chest x-ray for multidrug resistant tuberculosis. Choice E is incorrect because younger children have a paucity of symptoms or are asymptomatic when infected with tuberculosis.

17-23.   **The answer is C** (Chapter 70). Anxiety is incorrect as an anxious patient would not manifest a fever. Although misdiagnosis of pneumonia as tuberculosis, D, is a possibility, given the recent hospital admission, initiation of antituberculosis medications would have required some confirmatory studies. Choices B and E address a common concern when treating HIV patients and that is to determine whether the clinical presentation is due to HIV, opportunistic infection, or due to medications. Antituberculosis medications are associated with a number of undesired effects from affecting liver function to visual disturbances but seldom are they associated with fever and worsening of respiratory symptoms. Drug interactions do occur especially when multiple medications are simultaneously started or when new medications are added to a treatment regimen. It is important to review all medications a patient is currently taking and correlating the current symptoms to possible manifestations of drug interactions. Choice C, immune reconstitution disease, is seldom seen but plausible explanation for the symptoms described. The prevailing explanation for the symptoms is due to an improvement in immune function when antiretroviral medications are initiated and their effect manifests as an exuberant inflammatory response leading to symptoms that can be diagnostically difficult to differentiate between treatment failure, drug resistance, and medication noncompliance.

17-24. **The answer is C** (Chapter 72). Choices A and B urge maintaining an elevated respiratory rate to combat CO_2 retention and to match patient's level of ventilation prior to intubation. In this case, it is advisable to accept some level of hypoventilation to allow the patient to have adequate time to expire because of the airflow obstruction seen during the expiratory phase in acute asthma exacerbation. Ventilator strategies employ increasing airflow during inspiration and lowering respiratory rate. Choice D recommends a higher tidal volume that is not advisable in asthma exacerbation as this may predispose to barotraumas from intrinsic PEEP. Choice E addresses common misconceptions regarding ventilator management in asthmatic patients. In the acute phase of ventilator management for asthmatic patients with respiratory failure, low level of hypoventilation is acceptable and is termed "permissive hypoventilation." The goal of management should not be based solely on normalizing the arterial pH but evaluating the respiratory parameters such as airflow during expiration, degree of auto-PEEP, and expiratory volume. Many of these parameters are measured or calculated by modern mechanical ventilators and can be ascertained by the respiratory therapist. Choice C is the correct answer and is consistent with a permissive hypoventilation strategy.

17-25. **The answer is E** (Chapter 72). Choices A, B, and C are incorrect as these options describe this exacerbation as moderate despite evidence of hypoxemia and respiratory distress. Given the patients' level of distress

and fatigue after self-administering metered dose inhaled albuterol, beginning nebulized breathing treatments might be prudent as well as initiating steroids as soon as possible. Choice D is a reasonable approach to this patient and recognizes that this patient and fetus are at high risk; however, as with the previous choices, it does not mention fetal monitoring. Choice D is incorrect as it classifies this exacerbation as moderate. It does also include ipratropium as an adjunct that is category Class B that has not shown any teratogenicity in animals. Many feel this drug should be used with caution and weigh the benefits. Choice E is correct as it correctly classifies this as a severe exacerbation as notable by a PaO_2 <70 and a PCO_2 >35 indicating respiratory failure. The management expressed in choice E is reasonable considering the severity and also includes fetal monitoring that is recommended at 20 weeks.

17-26. **The answer is C** (Chapter 73). Choice D, administering 100% oxygen via non-rebreather, would be discouraged as this patient already has a blunted hypoxic drive and administering such a high concentration of oxygen can be deleterious. Choice A suggests administering albuterol, which may alleviate some of the bronchospastic component of his exacerbation but may not alleviate the work of breathing to a significant extent. Choice E, use of IV steroids, is a reasonable approach and will address the chronic inflammation of the airway but will not significantly address the work of breathing. Ipratropium bromide will also work on the bronchospastic component of this exacerbation but similarly not impact the work of breathing. Choice C is correct by suggesting utilization of noninvasive positive pressure ventilation as an accepted modality of mechanical ventilation. It significantly addresses the work of breathing and breathing treatments can be administered through a respiratory circuit.

17-27. **The answer is C** (Chapter 73). Albuterol is the mainstay of acute pharmacologic management of acute exacerbation of COPD. There is evidence for steroids in the acute setting.

Although studies have not shown a decrease in hospital admission, there is evidence that the initiation of steroids decrease ED revisits. Although there are sparse and conflicting results for the use of ipratropium for the acute management of COPD exacerbation, albuterol and ipratropium reverse airflow obstruction, which is one of the goals in management of these patients. There is evidence that the repeat administration of the combination of beta agonist and anticholinergics for asthma exacerbation is helpful, but these results have not been reproduced for COPD. There is currently no data to support administration of magnesium for acute exacerbation of COPD. Oxygen is used to reverse any hypercapnia and airflow obstruction but should be used judiciously particularly in patients who are home O_2 dependent.

17-28. **The answer is D** (Chapter 73). The GOLD (Global Initiative for Chronic Obstructive Lung Disease) does not recommend chronic oral corticosteroids use for COPD, but for acute exacerbation a 10-day course of prednisone 40 mg/day may decrease recurrence of exacerbations, and or hospitalization. There is no good evidence for oral magnesium supplementation as an adjunct for the management of acute exacerbation of COPD. The need for increasing home oxygen therapy would be based on baseline room air PaO_2 or pulse oximetry, not merely on admission for COPD exacerbation. Pulmonary rehabilitation may be helpful for persons severely limited by COPD, but physical therapy per se may not be a useful adjunct for improving respiratory function immediately after an exacerbation. Delivery of beta agonist via nebulizer has not been shown to be superior to metered dose inhaler administration.

17-29. **The answer is D** (Chapter 73). There is no close association of pets with COPD. A patient may have a history of atopy when exposed to pets, which can complicate their COPD, but there is no direct correlation. The severity of dyspnea with exertion is a key prognosticator of COPD severity. The

BODE index is a composite index that combines physiologic parameters such as forced expiratory volume in one second (FEV_1), 6-minute walk test, MRC dyspnea index, and body mass index as a higher body mass airflow dyspnea exercise capacity (BODE) index correlates with an increasing risk of death. Hemoptysis is a harbinger of various diseases including malignancy that can be seen in patients with COPD, who have a history of chronic smoking. The presence of ankle swelling may indicate that there is a problem with the patient's nutritional status or possibly that the patient has CHF. Occupational or environmental exposure can be correlated with disease etiology such as exposure to asbestos and asbestosis.

17-30. **The answer is B** (Chapter 69). The x-ray demonstrates a right-sided pleural effusion. The CT shows a moderate pleural effusion on the right and a small one on the left, which likely took time to develop. A history of acute onset fever and chills and night sweats points toward an infectious etiology such as pneumonia with empyema or atypical presentation of tuberculosis. A productive cough and fever would also point toward a more rapid course than is illustrated by the pleural effusion seen. Although postcardiotomy syndrome can cause an effusion, there are no sternal wires seen on this x-ray to indicate a recent coronary artery bypass surgery (CABG). Choice B is correct because it fits with the apparent process on chest x-ray and CT and once further history can be ascertained then a thoracentesis or thoracostomy to drain the fluid can be sent off for further diagnostic studies. Choice E is incorrect because the history would be suggestive of acute exacerbation of chronic bronchitis that would typically have a more benign appearance on chest x-ray.

17-31. **The answer is E** (Chapter 73). A prominent interstitial pattern could represent an exacerbation of CHF or interstitial fibrosis. A significantly elevated B-type hatriuretic peptide (BNP) would point toward CHF more than COPD exacerbation. Decubitus film is incorrect because they are useful in detecting the presence of pleural effusions. Choice B is incorrect because the clinical history points toward a process with a more indolent course such as CHF or COPD exacerbation as opposed to a pulmonary embolism. Determining whether or not there is a change in pulse oximetry after ambulation would indicate severity of hypoxia that could be due to any of various chronic respiratory or cardiac diseases rather than determining a specific etiology. Obtaining an arterial blood gas would determine the degree of hypoxemia and/or hypercarbia but will not point toward a specific etiology.

17-32.   The answer is B (Chapter 71). Chest x-ray is correct because based on the acute history, a pneumothorax is a diagnostic consideration. In addition, sudden onset of dyspnea is concerning for pulmonary embolism and a relatively clear chest x-ray or one with a Westermark sign or a Hampton hump will be helpful if present. Decubitus films would be helpful if a pleural effusion was a strong consideration. Physical examination revealed distant breath sounds and there was no mention of dullness on percussion. An arterial blood gas would reveal acute hypoxemia but would not point toward a specific etiology. A peak flow will give you an idea of expiratory flow but not clue you into the cause of compromised respiratory function. Last, pulmonary toilet has fallen out of favor. It was often used to relieve mucous plugging and would be less helpful if a pneumothorax is present.

17-33.   The answer is D (Chapter 71). Reexpansion pulmonary edema is more often seen in younger patients aged 20–39 years, and with larger pneumothoraces present for >72 hours that are rapidly expanded with suction. Pulmonary edema generally occurs on the side of the reexpanded lung. Treatment is supportive with aggressive volume resuscitation and sharply differs from treatment for cardiogenic pulmonary edema. Infection is rare at the thoracostomy site. There should be no contact between thoracostomy tube and conducting airways that may have copious secretions that can become inspissated.

17-34.   The answer is C (Chapter 65). This patient's advanced liver disease suggests that the findings can represent a sympathetic effusion/hydrothorax. Patients with significant cirrhosis and ascites often have impaired lymphatic drainage leading to pleural effusions. If patient is in respiratory distress and the etiology is unclear, determining whether the fluid is an exudate or a transudate would be helpful by comparing pleural fluid protein, lactate dehydrogenase (LDH) to serum protein, and LDH. If ratio of pleural protein to serum is >0.5 or pleural fluid LDH to serum LDH is >0.6, then the fluid is an exudate. Pneumonia is a possibility but is incorrect due to the insidious progression of symptoms, and lack of fever and cough make it slightly less likely. Acquired diaphragmatic hernias are rare and are seen usually after blunt or penetrating trauma. They usually occur on the left side owing to hepatic protection of the right diaphragm. Pulmonary embolism would typically have a more rapid onset.

17-35.   The answer is E (Chapter 71). The x-ray demonstrates a spontaneous pneumothorax on the right with a small hemothorax in an otherwise healthy young individual. Management of primary pneumothorax includes aspiration of pleural air either by needle thoracostomy or small catheter with or without Heimlich valve. A Hampton hump is a classic sign of pulmonary embolism with pulmonary infarction that is described as a pleural-based triangular wedge with base along the pleural surface and the top of the triangle pointing toward hilum. This is opposed to Westermark sign that is a sign of vascular oligemia distal to the location of a pulmonary embolism and is described as dilation of proximal pulmonary arteries and collapse of distal vessels. An atypical pneumonia would have a different radiographic appearance including patchy or subsegmental infiltrate. There is no evidence of cortical irregularities or displaced rib fractures on this chest radiograph and there is no history of trauma. Metabolic bone disease would likely manifest with some bony lesion either as lytic lesions or osteopenia.

17-36.   The answer is D (Chapter 71). This B-mode ultrasound of the chest demonstrates a lack of lung sliding. A finding that is apparent when there is a pneumothorax. A fluid such as blood is seen as a hypoechoic or black layering on ultrasound. Ultrasound is not an ideal study for identifying fractures. Abscesses have variable appearances on ultrasound.

Renal and Genitourinary Disorders
Questions

18-1. Which of the following statements about the pathophysiology of acute renal failure is TRUE?

(A) Damage to the nephrons from cytokine-mediated alteration of nitric oxide has been implicated in the pathophysiology of intrinsic renal failure and prerenal failure, but not postrenal failure.

(B) Intrinsic renal failure occurs when renal perfusion is decreased leading to ischemia of renal parenchyma.

(C) Patients with chronic hypertension require lower blood pressures to develop intrinsic renal failure when compared with patients without chronic hypertension.

(D) Tubular and glomerular function are not maintained in prerenal failure.

(E) Use of radiocontrast agents and aminoglycosides during a time of decreased renal perfusion does not lead to further renal injury in most cases.

18-2. Which of the following statements regarding radiocontrast-induced nephropathy is TRUE?

(A) It is an uncommon cause of in-hospital acute renal failure.

(B) It uncommonly occurs in patients with normal renal function.

(C) It usually results in permanent renal failure.

(D) Risk factors include chronic renal insufficiency, diabetes, older age, hypovolemia, and dose of contrast.

(E) The preventive role of bicarbonate infusion has been definitively proven in the literature.

18-3. Which of the following drugs is not usually implicated in crystal-induced nephropathy?

(A) Acyclovir
(B) Indinavir
(C) Phenytoin
(D) Sulfonamides
(E) Triamterene

18-4. Analysis of the urine from a patient with acute renal failure shows pigmented granular casts. What is the cause of the patient's acute renal failure?

(A) Acute glomerulonephritis
(B) Acute interstitial nephritis
(C) Acute tubular necrosis
(D) Prerenal azotemia
(E) Rhabdomyolysis

18-5. What is the best imaging modality for diagnosing the cause of acute renal failure in the emergency department (ED)?

(A) Computed tomography with intravenous contrast
(B) Computed tomography without intravenous contrast
(C) Intravenous pyelogram
(D) Magnetic resonance urography before and after diuretic use
(E) Renal ultrasound

18-6. Which of the following statements about vasopressor use in critically ill patients with renal failure is FALSE?

(A) Dopamine at low doses improves renal recovery and decreases mortality in critically ill patients with renal failure.

(B) Fenoldopam is considered by some experts as the agent of choice for hypertensive emergencies in patients with renal dysfunction.

(C) Fenoldopam is a dopamine and alpha-receptor agonist that increases blood flow to the renal cortex and outer medulla.

(D) Fenoldopam is titratable and reliably controls hypertension.

(E) Fenoldopam reduces mortality and provides renal protection in critically ill patients at risk for renal failure.

18-7. Which of the following is NOT an indication for emergent dialysis?

(A) Blood urea nitrogen (BUN) greater than 100 mg/dL

(B) Lithium poisoning

(C) Severe metabolic acidosis

(D) Uremic encephalopathy with seizures

(E) Uremic pericarditis

18-8. What is the most common organism responsible for dialysis catheter-related bacteremia?

(A) *Escherichia coli*

(B) *Pseudomonas aeruginosa*

(C) *Staphylococcus aureus*

(D) *Staphylococcus epidermidis*

(E) *Streptococcus pneumonia*

18-9. Which of the following is NOT a common complication of end-stage renal disease?

(A) Bleeding gastric and duodenal ulcers

(B) Pericarditis

(C) Peripheral neuropathy

(D) Subdural hematoma

(E) Uremic encephalopathy

18-10. What is the most common complication of hemodialysis?

(A) Air embolism

(B) Hyperphosphatemia

(C) Hypocalcemia

(D) Hypoglycemia

(E) Hypotension

18-11. What is the most common organism causing peritonitis in peritoneal dialysis patients?

(A) Anaerobic bacteria

(B) Gram-negative bacteria

(C) *S. aureus*

(D) *S. epidermidis*

(E) *Streptococcus* species

18-12. Which of the following antibiotics is the initial antibiotic of choice to treat a urinary tract infection in an HIV-positive patient?

(A) Cephalexin

(B) Ciprofloxacin

(C) Doxycycline

(D) Nitrofurantoin

(E) Trimethoprim/sulfamethoxazole

18-13. Which of the following correctly describes the radiologic findings on ultrasound or computed tomography associated with acute pyelonephritis?

(A) Areas of decreased density within the kidney that are ill defined, sometimes striated, or wedge-shaped

(B) Areas of decreased density within the kidney that are well defined

(C) Areas of gas within the kidney

(D) Diffusely enlarged kidney with perinephric stranding and no focal renal abnormalities

(E) No radiographic abnormalities

18-14. Which of the following signs or symptoms does NOT independently increase the probability of a urinary tract infection?

(A) Dysuria

(B) Fever

(C) Frequency

(D) Gross hematuria

(E) Vaginal discharge

18-15. A patient with a history of benign prostatic hypertrophy presents to the ED stating he has been unable to urinate normal volumes for 2 weeks. He is complaining of abdominal pain and mild shortness of breath. You place a Foley catheter to relieve his bladder obstruction. What is the minimum amount of time recommended to observe the patient in the ED for the development of postobstructive diuresis?

(A) 2 hours

(B) 4 hours

(C) 8 hours

(D) Patient does not need to be observed now that his obstruction has been treated

(E) Patient requires admission for 24 hours of observation

18-16. Patients placed on an alpha-adrenergic receptor blocker for the treatment of urinary retention need to be warned of what possible side effect?

(A) Bradycardia

(B) Erectile dysfunction

(C) Hypotension

(D) Tinnitus

(E) Urinary incontinence

18-17. An ill appearing male presents with severe scrotal pain. In addition to antibiotics, what is the appropriate management for this patient (Figure 18-1)?

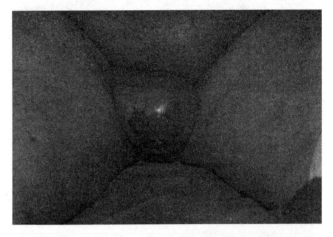

Figure 18-1. Reproduced with permission from Knoop KJ, Stack LB, Storrow AB, Thurman RJ: *The Atlas of Emergency Medicine,* 3rd Edition. Copyright © 2010 The McGraw-Hill Companies, Inc. Photo contributor: R. Jason Thurman, MD.

(A) CT of the abdomen and pelvis

(B) Incision and drainage in the ED

(C) Reduction of the hernia

(D) Surgical consultation

(E) Ultrasound of the scrotum

18-18. What is the most important diagnostic test for this patient (Figure 18-2)?

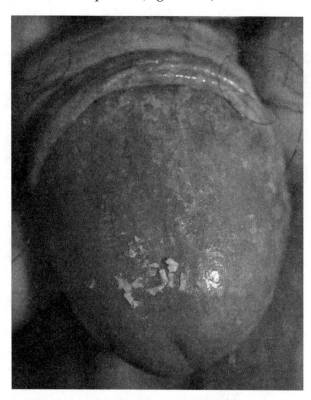

Figure 18-2. Reproduced with permission from Wolff K, Johnson RA: *Fitzpatrick's Color Atlas & Synopsis of Clinical Dermatology,* 6th Edition. Copyright © 2009 The McGraw-Hill Companies, Inc.

(A) Complete blood count (CBC)

(B) Erythrocyte sedimentation rate

(C) Glucose

(D) Rapid plasma reagin (RPR)

(E) Wound culture

18-19. Which of the following conditions requires emergent urologic consultation?

(A) Balanitis

(B) Balanoposthitis

(C) Paraphimosis

(D) Phimosis

(E) Posthitis

18-20. Nephrolithiasis is the most common misdiagnosis given to patients with what condition?

(A) Appendicitis

(B) Bladder cancer

(C) Glomerulonephritis

(D) Renal artery thrombosis

(E) Rupturing or expanding abdominal aortic aneurysm

18-21. Which of the following statements about urinary tract infections in patients with an indwelling Foley catheter is TRUE?

(A) Infections in patients with short-term indwelling catheters are usually caused by a single organism.

(B) Intermittent self-catheterization is associated with a higher risk of urinary tract infection compared with indwelling catheter.

(C) Pyuria is universal for patients with indwelling catheters for more than 30 days and diagnosis of urinary tract infection should not be made without the presence of other clinical symptoms or signs, such as fever, flank pain, or hematuria.

(D) Renal abscess is the most common complication of catheter-associated urinary tract infection with fever.

(E) The presence of Candida in the urine of a patient with an indwelling catheter is common and does not require treatment.

18-22. Which of the following patients with a ureteral stent can be discharged home with outpatient urology follow-up?

(A) A patient with flank pain and fever

(B) A patient with gross hematuria

(C) A patient with gross hematuria and syncope

(D) A patient with gross hematuria and hypotension

(E) A patient with mild flank pain, urgency, microscopic hematuria, and urinary incontinence

18-23. What is the most critical complication of injection therapy for the treatment of erectile dysfunction?

   (A) Localized hematoma
   (B) Penile pain
   (C) Priapism
   (D) Prolonged erection
   (E) Syncope

18-24. Which of the following conditions does NOT increase a patient's risk of developing nephrolithiasis?

   (A) Hyperparathyroidism
   (B) Inflammatory bowel disease
   (C) Neurogenic bladder
   (D) Pseudogout
   (E) Small bowel resection

Renal and Genitourinary Disorders
Answers and Explanations

18-1. **The answer is B** (Chapter 91). In prerenal failure, tubular and glomerular function is maintained. The most common cause of intrinsic renal failure, traditionally known as acute tubular necrosis and now called acute kidney injury, is ischemic acute renal failure. It occurs when renal perfusion is decreased so much that the kidney parenchyma suffers ischemic injury. During an ischemic insult from decreased renal blood flow, cytokine-mediated alteration of nitric oxide production and increased production of systemic vasoconstrictors cause worsening periglomerular vasoconstriction and further depress renal blood flow which, along with microvascular congestion, red blood cell trapping, and activation of the coagulation cascade, magnifies ischemic injury. During periods of depressed renal blood flow, the kidneys are especially vulnerable to further insult from nephrotoxic agents such as radiocontrast agents and aminoglycosides. Individuals with chronic hypertension develop altered renal autoregulation that establishes conditions under which renal ischemia can occur in spite of systemic blood pressures that would be normal, not low, for most patients.

18-2. **The answer is D** (Chapter 91). Radiocontrast-induced nephropathy is a common cause of in-hospital acute renal failure. It can occur in patients with normal renal function, either due to direct insult to the nephrons or in the setting of decreased renal blood flow from another cause, such as infection or dehydration. The typical course is an increase in creatinine over 3–5 days, followed by complete resolution. The beneficial role of bicarbonate has been suggested by some studies but remains controversial.

18-3. **The answer is C** (Chapter 91). Phenytoin, NSAIDs, diuretics, allopurinol, rifampin, and certain antibiotics can cause acute interstitial nephritis. Acyclovir, indinavir, sulfonamides, triamterene, and tumor lysis syndrome are causes of crystal-induced nephropathy.

18-4. **The answer is E** (Chapter 91). Microscopic examination of the urine is very useful in establishing the cause of renal failure. Acute glomerulonephritis will produce red cell casts in the urine. Acute interstitial nephritis will result in white cell casts and eosinophils in the urine. In acute tubular necrosis, the tubular epithelium breaks down and results in tubular epithelial cells and pigmented granular casts in the urine. Prerenal azotemia results in hyaline casts in the urine, although a few hyaline casts in a urine sample may be normal. Conditions that cause the filtration of pigmented proteins, such as myoglobinuria and hemoglobinuria, as you would see in rhabdomyolysis, will result in brown granular casts in the urine.

18-5. **The answer is E** (Chapter 91). Renal ultrasound is the test of choice for urological imaging in the setting of acute renal failure. Ultrasound has 90% sensitivity and specificity for detecting hydronephrosis due to obstruction without the radiation associated with computed tomography. In addition to identifying the presence of hydronephrosis, ultrasound can identify the presence of nephrolithiasis, renal size, and renal parenchymal disease, but cannot always detect the location of obstruction. A second study, noncontrast computed tomography, may be necessary to identify the location of obstruction. Noncontrast computed tomography has the same sensitivity and specificity as ultrasound for detecting hydronephrosis. Radionucleotide scans and magnetic resonance urography before and after diuretic use may be useful if functional obstruction is a consideration.

18-6. **The answer is A** (Chapter 91). Low (renal)-dose dopamine does not improve renal function or mortality and may increase urine output at the expense of increased medullary oxygen consumption. Fenoldopam (Corlopam) stimulates dopamine D1-like and alpha 2-adrenergic receptors, is easily titratable, works well in hypertensive emergencies, provides renal protection, and reduces mortality in critically ill patients at risk for or in renal failure.

18-7. **The answer is A** (Chapter 91). Indications for emergent hemodialysis are listed in Table 91–10. It is recommended to keep the BUN lower than 100 mg/dL. However, there is no absolute BUN value at which to dialyze a patient. Each patient should be evaluated by a nephrologist to assess the need for dialysis.

18-8. **The answer is C** (Chapter 93). Approximately 48% of patients with a dialysis catheter will develop bacteremia after 6 months. *S. aureus* is the most common organism responsible for catheter-related bacteremia, followed by gram-negative organisms. Vancomycin is the drug of choice because it effectively treats methicillin-resistant organisms and has a long half-life. An aminoglycoside should be added if a gram-negative organism is suspected.

18-9. **The answer is A** (Chapter 93). End-stage renal disease causes a number of complications in almost every organ system. Gastrointestinal complications include chronic constipation, gastritis, and increased gastrointestinal bleeding due to the bleeding

dyscrasias associated with uremia. However, the incidence of bleeding ulcers is the same as the general population. Pericarditis, usually from uremia, is a result of fluid overload, abnormal platelet function, and increased fibrinolysis. Other cardiovascular complications include accelerated atherosclerosis and myocardial infarction, hypertension, cardiac tamponade, congestive heart failure, and uremic cardiomyopathy. Peripheral neuropathy occurs in 60–100% of end-stage renal disease patients and does not respond to renal replacement therapy but does improve with renal transplant. Subdural hematomas are ten times more prevalent in hemodialysis patients than in the general population. End-stage renal disease patients with subdural hematomas can present without focal neurologic deficits, so a high degree of suspicion is required for any end-stage renal disease patient with a change in mental status. Uremic encephalopathy is a constellation of nonspecific neurologic symptoms and responds to renal replacement therapy. In contrast, dialysis dementia, which may present similarly to uremic encephalopathy, does not respond to hemodialysis and is progressive and eventually fatal. Other complications of end-stage renal disease include anemia, bleeding dyscrasias, autonomic dysfunction, immune suppression, and endocrine abnormalities.

18-10. **The answer is E** (Chapter 93). Hypotension occurs in up to 30% of hemodialysis treatments, usually caused by excessive ultrafiltration after underestimating the patient's ideal (dry) weight. Other complications that occur less frequently include air embolism, cerebral edema from dialysis disequilibrium, hemorrhage from accessing the vascular access site, hypercalcemia, hypermagnesemia, and hypoglycemia.

18-11. **The answer is D** (Chapter 93). Peritonitis is the most common complication of peritoneal dialysis. *S. epidermidis* from skin flora is the most common organism (40%) responsible for peritoneal dialysis-related peritonitis. Other organisms include

Streptococcus species (15–20%), Gram-negative bacteria (15–20%), *S. aureus* (10%), anaerobes (5%), and fungi (5%).

18-12. **The answer is B** (Chapter 94). Fluoroquinolones are the initial antibiotic of choice. Trimethoprim/sulfamethoxazole resistance is high in the HIV/AIDS population because of its use in *Pneumocystis carinii* prophylaxis. Most urinary tract infections in HIV/AIDS patients are caused by typical pathogens and sexually transmitted diseases (STD) organisms. Mycobacterium tuberculosis is an uncommon cause of urinary tract infection in the HIV/AIDS population.

18-13. **The answer is D** (Chapter 94). Pyelonephritis appears as diffusely enlarged kidneys with perinephric stranding and no focal renal abnormalities. Acute bacterial nephritis appears as ill-defined areas, sometimes striated or wedge-shaped, of decreased density. Renal abscesses appear as well-defined areas of decreased density. Emphysematous pyelonephritis is a rare gas-forming infection within the kidney that almost always occurs in diabetics (90%) and requires nephrectomy for effective treatment.

18-14. **The answer is E** (Chapter 94). Dysuria, frequency, gross hematuria, fever, and costovertebral angle tenderness are independently associated with a high likelihood of having a urinary tract infection. A patient with dysuria, frequency, or gross hematuria has a pretest probability of urinary tract infection that is too high to be ruled out by any test or exam findings, and the patient should be treated for urinary tract infection. The absence of dysuria or back pain has been shown to decrease the likelihood of urinary tract infection, especially in the presence of vaginal discharge.

18-15. **The answer is B** (Chapter 95). Postobstructive diuresis is a complication of urinary obstruction that occurs when the obstruction has been prolonged and has resulted in renal failure or volume overload. Postobstructive diuresis can result in significant volume loss

and hemodynamic instability. A minimum of 4 hours of observation is recommended before discharging a patient home. Admission is recommended for patients with persistent diuresis of 250 mL per hour for more than 2 hours, or 200 cc of urine output per hour over intake.

18-16. **The answer is C** (Chapter 95). Postural hypotension, especially with the first dose of an alpha blocking agent, is the most common side effect of alpha-adrenergic receptor blockade. Other side effects include syncope, tachycardia, priapism, dry mouth, blurred vision, and intraoperative floppy iris syndrome.

18-17. **The answer is C** (Chapter 96). Fournier's gangrene is a polymicrobial necrotizing fasciitis of the genitals that requires immediate wide surgical debridement and antibiotic coverage for Gram-positive, Gram negative, and anaerobic bacteria. Suspect Fournier's gangrene in alcoholics, diabetics, and patients with pain out of proportion to the physical findings. Ultrasound of the testes would be appropriate if hydrocele, orchitis, or epididymitis was suspected, but that is not what this image is showing. Oral antibiotics for 14 days are appropriate for epididymitis in an otherwise healthy, nontoxic patient.

18-18. **The answer is C** (Chapter 96). This patient has balanoposthitis that occurs commonly in diabetics. Balanitis, posthitis, and balanoposthitis may be the first presenting sign of diabetes mellitus and checking serum glucose is essential.

18-19. **The answer is C** (Chapter 96). Paraphimosis is the inability to reduce the proximal foreskin distally over the glans penis to its natural position. Prolonged venous engorgement can restrict arterial blood flow to the glans and cause ischemia and is a urologic emergency. Phimosis, the inability to retract the foreskin proximally to the glans penis is an emergency only if it results in urinary retention. Balanitis, inflammation of the glans, posthitis, inflammation of the foreskin, and balanoposthitis, inflammation of the glans and foreskin are inflammatory conditions caused by inadequate hygiene or colonization with Candida and are common in diabetics. These conditions are treated with cleansing and education on proper hygiene, antifungal creams, and antibiotics when appropriate.

18-20. **The answer is E** (Chapter 97). Ruptured or expanding abdominal aortic aneurysm is most commonly misdiagnosed as nephrolithiasis.

18-21. **The answer is A** (Chapter 98). Catheter-associated urinary tract infections are usually due to a single organism during short-term catheterizations, most commonly *E. coli*, *Klebsiella*, *Pseudomonas*, *Enterobacter*, and Gram-positive cocci. With long-term catheterization, catheter-associated urinary tract infections are usually polymicrobial from *E. coli*, *Proteus mirabilis*, *Pseudomonas*, *Morganella morganii* and *Candida* species. Catheter-associated *Candida* infections require removal of the catheter, and if symptomatic, treatment with an antifungal agent such as amphotericin B or fluconazole. Intermittent self-catheterization is associated with a lower rate of catheter-associated urinary tract infections. The occurrence of bacteriuria and pyuria among patients with long-term indwelling catheters is almost 100%. Treatment of bacteriuria or pyuria in cases of long-term catheter use should be limited to those patients with a clinical picture of urinary tract infection. Hematuria is a better indicator of infection than bacteriuria in these cases.

18-22. **The answer is E** (Chapter 98). Complications of ureteral stents include cystitis, pyelonephritis, sepsis, hematuria, obstruction, stent migration, flank pain, abdominal pain, vascular–ureter fistula, and irritative bladder symptoms such as frequency, urgency, dysuria, and urinary incontinence. Vascular–ureter fistula is a rare late complication and presents as gross hematuria with syncope or hypotension and requires aggressive resuscitation with intravenous fluids and emergent urologic consult. Stent migration or fragmentation is also one of

the less common complications and presents with obstructive or infectious signs including fever, hematuria, and pain and is a urologic emergency. Pyelonephritis or sepsis requires admission for intravenous antibiotics and urologic consult. Only patients with minor urinary tract infections (i.e., without fever, hypotension, or obstructive signs) or patients with symptoms of an irritative bladder can be safely discharged with outpatient urology follow-up.

18-23. **The answer is C** (Chapter 98). Injection therapy for erectile dysfunction can be intracavernosal or intraurethral. Agents used include alprostadil for both intracavernous and intraurethral or papaverine phentolamine for intracavernous injection. The mechanism involves vasodilation of the arteries and veins leading to corporal smooth muscle relaxation and penile erection. Priapism is the most critical complication as prolonged engorgement can lead to ischemia. Treatment of priapism consists of emergent urologic consult, narcotic analgesia, and injection of terbutaline, 0.25–0.5 milligrams subcutaneously into the deltoid, repeated in 30 minutes if needed. If this fails, corporal irrigation with phenylephrine or plain saline is required. If this fails as well, surgery may be required. Sickle cell patients with priapism require simple or exchange transfusion.

18-24. **The answer is D** (Chapter 97). Hyperparathyroidism, end-stage renal disease, and immobilization increase urinary calcium excretion and contribute to stone formation. Bowel disease and bowel resection promotes low urine volume and increases oxalate in urine, one of the solutes in calcium stones. Neurogenic bladder provides the urinary stasis required for stone formation. Gout, but not pseudogout, promotes hyperuricosuria. Twenty-five percent of patients with gout will develop uric acid kidney stones. Other risk factors for the development of nephrolithiasis include excess dietary meat, excess dietary sodium, family history, insulin resistance, dehydration, obesity, and renal tubular acidosis.

Resuscitation
Questions

19-1. What caused the majority of fatal dysrhythmias leading to sudden cardiac death?

(A) Brugada syndrome

(B) Commotio cordis, related to blunt trauma during athletics

(C) Congenital heart disease

(D) Dilated and hypertrophic cardiomyopathies

(E) Structural coronary artery abnormalities, including coronary atherosclerosis

19-2. Which of the following statements regarding sudden cardiac death and acute myocardial infarction (AMI) is TRUE?

(A) Autonomic tone plays no role in the heart's propensity to develop and sustain a serious ventricular dysrhythmia.

(B) Beta-blockade is not protective against sudden cardiac death in patients who have had AMI and have a low ejection fraction.

(C) Both sudden cardiac death and AMI are more likely to occur in summer rather than in climatic winter.

(D) Sudden cardiac death and AMI are more likely to occur in the evening hours prior to going to bed.

(E) Triggers of plaque rupture or thrombus formation likely affect the onset of ischemic cardiac events.

19-3. The findings in this ECG are most suggestive of which cardiac abnormality (Figure 19-1)?

(A) Acute anterior wall myocardial infarction (MI)

(B) Brugada syndrome

(C) Left bundle branch block

(D) Severe aortic stenosis

(E) Wolff–Parkinson–White syndrome

19-4. The outcome of resuscitation and the likelihood of survival are greatest when the initial cardiac rhythm is which of the following?

(A) Agonal rhythm

(B) Asystole

(C) Idioventricular rhythm

(D) Pulseless bradycardia

(E) Ventricular fibrillation (VF)

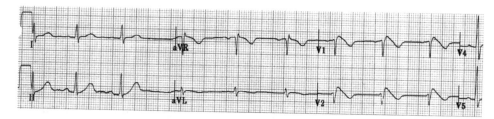

Figure 19-1. Reproduced with permission from Tintinalli JE, Stapczynski JS, Ma OJ, Cline DM, Cydulka RK, Meckler GD: *Tintinalli's Emergency Medicine: A Comprehensive Study Guide*, 7th Edition. Copyright © 2011 The McGraw-Hill Companies, Inc.

19-5. Proximal occlusion of which coronary artery is most likely to cause ischemia of both the sinoatrial (SA) and atrioventricular (AV) nodes, leading to bradycardia?

(A) Circumflex artery

(B) Left anterior descending artery

(C) Left main coronary artery

(D) Obtuse marginal branch

(E) Right coronary artery (RCA)

19-6. Stimulation of afferent vagal cardiac receptors during ischemia or infarction can trigger sympathetic inhibition, producing vasodilatation, bradycardia, and hypotension. This is known as:

(A) Bazett's equation

(B) Bezold–Jarisch reflex

(C) Lenegre disease

(D) Lev disease

(E) Preexcitation syndrome

19-7. Which of the following agents has been shown to be of protective value in patients at high sudden cardiac death risk?

(A) Amiodarone

(B) Atropine

(C) Encainide

(D) Flecainide

(E) Moricizine

19-8. A 67-year-old male suffers from recurrent ventricular dysrhythmias following an anterior wall MI. Which of the following treatments will have the greatest effectiveness at decreasing his mortality from sudden cardiac death?

(A) Amiodarone

(B) Beta-blockade

(C) Implantable cardioverter-defibrillator

(D) Pacemaker therapy

(E) Sotalol

19-9. The key to survival following cardiac arrest is:

(A) Depth of chest compression to 2 inches

(B) Early defibrillation

(C) Prolonged single rescuer cardiopulmonary resuscitation (CPR)

(D) Sodium bicarbonate therapy

(E) Ventilation with 100% oxygen

19-10. When approaching a collapsed victim in the out of hospital setting, after assessing the level of responsiveness, the next step should be:

(A) Administer ventilations

(B) Call for help

(C) Initiate an intravenous (IV)

(D) Stabilize the cervical spine

(E) Start chest compressions

19-11. A woman who is 39 weeks pregnant chokes on her steak dinner prior to collapsing to the floor. She is still conscious, but cannot speak and is turning blue. The preferred method of clearing her obstructed airway is:

(A) Chest thrust

(B) Endotracheal (ET) intubation

(C) Finger sweep

(D) Heimlich maneuver

(E) Laryngeal mask airway (LMA) placement

19-12. A near-term but low-birth-weight newborn has received tactile stimulation and blow by oxygen for a heart rate of 80. After 30 seconds of blow by oxygen, there has been no improvement. No meconium was noted. What is the next step?

(A) Chest compressions

(B) ET intubation and positive pressure ventilation

(C) ET intubation and aspiration for meconium

(D) LMA and ventilation

(E) Positive pressure ventilation with a bag-mask, at a rate of 40–60 breaths/min

19-13. As a rule of thumb, the appropriate depth of ET tube placement in a 3-kg infant as measured from the lips is:

(A) 5 cm

(B) 7 cm

(C) 9 cm

(D) 13 cm

(E) 17 cm

19-14. An intravenous (IV) line is required in a newborn infant. When placing the umbilical catheter, which of the following statements is TRUE?

(A) Ideal position for an umbilical catheter is in the inferior vena cava, above the liver and diaphragm, but below the heart.

(B) There are normally two umbilical veins and one umbilical artery.

(C) Umbilical vein access is contraindicated and should only be used as a last resort.

(D) Umbilical veins are ideal for fluid administration, but should never be used for medications.

(E) An umbilical vein is smaller than an umbilical artery.

19-15. What is the most common cause of primary cardiac arrest in children?

(A) Congenital heart disease

(B) Coronary artery disease

(C) Head injury

(D) Respiratory failure

(E) Toxicologic exposure

19-16. Which of the following statements is TRUE regarding the differences in an adult's and a child's airway?

(A) Hyperextension is acceptable for positioning prior to intubation in a child, but contraindicated in adults.

(B) The airway is higher in an adult than in a child.

(C) The airway is more anterior in an adult than in a child.

(D) The tongue and epiglottis are relatively larger compared to the airway in a child

than in an adult and are more likely to obstruct the airway.

(E) When an adult is supine, the prominent occiput causes flexion of the neck on the chest and occludes the airway, which does not happen in children.

19-17. A 6-year-old requires intubation for a severe exacerbation of asthma. Which of the following is TRUE regarding the ET tube selection?

(A) Only an uncuffed tube may be used in this patient.

(B) A curved (MacIntosh) blade should never be used in this age group.

(C) Preoxygenation should be avoided, as it may worsen airway spasm and constriction.

(D) The best predictor of ET tube size is a length-measuring device, such as the Broselow tape.

(E) The correct internal diameter of the ET tube is best chosen by measuring the end of the patient's little finger.

19-18. The correct procedure for accomplishing cardiopulmonary resuscitation in a 10-year-old child is as follows:

(A) Children of this age are treated as adults with respect to basic life support.

(B) Compress the lower half of the sternum with one hand, using the heel only.

(C) Current recommendations for ET drug use suggest a dose that is half of the IV dose.

(D) Monitor the brachial pulse for adequacy of compression.

(E) Use the two-thumb technique when two rescuers are present.

19-19. Which of the following is the current recommended drug for the treatment of supraventricular tachycardia (SVT) in children?

(A) Adenosine

(B) Amiodarone

(C) Calcium

(D) Magnesium

(E) Sodium bicarbonate

19-20. The most common medical cause of maternal death in pregnant women is:

(A) Homicide

(B) Infection

(C) Motor vehicle accidents

(D) Pregnancy-induced hypertension

(E) Pulmonary embolism

19-21. Which of the following statements is TRUE regarding the maternal cardiovascular system during pregnancy?

(A) A state of chronic respiratory acidosis develops during the first trimester of pregnancy due to lowered minute ventilation.

(B) Cardiac output decreases 30–45% below baseline at 20 weeks of gestation and does not return to normal until after delivery.

(C) Femoral and saphenous vein sites for IV access are recommended due to increased pelvic flow after 20 weeks of gestation, making them ideal sites for medication administration.

(D) Fetal physiology appears to be protective of severe hypoxia, with a left shift of the oxyhemoglobin dissociation curve relative to the mother.

(E) Pregnant women develop hypoxia less readily, and are more tolerant of apneic periods as compared to nonpregnant women of the same age.

19-22. A 23-year-old woman suffers a cardiac arrest in your emergency department (ED) from a suspected pulmonary embolism. She is 34 weeks pregnant. Resuscitative efforts are not going well. Which of the following is TRUE regarding perimortem cesarean section?

(A) Maternal CPR should be stopped as soon as the procedure is considered to avoid trauma to the infant.

(B) Perimortem cesarean section should not be considered after 4 minutes of maternal cardiac arrest.

(C) Prognosis for intact survival of the infant is best if delivery occurs within 5 minutes of cardiac arrest.

(D) The patient should be moved to an operating suite before the procedure is performed.

(E) The procedure is best performed using a horizontal, bikini-type incision.

19-23. Which of the following is the best choice regarding a diagnostic test to perform in a pregnant woman at 32 weeks of gestation with a suspected pulmonary embolism?

(A) Arterial blood gas.

(B) Chest radiograph.

(C) CT scan or ventilation perfusion scan.

(D) D-dimer.

(E) No diagnostic test is acceptable—simply treat the patient and admit for the duration of the pregnancy.

19-24. What is the most common cause of severe anaphylaxis reactions in the United States, accounting for 400–800 deaths per year?

(A) Beta-lactam antibiotics

(B) Blood transfusions

(C) Food allergies

(D) Hymenoptera

(E) Latex

19-25. A patient presents with pruritus, urticaria, and cutaneous flushing after eating a peanut butter sandwich. She rapidly progresses to a sense of fullness in the throat, chest tightness, and shortness of breath. Of the choices given, what is the single most important therapy to provide for her?

(A) Antihistamines

(B) Corticosteroids

(C) Dopamine

(D) Epinephrine

(E) Leukotriene inhibitors

19-26. A 50-year-old man with hypertension on a beta-blocker just received an IV beta-lactam antibiotic for a new pneumonia. The nurse calls you to the bedside for a suspected anaphylactic reaction to the antibiotic. The patient is hypotensive and remains so after receiving appropriate doses of epinephrine, steroids, diphenhydramine, and 2 L of crystalloid. Which if the following agents should you give him next?

(A) Cimetidine

(B) Fresh frozen plasma

(C) Glucagon

(D) Magnesium sulfate

(E) Terbutaline

19-27. A patient with known hereditary angioedema presents following a motor vehicle accident with shortness of breath, swelling of her lips, a sensation of swelling in her throat, and abdominal pain. She describes this as typical for an acute attack of angioedema. Which if the following is most likely to help her?

(A) Cimetidine

(B) Corticosteroids

(C) Diphenhydramine

(D) Epinephrine

(E) Fresh frozen plasma

19-28. A patient was seen at his doctor's office and prescribed cefaclor for a sore throat. Three days after completing the prescription, he comes to the ED complaining of malaise, arthralgias, arthritis, pruritus, hives, fever, and adenopathy. Which of the following is the most likely diagnosis?

(A) Angioedema

(B) Delayed hypersensitivity reaction

(C) Leukemia

(D) Serum sickness

(E) Viral illness

19-29. Select the TRUE statement regarding the evaluation and treatment of hemorrhagic shock.

(A) Bradycardia or lack of tachycardia is a rare and unusual finding in patients with intra-abdominal hemorrhage and hemoperitoneum.

(B) Elderly patients always develop a tachycardia in response to blood loss.

(C) Hypotension in the setting of head injury eliminates the need to look for occult hemorrhage.

(D) Urine output is especially helpful to follow in the initial assessment of the patient with acute hemorrhage.

(E) Young athletes may have such a robust response to hemorrhage that they will appear stable and not manifest tachycardia or hypotension even with significant hemorrhage.

19-30. For every liter of blood loss from hemorrhage, how many liters of crystalloid are required to restore normovolemia?

(A) 1/2

(B) 1

(C) 2

(D) 3

(E) 4

19-31. Which of the following statements is TRUE regarding the treatment of the patient in shock?

(A) Most patients in shock are normovolemic.

(B) Neuromuscular blocking agents should be avoided in shock.

(C) Optimizing hemodynamic endpoints with early goal-directed therapy is likely to reduce mortality.

(D) Vasopressors are equally effective when the vascular space is "full" or when it is depleted.

(E) The combination of sedatives and positive pressure ventilation is unlikely to affect blood pressure in the patient prior to volume resuscitation.

19-32. A patient presents in severe shock, and it is determined that bicarbonate therapy would be of benefit. What pH value, over time, should the arterial pH be corrected to?

(A) 6.90

(B) 7.05

(C) 7.15

(D) 7.25

(E) 7.40

19-33. The following vasopressor is a synthetic sympathomimetic that exerts potent inotropic and mild chronotropic activities. It increases myocardial contractility and systemic vasodilation with minimal changes in heart rate.

(A) Dopamine

(B) Dobutamine

(C) Epinephrine

(D) Norepinephrine

(E) Vasopressin

19-34. A 90-year-old man presents with a temperature of 103 F, BP of 78/45 mm Hg, altered mental status, and evidence of a urinary tract infection. After ensuring adequate fluid resuscitation, his blood pressure remains less than 90 mm Hg systolic. What agent should be used next?

(A) Dobutamine

(B) Dopamine

(C) Epinephrine

(D) Milrinone

(E) Vasopressin

19-35. According to the latest Advanced Cardiac Life Support (ACLS) manual, the first-line drug for the treatment of ventricular tachycardia (VT) or ventricular fibrillation is:

(A) Amiodarone

(B) Lidocaine

(C) Procainamide

(D) Propranolol

(E) Sodium bicarbonate

19-36. Long-term oral therapy with amiodarone is associated with which of the following side effects?

(A) Adrenal insufficiency

(B) Corneal deposits

(C) Impotence

(D) Retroperitoneal fibrosis

(E) Torsades de pointes

19-37. Which of the following agents is likely to increase serum digoxin levels and potentially lead to toxicity?

(A) Cholestyramine

(B) Dietary fiber

(C) Diltiazem

(D) Metoclopramide

(E) Penicillamine

19-38. Which of the following is TRUE regarding hyponatremia?

(A) Antidiuretic hormone (ADH) secretion is generally inhibited in most cases of hyponatremia.

(B) Seizures are unlikely to occur at a serum sodium level of 107 mEq/L

(C) Sodium in the human body is predominately an intracellular element.

(D) There is greater risk of brain damage from the treatment of hyponatremia than from the hyponatremia itself.

(E) Urinary sodium of 25 mEq/L is indicative that renal handling of sodium is appropriate in the setting of hyponatremia.

19-39. A patient presents with diabetic ketoacidosis (DKA). His initial measured glucose is 550 mg/dL. The measured sodium is 128 mEq/L. Using a normal glucose of 100 mg/dL, what is the corrected serum sodium value for this patient?

(A) 120

(B) 125

(C) 135

(D) 140

(E) 145

19-40. A 56-year-old male with chronic renal failure missed his hemodialysis yesterday. He presents with his wife complaining of weakness and lethargy. His serum potassium is 7.6 mEq/L. Which of the following agents acts by shifting the potassium from the extracellular space to the intracellular space?

(A) Calcium gluconate

(B) Furosemide

(C) Hemodialysis

(D) Insulin

(E) Sodium polystyrene sulfonate

19-41. A 47-year-old man suffers a right ventricular and inferior wall infarction. Which of the following is MOST LIKELY to occur as a complication of this heart attack?

(A) Aortic valve failure

(B) Flash pulmonary edema

(C) Left bundle branch block

(D) Right bundle branch block

(E) Second-degree AV block

19-42. A 72-year-old woman presents for evaluation of an ingrown toenail. On physical exam, her heart rate is 42 and AV block is noted on her ECG. Her blood pressure is 165/85, her mental status is normal, and she has no other complaints. Of the following, which is the best course of action?

(A) Atropine 1 mg IV

(B) Epinephrine 1:1000, 0.3 mg IV

(C) Glucagon 0.1 mg test dose, followed by 1 mg IV

(D) Isoproterenol drip

(E) Place pacing pads on the patient and observe her pending admission.

19-43. A 75-year-old man is diagnosed with sick sinus syndrome. What is the most important and appropriate initial therapy?

(A) Atropine

(B) Diltiazem

(C) Increase fluids and acetaminophen as needed

(D) Metoprolol

(E) Permanent pacemaker placement

19-44. Which of the following statements is TRUE regarding therapy with adenosine?

(A) Adenosine has a prolonged antiarrhythmic effect.

(B) Adenosine is approved for use in Wolff–Parkinson–White syndrome when the QRS complex is narrow.

(C) Adenosine is unlikely to produce chest pain and flushing as a side effect.

(D) Adenosine is unsafe in pregnancy.

(E) Adenosine should never be used in patients with reentrant SVTs and chest pain or hypotension.

19-45. A patient is brought in by emergency medical services breathing 60% oxygen by face mask. What is his estimated PaO_2?

(A) 100 mm Hg

(B) 150 mm Hg

(C) 240 mm Hg

(D) 360 mm Hg

(E) 390 mm Hg

19-46. Which of the following conditions is associated with a normal oxygen saturation reading as measured by pulse oximetry, without a falsely elevated or falsely lowered result?

(A) Carbon monoxide exposure

(B) Cyanide poisoning

(C) Hypothermia

(D) Severe anemia

(E) Toxic hemoglobins

19-47. Select the TRUE statement regarding lactic acid in the blood.

(A) Early lactate clearance in shock is predictive of a lower survival rate.

(B) Elevated lactate levels are predictive of mortality with shock.

(C) Lactate levels are accurate from an arterial sample, but should not be measured in a venous sample.

(D) The blood pressure and heart rate are better markers of shock than serum lactate.

(E) Type B lactic acidosis is a consequence of tissue hypoperfusion.

19-48. Select the TRUE statement regarding acid–base balance.

(A) A normal or high pH excludes acidosis.

(B) Arterial and venous samples for pH and CO_2 content in normal patients and in patients with DKA correlate well, implying that venous blood may be used for acid–base evaluation.

(C) Compensatory mechanisms for acid–base disorders will generally return the blood pH to normal.

(D) Respiratory acid–base disorders are primarily due to changes in the concentration of bicarbonate in the blood.

(E) Serum pH is always the most important value from the blood gas for diagnosis and management of acid–base disorders, and therefore should always be measured arterially.

19-49. A patient presents in severe DKA, with a pH on blood gas of 6.8. His serum potassium is measured at 3.7 mEq/L. The normal value ranges from 3.5 to 5.0 mEq/L. Which of the following statements is CORRECT?

(A) The total body potassium will be high, and the patient should undergo corrective measures immediately.

(B) The total body potassium is high, but no action is required as this is clinically insignificant.

(C) The total body potassium is low, but no action is required as this is clinically insignificant.

(D) The total body potassium level is low, and this should be addressed as pH is corrected.

(E) The total body potassium is normal as indicated by the normal serum level.

Resuscitation
Answers and Explanations

19-1. **The answer is E** (Chapter 12). Structural coronary artery abnormalities and their consequences (e.g., myocardial ischemia and infarction) are associated with 80% of fatal arrhythmias.

19-2. **The answer is E** (Chapter 12). Both sudden cardiac death and AMI are most likely to occur within the first few hours after awakening from sleep, at a time when there is increased sympathetic stimulation. Beta-blockade appears to protect against sudden cardiac death, particularly in patients with known coronary artery disease who have had an AMI and have a low ejection fraction. In addition, both sudden cardiac death and AMI are much more likely to occur during climatic winter rather than during summer. These and other epidemiologic and experimental findings suggest that neurophysiological factors, such as autonomic tone, may alter the heart's propensity to develop and sustain a serious ventricular dysrhythmia. An alternative possibility is that there are factors external to the atherosclerotic plaque, such as triggers of plaque rupture or thrombus formation, which may affect the onset of ischemic cardiac events.

19-3. **The answer is B** (Chapter 12). Twelve-lead ECG typical of Brugada syndrome shows characteristic downsloping ST-segment elevation in leads V_1 and V_2 and QRS morphology resembling a right bundle branch block.

19-4. **The answer is E** (Chapter 12). The likelihood of survival is relatively high (up to 60%) if the initial rhythm is VT or VF, especially if the VF is "coarse."

19-5. **The answer is E** (Chapter 12). Proximal occlusion of the RCA can cause ischemia and/or infarction of both the SA and AV nodes, because in humans, the SA node is supplied by a branch from the proximal RCA in 55% of the time, and the AV node receives its nourishment from a branch of the distal RCA 90% of the time. Ischemia or infarction of the AV node can disrupt normal conduction, causing bradycardia as a consequence of AV block.

19-6. **The answer is B** (Chapter 12). Autonomic disturbances have been documented in the majority of patients with AMI, especially during the first 30–60 minutes after coronary artery occlusion. Stimulation of afferent vagal cardiac receptors, particularly those located in the posterior left ventricle, during ischemia or infarction can trigger sympathetic inhibition producing vasodilation, bradycardia, and hypotension (the Bezold–Jarisch reflex). Activation of this reflex may explain the higher incidence of nausea and vomiting in patients with inferior (69%) infarction compared to anterior (29%) infarction.

19-7. **The answer is A** (Chapter 12). The Cardiac Arrhythmia Suppression Trial (CAST) showed that potent Class I sodium channel-blocking antidysrhythmic drugs (encainide, flecainide, and moricizine) are proarrhythmic and paradoxically increase the odds of developing sudden cardiac death, as compared with placebo, in patients at relatively low risk for death. Conversely, Class III agents (amiodarone, sotalol) and/or beta-blockers may be of some protective value in patients at high sudden cardiac death risk.

19-8. **The answer is C** (Chapter 12). The benefits of beta-blockade, sotalol, and amiodarone in decreasing mortality from sudden cardiac death pale in comparison with the protective effects of the implantable cardioverter-defibrillator on high-risk patients.

19-9. **The answer is B** (Chapter 12). Ventricular tachydysrhythmias are the most common cause of sudden cardiac death in adults. Defibrillation is the most effective treatment for VT and VF. The effectiveness of defibrillation diminishes rapidly over time, and unless treated promptly, VF becomes less coarse and eventually converts to the less treatable rhythm of fine VF or asystole. Adding field ACLS capability appears to affect survival from out-of-hospital cardiac arrest favorably, although the degree of benefit is relatively minimal compared to the powerful effect of early defibrillation.

19-10. **The answer is B** (Chapter 13). Once the patient is reached, determine the patient's level of responsiveness to noxious stimuli. If the individual does not respond, get help first before starting ventilations and chest compressions.

19-11. **The answer is A** (Chapter 13). The chest thrust maneuver for foreign body airway obstruction is used primarily in morbidly obese patients or patients in the late stages of pregnancy when the rescuer cannot reach around the patient's abdomen to perform the Heimlich maneuver.

19-12. **The answer is E** (Chapter 14). The apneic and/or bradycardic (<100 beats/min) newborn should initially receive tactile stimulation and have blow-by oxygen administered. If these maneuvers are unsuccessful after 30 seconds, positive pressure ventilation should be initiated, beginning with bag-mask ventilation. Use a mask with a tight seal, and ventilate at 40–60 breaths/min.

19-13. **The answer is C** (Chapter 14). An accurate rule of thumb for proper tube placement is add 6 to the newborn's weight (in kilograms) and place ET tube centimeter marker at that number at the newborn's lip edge. Hence, the proper ET tube placement for a 3-kg newborn is 9 cm (6 + 3) at the lips.

19-14. **The answer is A** (Chapter 14). The umbilical vein is the recommended access in the newborn. The vein is easily identified from the two umbilical arteries because it is larger with a thinner wall. The ideal position for the umbilical venous catheter is in the inferior vena cava above the liver and diaphragm, but below the heart, at the T-7 to T-8 level.

19-15. **The answer is D** (Chapter 15). One major difference between adult and pediatric cardiopulmonary arrest is the cause of the arrest. The most common cause of primary cardiac arrest in adults is coronary artery disease. Respiratory failure and shock are more common causes among children and infants.

19-16. **The answer is D** (Chapter 15). A child's airway is much smaller than an adult's. Anatomic and functional differences are more pronounced in infants and young children. The airway is higher and more anterior in a child than in an adult. The tongue and epiglottis are relatively larger and thus more likely to obstruct the airway. When a child is supine, the prominent occiput causes flexion of the neck on the chest and occludes the airway, which can be corrected by mild extension of the neck to the sniffing position. Overextension or hyperextension, acceptable for adults, causes obstruction and may kink the trachea, because the cartilaginous support is poor.

19-17. **The answer is D** (Chapter 15). For two reasons, the curved (MacIntosh) blade is rarely used in children younger than 4 years. First, the relatively large and flaccid epiglottis is not effectively displaced by pulling on it indirectly from the vallecular space. Second, an exact-size blade must be used to fit the curvature of the tongue. Therefore, a straight (Miller) blade is preferred. The straight blade is inserted in the midline with the tip underneath the epiglottis, such that the epiglottis is directly lifted up to allow tracheal visualization. ET tube sizes vary with a patient's age. An often-quoted rule is that the correct internal diameter tube size is approximately the same size as the end of the patient's little finger. However, this tenet has been disproved. The age-based formula, (age + 16)/4, remains a better predictor of correct ET tube size for children. The best predictor of ET tube size is a length-based measuring device. Cuffed or **uncuffed tubes are used for children up to 7** or **8 years old** (tube size, 2.5–5.5 mm), because in children (unlike adults), the subglottic trachea is the narrowest spot of the trachea and forms a seal around the uncuffed ET tube in this age group. In patients older than 8 years, the vocal cords are the narrowest part to the airway, and a cuff is needed to provide an adequate seal for positive pressure ventilation. When cuffed tubes are used in younger children, the exacting selection of an uncuffed tube becomes unnecessary. Use of a cuffed tube does require monitoring of the cuff pressure as well as proper positioning to ensure the cuff is below the vocal cords.

19-18. **The answer is A** (Chapter 15). Children >8 years old are treated as adults with respect to basic life support. Although the ideal ET doses for drugs other than epinephrine have never been studied in children, current recommendations support the use of two to three times the respective IV dose. Other foils are true for younger children and infants only.

19-19. **The answer is A** (Chapter 15). Adenosine (0.1 mg/kg) is the current recommended drug for SVT in children. This dose can be doubled if the first dose is unsuccessful.

19-20. **The answer is E** (Chapter 16). Pulmonary embolism is the most common *medical* cause of death in pregnant women, trauma (homicide) is the most common overall cause of maternal death. Interpersonal violence indicators should be examined in all pregnant patients as a preventive measure.

19-21. **The answer is D** (Chapter 16). The fetal oxyhemoglobin dissociation curve is shifted to the left relative to the maternal oxyhemoglobin dissociation curve because of the greater affinity of hemoglobin F for oxygen. Thus, at any partial pressure of oxygen (Po_2), fetal hemoglobin will bind oxygen more strongly, resulting in greater saturation. Fetal Po_2 does not fall significantly unless maternal Po_2 falls below 60 mm Hg. Cardiac output increases to 30–45% above baseline levels by the 20th week of gestation and remains at that level until delivery. Poor venous flow compromises the delivery of medications administered through infradiaphragmatic sites, such as the femoral or saphenous vein. Therefore, femoral or saphenous venous sites are not recommended for IV access during the resuscitation of a pregnant patient with greater than 20 weeks of gestation. Compression of the aorta also occurs, causing diminished distal blood flow. A state of chronic respiratory alkalosis develops during the first trimester of pregnancy due to increased minute ventilation secondary to increased tidal volume and mild progesterone-stimulated hyperventilation. Pregnant patients develop hypoxia more quickly and are less tolerant of apneic periods than nonpregnant patients.

19-22. **The answer is C** (Chapter 16). Prognosis for intact survival of the infant is best if delivery occurs within 5 minute of maternal arrest. If the 5-minutes time frame has been exceeded, a perimortem cesarean section is still recommended. The patient should not be moved to an operating suite, as this wastes time. **It is not necessary and only delays a potentially lifesaving procedure to evaluate fetal viability before initiation of the cesarean section.** Maternal CPR should be continued throughout the procedure and for a brief time afterward, as successful maternal resuscitation may occur once aortocaval obstruction is relieved. A vertical midline (classic) incision is made from 4 to 5 cm below the xiphoid process to the pubic symphysis through the abdominal wall. The rectus muscles may be separated with blunt dissection, and the peritoneum is entered with a midline incision that is continued superiorly and inferiorly to allow visualization of the uterus.

19-23. **The answer is C** (Chapter 16). When pulmonary embolism is suspected, empiric treatment with heparin should be started immediately, especially if the patient is hypoxic or hemodynamically unstable. Once treatment has begun, a CT scan or ventilation-perfusion scan should be obtained to confirm the diagnosis. D-dimer concentrations increase progressively throughout normal pregnancy and an elevated D-dimer level is not a helpful screen for the diagnosis of venous thromboembolic disease during pregnancy. Chest radiograph and ABG are not sensitive and are nonspecific.

19-24. **The answer is A** (Chapter 27). β-Lactam antibiotics are estimated to cause 400–800 deaths in the United States annually, with a systemic allergic reaction occurring in 1 per 10,000 exposures. Hymenoptera stings constitute the next most common cause of anaphylaxis, with fewer than 100 deaths in the United States annually. Pediatric surveillance studies have shown food allergy to be a very common cause of anaphylaxis in children. Latex hypersensitivity is also increasing in prevalence in the general population, with a resultant risk for anaphylaxis.

19-25. **The answer is A** (Chapter 27). With *suspected* anaphylaxis, the single most important step in treatment is the rapid administration of epinephrine. Moreover, with this rapid administration, many of the secondary measures discussed below may not be necessary. Emergency management starts with the ABCs (airway, breathing, circulation) of resuscitation. The first-line therapies for anaphylaxis (e.g., epinephrine, IV fluids, and oxygen) have immediate effect during the acute stage of anaphylaxis. Vital signs, IV access, oxygen administration, cardiac monitoring, and pulse oximetry measurements should be initiated immediately.

19-26. **The answer is C** (Chapter 27). Concurrent use of β-blocking drugs by the patient is a risk factor for severe prolonged anaphylaxis. In one study, three of five patients who had severe protracted reactions were being treated with β-blocking drugs. For patients taking β-blockers with hypotension refractory to fluids and epinephrine, glucagon should be used in a dose of 1 mg IV every 5 minutes until hypotension resolves, followed by an infusion of 5–15 µg/min.

19-27. **The answer is E** (Chapter 27). Hereditary angioedema is an autosomal dominant disorder with a characteristic complement pathway defect: low levels of C1 esterase inhibitor or elevated levels of dysfunctional C1 esterase inhibitor with low levels of C4 between acute attacks. Reactions often involve the upper respiratory tract and gastrointestinal tract. Attacks can last from a few hours to 1–2 days. Minor trauma often precipitates a reaction. Many of the typical treatments for allergic reactions, such as epinephrine, steroids, and antihistamines, are ineffective. Prophylaxis of acute attacks may be possible with attenuated androgens, such as stanozolol 2 mg/day or danazol 200 mg/day. Acute attacks can be shortened by C1 esterase inhibitor (C1-INH inhibitor) replacement by a concentrate. Successful treatment with fresh frozen plasma has also been reported and may be tried if C1-INH inhibitor is not available. Treatment of patients is complex and best done in coordination with the appropriate specialist.

19-28. **The answer is D** (Chapter 27). Serum sickness usually begins in the first or second week after the administration of the drug and can take many weeks to subside after drug withdrawal. Generalized malaise, arthralgias, arthritis, pruritus, urticarial eruptions, fever, adenopathy, and hepatosplenomegaly are common signs and symptoms. Drug fever may occur without other associated clinical findings and may also occur without an immunologic basis. Circulating immune complexes are probably responsible for the lupus-like reactions caused by some drugs. Cytotoxic reactions, such as penicillin-induced hemolytic anemia, can occur. Skin eruptions include erythema, pruritus, urticaria, angioedema, erythema multiforme, and photosensitivity. Severe reactions, such as those seen in Stevens–Johnson syndrome and toxic epidermal necrolysis, may also occur. Pulmonary complications, including bronchospasm and airway obstruction, can occur.

19-29.   The answer is E (Chapter 26). Patients with excellent baseline physiological status (e.g., young athletes) may have such a robust compensatory response to hemorrhage that they appear stable and do not manifest tachycardia or hypotension even with significant hemorrhage. Signs of peripheral hypoperfusion and subtle mental status alterations may be the only clues that the severity of hemorrhage is greater than predicted based on hemodynamic parameters. Elderly patients may not develop a tachycardic response to blood loss due to underlying heart disease or medications such as β-adrenergic blockers. Bradycardia or lack of tachycardia may occur in about 30% of patients with intra-abdominal hemorrhage from increased vagal tone in response to hemoperitoneum. In a pregnant trauma patient, compression of the inferior vena cava by the gravid uterus can decrease central venous return and worsen hypotension and tachycardia in the setting of less severe hemorrhage. Systemic hypoperfusion usually results in decreased urine output due to renal hypoperfusion and compensatory fluid reabsorption. Urine output is not helpful in the initial assessment of the patient with acute hemorrhage but over time helps assess response to resuscitation. Hypotension in the setting of trauma does not always indicate hemorrhage. Other life-threatening conditions, such as primary myocardial dysfunction, airway compromise, hypoxemia due to lung injury, pericardial tamponade, tension pneumothorax, spinal cord injury, and toxicologic syndromes, should be kept in mind. However, hypotension always warrants a careful search for occult hemorrhage.

19-30.   The answer is D (Chapter 26). This is the physiologic basis for the 3:1 ratio for isotonic crystalloid volume replacement: for each given quantity of blood lost, three times that amount of isotonic crystalloid is required to store intravascular volume because, at best, about 30% of the infused fluid stays intravascular. Based on this rule, a loss of 1 L of blood (about 15–20% of total circulating blood volume) would require about 3 L of isotonic crystalloid to restore normovolemia.

19-31.   The answer is C (Chapter 25). Fluid resuscitation begins with isotonic crystalloid. The amount and rate of infusion are determined by an estimate of the hemodynamic abnormality. Most patients in shock have either an absolute or relative volume deficit. The exception is the patient in cardiogenic shock with pulmonary edema. Respiratory muscles are significant consumers of oxygen during shock and contribute to lactate production. Mechanical ventilation and sedation allow for adequate oxygenation, improvement of hypercapnia, and assisted, controlled, synchronized ventilation—all of which decrease the work of breathing and improve survival. SaO_2 should be restored to greater than 93% and ventilation controlled to maintain a $PaCO_2$ 35–40 mm Hg. Normalizing pH above 7.3 by hyperventilation is not beneficial. Neuromuscular blocking agents should be used as adjuncts to further decrease respiratory muscle oxygen consumption and preserve DO_2 to vital organs. Vasopressors are most effective when the vascular space is "full" and least effective when the vascular space is depleted. Sedatives used to facilitate intubation may cause arterial vasodilatation, venodilation, and myocardial suppression and result in hypotension. Positive pressure ventilation reduces preload and cardiac output. The combination of sedative agents and positive pressure ventilation can lead to hemodynamic collapse. Consider volume resuscitation or application of vasoactive agents prior to intubation and positive pressure ventilation. Application of an algorithmic approach to optimize hemodynamic endpoints with early goal-directed therapy (EGDT) in the ED reduces mortality by 16% in patients with severe sepsis or septic shock. EGDT has been validated in both septic and nonseptic populations.

19-32. **The answer is D** (Chapter 25). Many clinicians remain uncomfortable withholding bicarbonate if metabolic acidosis is severe. A compromise position is to partially correct the metabolic acidosis over time to an arterial pH 7.25.

19-33. **The answer is B** (Chapter 24). Dobutamine (Dobutrex) is a synthetic sympathomimetic drug that exerts potent inotropic and mild chronotropic activities. Dobutamine is formulated as a racemic mixture with β_1- and β_2-adrenergic and α-adrenergic agonist activities that are offset by α-adrenergic antagonist activity. The net result is an increase in myocardial contractility and systemic vasodilation, with minimal changes in heart rate. Doses of up to 20 μg/kg/min will increase cardiac output, decrease peripheral vascular resistance, and decrease pulmonary occlusive pressures. Conversely, doses larger than 20 μg/kg/min will increase the heart rate and induce arrhythmias.

19-34. **The answer is B** (Chapter 24). Dopamine is indicated for reversing hemodynamically significant hypotension caused by MI, trauma, heart failure, and renal failure when fluid resuscitation is unsuccessful or not appropriate. Like norepinephrine, it is considered first-line therapy for septic shock. Dopamine is used to increase cardiac output, blood pressure, and peripheral perfusion. It should not be used at low doses solely for the purpose of renal protection or to increase urine output.

19-35. **The answer is A** (Chapter 23). Lidocaine is used in the treatment of ventricular arrhythmias and ectopy. In the most recent ACLS guidelines, it is considered second line to amiodarone for the treatment of VF and pulseless VT.

19-36. **The answer is B** (Chapter 23). Long-term oral therapy is associated with thyroid disorders, pulmonary fibrosis, skin discoloration, hep-

atic dysfunction, corneal infiltrates, and other conditions. Before long-term treatment, patients need baseline ophthalmologic and pulmonary function tests.

19-37. **The answer is C** (Chapter 23). Several drug interactions can increase serum digoxin levels, including amiodarone, verapamil, nifedipine, diltiazem, flecainide, quinidine, erythromycin, and tetracycline. In contrast, cholestyramine, metoclopramide, penicillamine, and dietary fiber may result in decreased serum digoxin levels.

19-38. **The answer is D** (Chapter 21). Antidiuretic hormone (ADH) release occurs in almost all hyponatremic conditions. The brain has two mechanisms to protect against fluid shifts secondary to hyponatremia: (1) an increase in hydrostatic pressure causes movement of interstitial fluid into the cerebrospinal fluid and (2) the loss of cellular $[Na^+]/[K^+]$ and organic osmolytes decreases the osmotic gradient. While adaptive changes protect the brain from excessive swelling, they also render it susceptible to volume depletion during correction of the fluid and electrolyte problem. There is often greater risk of brain damage during treatment than from the hyponatremia itself. The rate of rise of intracellular potassium and organic osmolytes in the brain during correction of the hyponatremia occurs much more slowly than the rate of loss of these substances during the development of the problem. If correction of hyponatremia occurs more rapidly than the brain can recover solute, the higher plasma osmolality may result in a fluid shift out of cells and injury to the brain. This is referred to as the *osmotic demyelination syndrome* or *central pontine myelinolysis*. The total body $[Na^+]$ content is between 40 and 50 mEq/kg. It is found predominantly in the extracellular fluid (ECG) space (98%), with a concentration of approximately 140 mEq/L. A urine $[Na^+]$ <10 mEq/L usually indicates that the renal handling of $[Na^+]$ is intact and that the effective arterial blood volume is contracted. In contrast, a urine $[Na^+]$ >20 mEq/L often indicates intrinsic renal tubular damage or a natriuretic response to hypervolemia. Seizures are quite likely at [Na^+] of 113 mEq/L or less.

19-39.   The answer is C (Chapter 21). Hypertonic hyponatremia occurs when large quantities of osmotically active solutes accumulate in the ECF space. In this setting, there is a net movement of water from the ICF to the ECF, thereby effectively diluting the ECF [Na^+]. The most common cause of this is hyperglycemia. Each 100 mg/dL increase in plasma glucose decreases the serum [Na^+] by 1.6–1.8 mEq/L.

19-40.   The answer is D (Chapter 21). Insulin shifts the potassium intracellularly. Calcium stabilizes the cardiac membrane. Furosemide, hemodialysis, and sodium polystyrene eliminate potassium from the body.

19-41.   The answer is E (Chapter 22). The AV node is under the surface of the right atrial endocardium. The AV node receives its blood supply from the right coronary artery in 90% of individuals or from left circumflex artery in the other 10%. This accounts for the common occurrence of AV conduction disturbances with acute inferior MIs.

19-42.   The answer is E (Chapter 22). In general, emergent treatment of bradycardia is not required, unless (1) the heart rate is slower than 50 beats/min and there is clinical evidence of hypoperfusion or (2) the bradycardia is due to structural disease of the infranodal conducting system (transient or permanent) that has a risk of progressing to complete AV block. The first group of patients requires immediate treatment during assessment of the etiology of the bradycardia and consideration of whether internal pacing will be required. The second group of patients does not always require immediate treatment but should be monitored closely, with therapy readily available, while arrangements are made for further evaluation and possible internal cardiac pacing.

19-43.   The answer is E (Chapter 22). Sick sinus syndrome is an indication for a permanent pacemaker. Pharmacologic treatment of atrial tachyarrhythmias carries the risk of aggravating preexisting AV block or sinus arrest. Therefore, most patients should have pacemaker implantation before drug therapy is begun.

19-44.   The answer is B (Chapter 22). Adenosine, an ultra-short-acting (20 seconds) agent with a half-life of 10 seconds, produces AV block and has been observed to convert over 90% of reentrant SVT. This is the only Class 1 pharmacologic therapy for treatment of SVT. Adenosine **must be given in a large vein,** preferably in the antecubital space. At least 50% of patients experience distressing, but transient, side effects that include facial flushing or chest pain and should be advised of this possibility before treatment. Because adenosine possesses no sustained antiarrhythmic effect, subsequent ectopic beats can reinitiate the arrhythmia, and early recurrences of SVT are seen in up to 25% of patients. The major advantage of adenosine is its ultrashort effect and its lack of hypotensive or myocardial depressive activity. Adenosine is also safe and effective in unstable patients (chest pain and/or hypotension) with reentrant SVT. It is safe in pregnancy. In addition, it is not contraindicated in the presence of WPW syndrome, when the QRS complex is narrow.

19-45.   The answer is D (Chapter 22). An expected PaO_2 when a patient is given oxygen can be estimated by multiplying the actual delivered percentage of oxygen by 6. Thus, a patient getting 60% oxygen would be expected to have a PaO_2 of about 60×6, or 360 mm Hg.

19-46.   The answer is D (Chapter 22). Pulse oximetry is not a substitute for blood gas analysis as it is solely a measure of the percentage of hemoglobin that is saturated with oxygen (SaO_2) using infrared light absorption. It gives no information about pH, $PaCO_2$, bicarbonate measurements, hemoglobin, or oxygen content (PaO_2) of the blood. A patient with severe anemia could have a normal

SaO$_2$, yet very low oxygen content. Limitations associated with pulse oximetry include falsely elevated saturation readings in the presence of toxic hemoglobins and cyanide and falsely low readings in the presence of impaired local perfusion, arteriovenous grafts, hypothermia, vasopressor use, fluorescent light and a few nail polishes. Fetal hemoglobin absorbs light, at the same spectrum as normal hemoglobin and gives accurate values.

19-47. **The answer is B** (Chapter 22). Lactate is an excellent marker of hypoperfusion and global anaerobic metabolism and can be measured from either an arterial or venous source. Lactate measurement is readily available on most blood gas analyzers and serves as a far better marker of shock than traditional vital signs. Lactate levels are predictive of mortality in a variety of shock states, including trauma and sepsis. A serum lactate >4 mmol/dL is associated with a 28% mortality rate in patients with signs and symptoms suggestive of infection. Clearance of lactate correlates with mortality and is often used as a resuscitation endpoint for patients in shock. Early lactate clearance is predictive of survival in patients with severe sepsis and septic shock and clearance within 48 hours is associated with survival following injury. There are two types of lactic acidosis. Lactic acidosis as a consequence of tissue hypoperfusion is referred to as type A. Type B lactic acidosis is not a consequence of tissue hypoxia and can be seen in hepatic failure, with certain drugs like alcohol and metformin, and also with inborn errors of metabolism.

19-48. **The answer is B** (Chapter 19). Although acidemia is diagnostic of acidosis and alkalemia of alkalosis, a normal or high pH does not exclude acidosis and a normal or low pH does not exclude alkalosis. Acid–base disturbances are further classified as respiratory or metabolic. Respiratory acid–base disorders are due to primary changes in PCO$_2$, and metabolic disorders reflect primary changes in [HCO$_3^-$]. Normal compensatory responses to each primary acid–base disturbance have been established through careful study and are presented later in this chapter. It is important to note that compensatory mechanisms return the pH toward, but not completely to, normal. The fact that compensatory mechanisms cannot become complete is evident when one considers that complete compensation would necessarily remove the (physiologic) stimulus driving the compensation. Blood samples for acid–base evaluation are traditionally obtained by arterial puncture, but in certain clinical conditions, venous blood may be used instead. Arterial and capillary values of pH and CO$_2$ content in normal patients and those with DKA correlate well. Correlations between arterial and venous pH and between arterial and venous bicarbonate concentrations in ED patients with DKA are also high. The correlation between venous and arterial blood gas values in patients with severe shock remains uncertain, but in other circumstances, the use of venous gas values seems reasonable. Inexperienced clinicians frequently resort to arterial blood gas (ABG) determination as a means to "know" the pH. However, the pH per se is often the least important value for diagnosis and management. When respiratory status is not compromised (which should be presumed only with caution), the pH can be calculated with the aid of the Kassirer-Bleich equation from the venous [HCO$_3^-$] alone.

19-49. **The answer is D** (Chapter 19). The serum [K$^+$] level is affected by metabolic acidosis. The movement of H$^+$ into cells is associated with extrusion of K$^+$. Changes in [K$^+$] are more substantial in inorganic acidosis, although elevated serum [K$^+$] are typically seen in DKA. In general, for each 0.10 decrease in the pH, serum [K$^+$] will increase by approximately 0.5 mEq/L. A low or normal serum [K$^+$] in a patient with acidosis likely reflects severe intracellular K$^+$ depletion. As the acidosis is corrected, serum [K$^+$] should fall, possibly to levels that may produce clinical sequelae.

Special Situations
Questions

20-1. During the resuscitation and ultimate death of a child in the emergency department (ED), the family-centered and team-oriented approach would encourage that the family be:

(A) In a quiet and private waiting area of the ED and notified of death

(B) Notified of death by chaplain or social services

(C) Outside of the ED for fear of violent reprisals

(D) Present during the resuscitation and encouraged to remain with their child after death

(E) Under direct supervision of security or local law enforcement

20-2. Which of the following is TRUE regarding sexual assault?

(A) Most victims of sexual assault will have no physical exam findings.

(B) Most victims will have a genital injury on gross physical exam.

(C) The use of weapons during a sexual assault is frequently reported.

(D) Victims are equally composed of men and women.

(E) Victims infrequently know their perpetrators.

20-3. A 28-year-old male presents to the ED agitated. Initial attempts of comforting and placing limits on the agitated patient have failed, and the patient's behavior has escalated into physical aggression. The most appropriate next step is:

(A) Another verbal response

(B) Leaving the patient alone for 30 minutes to "cool off"

(C) Negotiation with the patient

(D) Proceed to physical restraints and chemical sedation

(E) Transfer the patient to a facility with higher level of care

20-4. A 23-year-old female presents to the ED requesting a "rape exam." She states that she was at a party then remembers waking up in a stranger's bed. She has no recollection of the events between the party and waking up. Which of the following queries are irrelevant with respect to the evidentiary exam?

(A) Are you on birth control?

(B) Describe your sexual activity for the last year.

(C) Describe the surroundings of where you woke up.

(D) Do you have a history of drug or alcohol use in the past month?

(E) Is there any rectal or vaginal soreness?

20-5. The incidence of endocarditis in intravenous drug users is reported to be 40 times that of the general population with the majority of cases involving the right side of the heart and the tricuspid valve. The organism that is most commonly implicated in these patients is

(A) *Haemophilus parainfluenzae*

(B) *Pseudomonas aeruginosa*

(C) *Staphylococcus aureus*

(D) *Streptococcus pneumoniae*

(E) *Streptococcus viridans*

20-6. A 32-year-old female was sexually assaulted within the past 24 hours. On physical exam, there was no evidence of injury. The following is correct in regard to HIV transmission and postexposure prophylaxis.

(A) Avoid asking questions regarding the patient's risk factors for HIV.

(B) Avoid obtaining information about the assailant's risk for HIV.

(C) Do not obtain an HIV test, as you are unable to provide counseling follow-up.

(D) If postexposure prophylaxis for HIV is indicated, administer therapy immediately.

(E) Obtain routine baseline blood work including a CBC, chemistries, and liver function tests before administering therapy.

20-7. A 27-year-old female presents to your ED in the evening hours on a Saturday. She complains of headache and states she drank a few beers. She has several bruises on her face that she states were from a fall 2 days earlier, and she recently ran out of her antidepressant medication. She appears mildly anxious but has normal vital signs. During your interview and when informed that her urine pregnancy is positive, she demands to leave the department and asks for her "paperwork." Which of the following would most influence your decision to hold the patient in the ED and declare that she does not have capacity?

(A) History of psychiatric illness

(B) Determination that assault caused the bruising to the face

(C) Positive urine pregnancy test

(D) Presence of her husband who is willing to drive her home

(E) Triage alcohol breathalyzer reading of 0.24%

20-8. A 6-year-old male presents to the ED with his mother complaining of an "itch" in the hole in his bottom. On review of systems, the mother has noticed an increase in bedwetting, nightmares, and vague abdominal complaints for the past few weeks. Today, the mother noted a strong odor coming from the child's urogenital region. On further investigation, the mother states that her child has been going to a new day care program. The physical exam results show no abnormal physical findings. Choose the next best step.

(A) Contact child life specialists for developmental support with her 6-year-old.

(B) File a report for child sexual abuse with child protective services.

(C) File a report for child sexual abuse with the local law enforcement agency.

(D) File a report for suspected child sexual abuse with child protective services and the local law enforcement agency.

(E) Treat the patient for pinworms and arrange follow-up with the primary physician.

20-9. Which of the following is most responsible for improving solid organ transplant viability during the past 20 years?

(A) Better infection control

(B) Improved techniques for immunosuppression

(C) Improved technique in transplantation

(D) Improved technology in obtaining the organ

(E) More aggressive organ harvesting

20-10. A 7-month-old female is brought to the ED by her grandmother with irritability. The grandmother states that she arrived to the house while the patient was napping and found her difficult to arouse, inconsolable while awake, and less interactive than normal. When the father arrives, he states that before her nap he had taken the child to the park where she had fallen but was otherwise fine. On physical exam, the patient is lethargic and has multiple ecchymoses in varying stages of healing on her abdomen and buttock region. On further exam, there is mild swelling and tenderness on the posterior aspect of the patient's head. When the father is asked about the ecchymoses, he states that the patient sustained the injuries while playing at the park 3 days ago (Figure 20-1). Which of the following statements is correct?

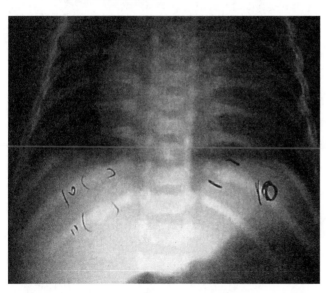

Figure 20-1. Reproduced with permission from Tintinalli JE, Stapczynski JS, Ma OJ, Cline DM, Cydulka RK, Meckler GD: *Tintinalli's Emergency Medicine: A Comprehensive Study Guide*, 7th Edition. Copyright © 2011 The McGraw-Hill Companies, Inc.

(A) A negative workup in the past for physical abuse is reassuring.

(B) Delay in seeking care by the father is a convincing indicator that intentional abuse occurred.

(C) Discordant stories by caregivers may be an indicator of intentional abuse.

(D) The history of trauma is consistent with the pattern of injury.

(E) The imaging priority in this patient is a skeletal survey.

20-11. A 63-year-old man received a cadaveric kidney transplant for end-stage renal disease due to diabetic nephropathy approximately 8 weeks ago. The patient presents to the ED with 3 days of decreased urine output, tenderness over the graft site, and a potassium level of 5.6 mEq/L (baseline, 4.8 mEq/L posttransplant). Vital signs include a blood pressure of 185/98 mm Hg, heart rate of 92 beats/min, and a temperature of 100°F (37.8°C). Given this patient's presentation, which of the following would be the most likely diagnosis?

(A) Acute renal artery occlusion

(B) Infection from cytomegalovirus (CMV)

(C) Medication noncompliance

(D) *S. aureus* bacteremia

(E) Urinoma

20-12. Which of the following are recognized characteristics of intimate partner violence?

(A) Financial constraints

(B) Mutual combatants

(C) Progressive social isolation

(D) Restrictive custody agreements

(E) Outbursts

20-13. A 62-year-old female who underwent liver transplantation a year earlier due to hepatitis C cirrhosis presents to the ED with fever, confusion, and new onset ascites. Her transplant medications include prednisone and tacrolimus. The patient was stable until 2 weeks ago when she was exposed to an upper respiratory infection. She presented to her primary care physician and was given pseudoephedrine, azithromycin, and an antitussive. What is the most likely etiology to this patient's hepatic encephalopathy?

(A) Acute hepatitis C

(B) Disappearing duct syndrome

(C) Portal vein thrombosis

(D) Primary graft failure

(E) Tacrolimus toxicity

20-14. Which of the following patients is at highest risk for intimate partner violence?

(A) 22-year-old college student living with a roommate in student housing

(B) 23-year-old postpartum female renting an apartment

(C) 35-year-old divorced mother of two who owns her own home

(D) 38-year-old pregnant female who lives with her parents

(E) 42-year-old male in a relationship with another male living in their own home

CHAPTER 20

Special Situations
Answers and Explanations

20-1. The answer is D (Chapter 297). The resuscitation and death of a child is one of the most traumatic experiences for a family. In addition, it presents particular and difficult challenges for the emergency medicine practitioner and the ED. The "family-centered and team-oriented approach" to the death of a child was developed by the American Academy of Pediatrics and the American College of Emergency Physicians as a method to ease the pain of the loss of a child and offer techniques for the emergency medicine practitioner and department to facilitate this in a compassionate and caring manner utilizing the resources of the department. This approach encourages that family be present during the resuscitation of a child, and encourages the presence of the family after the pronouncement of death. The presence of the family or parents should not be viewed as a distraction but rather as one of mutual support, allowing for earlier grieving and recovery.

20-2. The answer is A (Chapter 291). Sexual assault is a significant public health problem with a staggering number of victims in the United States. Although the rates of sexual assault are highest in females, males account for about 5–10% of victims of sexual assault. The assailant in sexual assaults is usually a single person and frequently knows the victim. Although some type of force is used in most sexual assaults, force with weapons is less commonly used. It is critical to remember that most sexually assaulted victims have little or no evidence of physical harm on gross physical exam. Half or less of the victims of sexual assault will have a non-toluidine dye evident genital injury. The most common injury seen in sexual assault is light bruising, most frequently located on limbs and face.

20-3. The answer is D (Chapter e293.1). The anxious, defensive, aggressive, and violent patient presents a difficult situation for the emergency medicine provider and the ED. Initial responses of listening and comforting the patient can often defuse the situation. Setting limits for these patients can often provide the next line of intervention and prevent further escalation by defining what is and what is not acceptable behavior. When these have failed and the patient has further escalated the situation into physical aggression, the patient should be restrained by trained personnel and given chemical sedation. Seclusion is another technique with potential for deescalation but may not always be applicable. "The best predictor of future violent behavior is past violent behavior."

20-4. The answer is B (Chapter 291). The history is important when it comes to evaluating for physical and psychological injuries, guiding ED treatment, evaluating for the need of postexposure prophylaxis and helping in the collection of appropriate evidence for the evidentiary exam. Critical information for the evidentiary exam includes many questions that are explicit in regard to the assault. Some important question may include the presence of rectal intercourse or soreness. This finding has been associated with higher incidence of STD transmission including HIV. A patient on birth control has a different risk of pregnancy compared with someone who is not. Alcohol and drug use may affect the ability to detect "date rape" drugs and the location of the rape may help in obtaining corroborating evidence in the alleged assault. The sexual practices of a patient more than 5 days before the alleged assault will not change the postexposure treatment guidelines or patient follow-up recommendations of the Centers for Disease Control and Prevention (CDC).

20-5. **The answer is C** (Chapter 294). The intravenous street drug users present another special but all too common situation in the ED. These patients are prone to various infections due to underlying disease such as HIV, poor health, or little medical care. The incidence of endocarditis is 40 times that of the general population. The right side of the heart and the tricuspid valve are more commonly involved, and the most commonly implicated organism is *S. aureus*. Antibiotic options should consider that up to two-thirds of these cases with *S. aureus* in large urban areas have methicillin resistance.

20-6. **The answer is D** (Chapter 291). Postexposure prophylaxis against HIV is clearly supported by the CDC in sexually assaulted victims. The factors involved in whether to initiate or withhold HIV prophylaxis are dependent on each case. Knowledge of the characteristics associated with increase risk of HIV both in the assailant and in transmission is paramount. The characteristics of increased HIV transmission include anal intercourse; bleeding with penetration of vaginal, anal, or oral orifices; a perpetrator with uncontrolled HIV or a high viral load and open genital sores on the victim or assailant. These recommendations are primarily used in situations where the rape has occurred within 72 hours of the victim's presentation. Routine laboratory collection is not indicated but should be done if clinically indicated. If HIV prophylaxis is indicated, it should be given immediately without waiting for baseline laboratory or culture results to be returned. It is important to reassure victims of sexual assault that there is no

evidence of increased rates of HIV/STI than demographically matched patients in sexual assault cases.

20-7. **The answer is E** (Chapter 298). The determination of capacity can be one of the most difficult situations for the emergency provider. Patients often present to the ED for various reasons and often seeking help for a social or safety situation. Many factors are considered when making a decision of capacity, and these include communication and understanding, as well as underlying illness. The history by the emergency provider is often times the sole determinant of capacity, and in cases of incapacity, documentation must clearly support the decision. Poor judgment should not be mistaken for lack of capacity. In this case, a history of psychiatric illness would not automatically cause one to be incapacitated, nor would a positive pregnancy test. History of assault and bruising also would not necessarily remove one's capacity, except if there was concern for an underlying brain injury. In this case, the alcohol breathalyzer reading of 0.24% gives a clear indication of alcohol intoxication, which would impair the patient's ability to give a history or comprehend what is being asked of her. The intoxication associated with the unclear presentation would give the provider the ability to declare the patient with a lack of capacity and hold them in the ED until sober, so that a complete history is obtained and a safe discharge is ensured. Note that laws vary from state to state and it is paramount to understand the law in your state of practice.

20-8. **The answer is D** (Chapter 290). Any significant and precipitous change in a child's behavior should alert a parent or care provider to the potential of sexual assault or physical abuse and/or neglect. Similar to adults, the absence of physical findings does not exclude sexual abuse. Signs of sexual abuse may be related to urogenital complaints or behavioral issues such as genital fondling, provocative behavior, encopresis, regression, and nightmares. Longstanding and vague physical complaints are seen in chronically sexually abused children. It is critical to remember that physicians are required by law to report every case of suspected child abuse (sexual, physical, or neglect). The health care provider is required to notify both child protective services and local law enforcement agencies. Every state has this requirement and it is the role of these agencies to pursue an investigation and assure the safety of the child at home.

20-9. **The answer is B** (Chapter 295). In the past 15 years, transplanted organs have become significantly more viable and common. Advances in communication, travel, and notification of available organs have also significantly improved organ retrieval and, hence, the number of transplantations in the last 20 years. Despite these advances, the single most important factor in organ survival has been the improvement in immunosuppressive technology. This improvement has allowed transplanted organs to maintain their viability and function. Unfortunately, as immunosuppression has improved, the biggest challenges in organ survival currently include infection and malignancy.

20-10. **The answer is C** (Chapter 290). Regardless of the etiology, there is significant concern in this child for an intracranial injury given her altered mental status, lethargy, and evidence of head trauma. In this case, the treatment priority is a head CT over any other radiological study based on clinical presentation. While historical data may raise suspicion of intentional trauma, patient stabilization is the priority of the provider over the diagnosis of intentional child abuse. Once the patient is considered stable, a skeletal survey, screening blood work, and historical information should be obtained in the case where child abuse is suspected. Suspicious historical information can include inconsistent stories between caregivers, delay in care, and a history of multiple traumatic events in the past. Knowledge of normal development in children is critical for the adequate assessment of the likelihood of injury patterns. In this case, it is suspicious that a 7-month-

old would be mobile enough to sustain the bruises, swelling, and tenderness noted on physical exam. Given this nondevelopmentally appropriate ecchymosis and delay to care, there is a high suspicion for intentional trauma. The lack of familiarity of developmental milestones has led to many cases of child abuse not being recognized on the initial visits, requiring multiple repeat visits for final diagnosis.

20-11. **The answer is B** (Chapter 295). In this case, an 8 week post transplant patient is exhibiting signs of transplant organ rejection identified by decreased urine output, pain over the transplant site, and an elevated potassium level. From 1 to 6 months posttransplant, CMV is the most important organism affecting the long-term viability of transplanted solid organs. CMV can infect a transplanted organ at any time after transplantation. Immunosuppression, which is typically maximized in the first 1.5 months after transplantation, contributes to the early appearance of CMV. Given that infection is the most common cause of organ demise in all transplants, it is reasonable to consider *S. aureus.* However, these nosocomial organisms generally cause infection in the first month after transplantation when immunosuppression is at its highest levels. Acute renal artery occlusion occurs more precipitously than described in this case. A urinoma can present with similar symptoms but usually occurs within the first 2 weeks after transplantation. Medication noncompliance is unlikely since transplant patients are under vigilant care of the transplant service during the first months after transplantation and have routine testing to monitor immunosuppressive levels.

20-12. **The answer is D** (Chapter 292). Intimate partner violence and abuse has replaced the terminology for spousal abuse, partner abuse, and domestic violence. It is important to recognize that the definition of "partner" is not restricted to traditional concepts of marriage or domestic partners, but includes previous relationships, relationships with children in common, and same sex relationships. The key concept in intimate partner violence and abuse is that it encompasses psychological and physical behaviors that are demeaning and assaultive in order to control a relationship. Behaviors that are included in the definition of intimate partner violence and abuse include physical injury, sexual assault, progressive social isolation, stalking, deprivation, intimidation, manipulation, and threats.

20-13.   **The answer is E** (Chapter 295). Immunosuppressive agents are the cornerstone of posttransplant longevity, but these same agents can be toxic at high levels. In this case, the patient was recently placed on a macrolide (azithromycin), which can increase serum concentrations of immunosuppressive agents such as tacrolimus and cyclosporine. Inappropriate levels of these medications can precipitate graft rejection in an otherwise healthy organ. Although acute hepatitis C, disappearing duct syndrome, portal vein thrombosis, and primary graft failure can also lead to liver transplant rejection, the most likely cause in this case is medication toxicity due to an interaction between the macrolide and the immunosuppressive medications.

20-14.   **The answer is B** (Chapter 292). While intimate partner or interpersonal violence has no boundaries or absolutes, there are demographics of patients who are more likely to be victim of it. Screening for these risk factors can change these patients' lives. Intimate partner violence and abuse is classically seen in females. Risk factors in patients with abuse include being female, age between 22 and 24 years old, having a low income, living in rental housing, and being separated versus being divorced or married. Pregnancy and the postpartum period have been seen as one of the highest risk times for intimate partner violence. Unfortunately, childhood experiences predict future encounters, and females who have been sexually or physically abused as children have high risk of future abuse. Females are twice as likely to report abuse to a health care professional versus law enforcement. Failure to recognize victims of intimate partner abuse and violence may have devastating consequences.

Toxicologic Emergencies
Questions

21-1. A 22-year-old woman presents to the emergency department after an acute overdose of approximately 10 g of acetaminophen 4 hours ago. How long after her ingestion do you expect to see laboratory evidence of hepatic injury?

(A) 0–6 hours

(B) 6–12 hours

(C) 18–24 hours

(D) 72–96 hours

(E) >96 hours

21-2. A 17-year-old boy presents to the emergency department after a fight with his girlfriend. He ingested 50 non enteric-coated adult aspirin tablets 1 hour ago. He is crying but otherwise provides an accurate history of his ingestion. What is the most likely acid–base disturbance to see on his initial arterial blood gas?

(A) Acute respiratory alkalosis and alkalemia

(B) Acute respiratory acidosis and acidemia

(C) Acute respiratory alkalosis, metabolic acidosis, and alkalemia

(D) Acute respiratory alkalosis, metabolic acidosis, and acidemia

(E) Metabolic acidosis, compensatory respiratory alkalosis, and acidemia

21-3. In a poisoned patient with an increased anion gap metabolic acidosis, what etiology is likely with the additional finding of calcium oxalate crystals in the urine?

(A) Ethanol

(B) Ethylene glycol

(C) Isopropyl alcohol

(D) Methanol

(E) Propylene glycol

21-4. In patients with acute labetalol toxicity, which antidote may produce dramatic improvement in heart rate and blood pressure?

(A) Calcium

(B) Flumazenil

(C) Glucagon

(D) Lidocaine

(E) Octreotide

21-5. A 35-year-old man presents with a hydrofluoric acid burn to this right index and middle finger. He is complaining of severe pain in the region, but very little is seen on physical exam other than slight discoloration of the nails. What is the antidote in this case?

(A) Calcium gluconate

(B) Dimercaprol

(C) Flumazenil

(D) Octreotide

(E) Sodium bicarbonate

21-6. A 5-year-old child is brought to the emergency department from a house fire. The child is hypotensive and severely acidemic with a high serum lactate. Which of the following is the definitive antidote for this child?

(A) Acetylcysteine

(B) Amyl nitrite

(C) Methylene blue

(D) Hydroxocobalamin

(E) Pyridoxine

21-7. A child is undergoing endoscopy and procedural sedation for a swallowed coin. The child suddenly becomes acutely cyanotic. The pulse oximetry on ambient air is 89%. The initial blood gas reveals pH 7.34, PCO_2 32 mm Hg, PO_2 117 mm Hg, and HCO_3 22 mEq/L. Which of the following agents was the most likely cause of this patient's condition?

(A) Benzocaine

(B) Ethylene oxide

(C) Etomidate

(D) Fentanyl

(E) Lorazepam

21-8. A 54-year-old woman presents to the emergency department following an acute drug overdose. She is awake with warm, flushed skin and has bibasilar rales. Vital signs reveal BP, 89/56 mm Hg; P, 45 bpm; RR 18 bpm; and T 36°C. Her electrocardiogram (ECG) demonstrates a wide complex bradycardia with no P waves. Laboratory studies are potassium, 4.2 mEq/L; bicarbonate, 24 mEq/L; creatinine, 0.8 mg/dL; and glucose, 386 mg/dL. What is the most likely drug responsible for her condition?

(A) Clonidine

(B) Digoxin

(C) Lisinopril

(D) Propranolol

(E) Verapamil

21-9. A 25-year-old man presents to the emergency department with acute chest pain 30 minutes after smoking crack cocaine. His ECG shows sinus tachycardia and no evidence of acute ischemia. His chest x-ray is normal. His initial troponin is normal. Which of the following treatments would you use first in the management of his chest pain?

(A) Diazepam

(B) Heparin

(C) Metoprolol

(D) Morphine

(E) Nitroglycerin

21-10. Which of the following anticonvulsant drugs is most likely to require cardiac monitoring following acute oral overdose in adults?

(A) Carbamazepine (Tegretol)

(B) Levetiracetam (Keppra)

(C) Phenytoin (Dilantin)

(D) Topiramate (Topamax)

(E) Valproic acid (Depakote)

21-11. Which of the following drugs or intoxicants is most likely to be adsorbed by activated charcoal?

(A) Bleach (sodium hydroxide)

(B) Iron

(C) Kerosene

(D) Lithium

(E) Methyl salicylate

21-12. A 40-year-old man presents to the emergency department requesting a medical refill for his clonidine. He is also complaining of abdominal cramping, nausea, diarrhea, and flu-like symptoms. What is the most likely drug this patient is also abusing?

(A) Cocaine

(B) Ketamine

(C) Khat

(D) Methamphetamine

(E) Oxycodone

21-13. A young woman with a history of bipolar disease and taking lithium develops ataxia, tremor, and confusion over the past several days. What is the initial treatment of choice to enhance the elimination of lithium?

(A) Charcoal hemoperfusion

(B) Hemodialysis

(C) Normal saline

(D) Sodium bicarbonate

(E) Whole bowel irrigation

21-14. A patient is brought in the emergency department by emergency medical services (EMS) for altered mental status. Initial laboratory studies demonstrate a normal pH, a large osmolar gap, normal glucose, elevated serum creatinine, a normal BUN, and a large amount of urine ketones. What is the likely cause of this patient's condition?

(A) Diabetic ketoacidosis

(B) Ethanol

(C) Ethylene glycol

(D) Isopropyl alcohol

(E) Methanol

21-15. A 45-year-old man presents to the emergency department for a medication refill. The patient has a known history of venous thromboembolism for which he takes warfarin 5 mg each evening. He has an incidental finding of an elevated INR of 6.0. He has no signs of spontaneous bleeding. What is the appropriate course of management in this patient?

(A) 1 mg intravenous vitamin K

(B) 3 mg oral vitamin K

(C) 6 units fresh-frozen plasma

(D) Hold evening's dose of warfarin therapy and provide 2.5 mg oral vitamin K

(E) Hold the next dose of warfarin therapy with no vitamin K

21-16. Which of the following is an indication for intravenous hypertonic sodium bicarbonate in the setting of acute cyclic antidepressant overdose?

(A) Coma

(B) QRS prolongation >100 msec

(C) QTc prolongation >500 msec

(D) Seizures

(E) Urine pH <7.5

21-17. Which of the following clinical features best distinguishes serotonin syndrome from neuroleptic malignant syndrome (NMS)?

(A) Altered mentation

(B) Clonus

(C) Hyperthermia

(D) Onset >24 hours

(E) Rigidity

21-18. A 35-year-old farmer has an acute exposure to an unknown pesticide and presents with nausea, vomiting, and diarrhea. On examination, you notice miosis, bradycardia, and wheezing. His pulse oximetry reads 92% on room air. Which of the following antidotes is most appropriate as the first step in managing this patient?

(A) Atropine

(B) Lorazepam

(C) Methylene blue

(D) Physostigmine

(E) Pralidoxime

21-19. A 2-year-old girl is found by her parents after an ingestion of lamp oil and is brought to the emergency department. Which of the following best describes pediatric exposures to volatile hydrocarbons?

(A) Approximately 50% of children develop abnormalities on chest x-ray by 4 hours.

(B) Children always require overnight monitoring due to the high risk of delayed pulmonary edema.

(C) Children can be discharged home after 6 hours with a normal chest x-ray, no hypoxia, and clear lung sounds.

(D) Prophylactic antibiotics are recommended to prevent pneumonia.

(E) Steroids have demonstrated improved outcomes in these cases.

21-20. A 22-year-old woman presents to the emergency department from a party after having recurrent seizures. She continues to demonstrate significant altered mentation and seizures despite benzodiazepine therapy. There is a history of taking Ecstasy (MDMA). Her head CT is negative. What is the most likely cause of her seizures?

(A) Hypercalcemia
(B) Hypermagnesemia
(C) Hypoglycemia
(D) Hypokalemia
(E) Hyponatremia

21-21. A 2-year-old girl presents to the hospital approximately 30 minutes after ingesting her mother's prenatal vitamins with iron. Which of the following suggests that this child can be safely discharged home?

(A) Normal serum potassium level
(B) Patient asymptomatic for 6 hours
(C) Serum glucose <150 mg/dL
(D) TIBC <serum iron level
(E) White blood cell (WBC) <15,000/mm^3

21-22. An adolescent male presents to the hospital after consuming several "energy drinks" containing large amounts of caffeine. What clinical findings are consistent with acute caffeine intoxication?

(A) Coma, respiratory depression, miosis
(B) Hypertension, miosis, diaphoresis
(C) Hypotension, hyperkalemia, bradycardia
(D) Vomiting, hallucinations, hyperglycemia
(E) Wide pulse pressure, hypokalemia, tachycardia

21-23. A mother brings her 18-month-old child to the emergency department for an evaluation of an upper respiratory infection. The mother has been treating his symptoms with diphenhydramine. The child is sleepy with dilated pupils and tachycardic with warm, flushed skin. He has had a decrease in urine output throughout the day. What toxidrome has this infant developed?

(A) Antimuscarinic
(B) Cholinergic
(C) Opiate
(D) Sedative–hypnotic
(E) Sympathomimetic

21-24. A young woman with a history of atrial tachydysrhythmias presents to the hospital following a syncopal episode. The initial ECG demonstrates an HR, 45 bpm; QRS, 94 msec; and QTc, 610 msec. What beta-adrenergic antagonist is this patient likely taking for her underlying heart condition?

(A) Atenolol
(B) Labetalol
(C) Metoprolol
(D) Propranolol
(E) Sotalol

21-25. A 56-year-old woman presents after an acute overdose of clonidine. When do you expect to see the onset of symptoms based on the time of his ingestion?

(A) <1 hour
(B) 3–6 hours
(C) 6–12 hours
(D) 12–24 hours
(E) >24 hours

21-26. Which of the following is the most appropriate antidote for patients with recurrent hypoglycemia following an acute sulfonylurea overdose after they have received dextrose?

(A) Carboxypeptidase
(B) Diazoxide
(C) Glucagon
(D) Octreotide
(E) Streptozotocin

21-27. A 25-year-old man presents to the emergency department following an acute overdose of digoxin. At what serum potassium level are digoxin Fab fragments indicated in this patient?

(A) 2.0 mEq/L

(B) 2.5 mEq/L

(C) 4.0 mEq/L

(D) 4.5 mEq/L

(E) 5.5 mEq/L

21-28. Which of the following is the most appropriate initial therapy for envenomation by the organism shown in Figure 21-1?

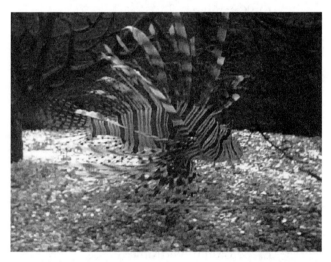

Figure 21-1. Used with permission from G. Patrick Daubert, MD.

(A) Acetic acid

(B) Antivenom

(C) Ice

(D) Meat tenderizer

(E) Warm water immersion

21-29. A young woman is brought to the emergency department from a house fire. Which of the following is the greatest risk factor for developing neuropsychologic sequelae from her carbon monoxide poisoning?

(A) Carboxyhemoglobin level >20%

(B) Headache

(C) Metabolic acidosis

(D) Soot in nose and mouth

(E) Syncope

21-30. A 2-year-old child is brought to the emergency department after swallowing a button battery. Plain film chest x-ray reveals the object in the esophagus just superior to the carina. What is the most appropriate management?

(A) Admit for observation

(B) Induce vomiting (i.e., administer ipecac)

(C) Observe for 6 hours; if no symptoms, discharge home with repeat x-ray in 24 hours

(D) Urgent endoscopy for removal

(E) Whole bowel irrigation with polyethylene glycol (GoLytely)

21-31. An 18 year old male presents to the emergency department after an acute rattlesnake bite to his right hand. His hands are shown in Figure 21-2. Which of the following is the first step in the management of this patient's envenomation?

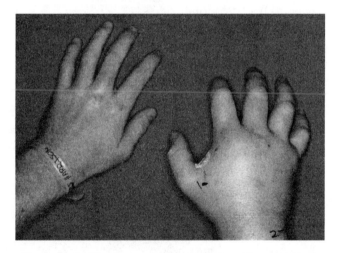

Figure 21-2. Reproduced with permission from Knoop KJ, Stack LB, Storrow AB, Thurman RJ: *The Atlas of Emergency Medicine*, 3rd Edition. Copyright © 2010 The McGraw-Hill Companies, Inc. Photo contributor: Edward J. Otten, MD.

(A) Antivenom

(B) Cryoprecipitate

(C) Fresh-frozen plasma

(D) Plasmapheresis

(E) Vitamin K

21-32. A 3-year-old child presents to the hospital in status epilepticus. The parents found the child convulsing with an open bottle of isoniazid. Which of the following is the definitive therapy to stop his seizures?

(A) Isoniazid Fab fragments

(B) Lorazepam

(C) Naloxone

(D) Physostigmine

(E) Pyridoxine

21-33. A 16-year-old boy is brought to the emergency department for altered mentation. He is visually hallucinating, has rotary nystagmus, and a positive phencyclidine on a urine drugs of abuse screen. What is the most likely drug this patient is abusing?

(A) Cocaine

(B) Dextromethorphan

(C) Ecstasy (MDMA)

(D) Oxycodone

(E) Toluene

21-34. A 56-year-old woman comes to the hospital 10 hours after the ingestion of several mushrooms picked from her yard. She has profuse vomiting and mild diarrhea. Her liver enzymes are elevated and she has an elevated INR. Which of the following is the most likely mushroom ingested?

(A) *Amanita phalloides*

(B) *Cortinarius orellanus*

(C) *Gyromitra esculenta*

(D) *Psilocybin cubensis*

(E) *Tricholoma equestre*

21-35. After the administration of prochlorperazine (Compazine), a patient develops sudden contractions of the neck and jaw. His mental status remains normal. Which of the following drugs is the most appropriate therapy in the patient?

(A) Droperidol

(B) Diphenhydramine

(C) Flumazenil

(D) Naloxone

(E) Physostigmine

21-36. A 28-year-old man presents to the emergency department by EMS for agitation, tachycardia, hypertension, diaphoresis, and tremor. His roommate stated that the patient recently lost his job and is in financial difficulty. What drug was this patient likely using that he has now discontinued?

(A) Cocaine

(B) Dextromethorphan

(C) GHB

(D) Heroin

(E) Ketamine

21-37. A 42-year-old man with schizophrenia presents with a 4-day history of worsening mental status and fevers. Upon presentation, he is altered and agitated, hyperthermic, tachycardic, hypotensive, and has muscular rigidity. What is the most likely diagnosis in this patient?

(A) Amphetamine withdrawal

(B) Bupropion overdose

(C) Malignant hyperthermia

(D) Neuroleptic malignant syndrome

(E) Serotonin syndrome

21-38. A 15-year-old girl presents with complaints of diffuse headache and neck stiffness. Her lumbar puncture demonstrates a normal opening pressure with an elevated WBC count. The cerebrospinal fluid (CSF) glucose is normal and the CSF protein is slightly elevated. Her CSF Gram stain and cultures are negative. What medication use is associated with the above findings?

(A) Acetaminophen

(B) Colchicine

(C) Hydrocodone

(D) Ibuprofen

(E) Tramadol

21-39. A 43-year-old man presents in a coma. His pupils are dilated, nonreactive with papilledema. Investigational studies reveal a wide anion gap acidosis, a normal osmolar gap, and a normal renal function. Which of the following overdoses is the most likely cause of this patient's condition?

(A) Acetaminophen

(B) Ethylene glycol

(C) Iron

(D) Methanol

(E) Theophylline

21-40. A 2-year-old child presents after ingesting several pellets of D-Con rat poison containing brodifacoum. The child's evaluation 2 hours after the ingestion is unremarkable. What is the appropriate management of this child?

(A) Admit to the hospital for observation

(B) Discharge home on oral vitamin K for the next 2 weeks

(C) Discharge home with no vitamin K or lab studies at this time

(D) Immediately administer 10 mg vitamin K

(E) Send PT/INR and discharge home after 6 hours of observation if the labs are normal

Toxicologic Emergencies
Answers and Explanations

21-1. **The answer is C** (Chapter 184). The clinical course of acute acetaminophen poisoning is described in four stages. Nausea and vomiting predominate in the first 1–12 hours. Laboratory indices of liver injury and function are normal during this period. The onset of liver injury generally occurs 18–24 hours after an acute ingestion. Peak transaminase elevation occurs 72–96 hours after ingestion with hepatic regeneration in days to weeks following. No long-term hepatic sequelae are known to occur after acetaminophen poisoning.

21-2. **The answer is C** (Chapter 183). Salicylates act directly on the respiratory center in the brainstem, causing hyperventilation and respiratory alkalosis. In addition, salicylates interfere with the citric acid cycle limiting adenosine triphosphate (ATP) production and generating lactate. Due to increased catecholamines and an increased utilization of glucose, fatty acid metabolism increases leading to ketoacidosis. Finally, salicylates are weak acids and contribute to the acidosis through direct proton donation. These factors contribute to increased ventilation through compensation but would not be expected to cause alkalemia (overcompensation). Although the metabolic acidosis begins in the earliest stages of salicylate toxicity, the respiratory alkalosis predominates initially, leaving the patient with a respiratory alkalosis, metabolic acidosis, and alkalemia. Adolescents or adults presenting with respiratory acidosis early after a salicylate overdose likely have a coingested CNS depressants, experience salicylate-induced acute lung injury,

or have underlying respiratory disease. The combination of acute respiratory alkalosis, metabolic acidosis, and acidemia is an ominous finding, indicating a life-threatening salicylate overdose.

21-3. **The answer is B** (Chapter 179). Oxalic acid is a final pathway in metabolism of ethylene glycol. Calcium oxalate monohydrate crystals are found in approximately 60% of patients poisoned with ethylene glycol. They are often prism or needlelike in shape. Ethanol does not produce specific urine abnormalities. Isopropyl alcohol is metabolized to acetone by alcohol dehydrogenase. Acetone may be detected in the urine as a ketone. Methanol may also produce ketoacids but does not produce oxalate crystals. Propylene glycol is a common medicinal diluent and can lead to hypotension, asystole, and lactic acidosis but does not produce specific urinary findings.

21-4. **The answer is C** (Chapter 188). In acute overdose of beta-adrenergic antagonists, glucagon has been shown to increase contractility, restore sinus node function after sinus node arrest, increase AV nodal conduction time, and improve survival. Calcium is used as an antidote in acute calcium channel antagonist poisoning or acute hydrofluoric acid poisoning. Flumazenil is a benzodiazepine antagonist. Lidocaine is expected to be used in drug or toxin-induced dysrhythmias but is not specific to beta-antagonist poisoning. Octreotide is used in the treatment of sulfonylurea or meglitinide-induced hypoglycemia.

21-5. **The answer is A** (Chapter 211). Hydrofluoric acid is a weak acid that contributes little toxicity from its acid–base status but rather from the highly electronegative fluoride ion. Topical or parenteral calcium gluconate therapy is currently the preferred method of detoxifying the fluoride ion. Dimercaprol (British Anti-Lewisite) is a chelating agent most commonly used for arsenic and lead poisoning. Flumazenil is a benzodiazepine antagonist. Octreotide is used in the treatment of sulfonylurea or meglitinide-induced hypoglycemia. Sodium bicarbonate is likely to be used in the setting of sodium channel blockade such as seen with acute cyclic antidepressant poisoning or used in the enhanced elimination of weak acids such as aspirin.

21-6. **The answer is D** (Chapter 198). This patient's presentation is consistent with cyanide poisoning. Hydroxocobalamin is the preferred antidote for cyanide poisoning. Sodium thiosulfate would also be appropriate and is often used synergistically with hydroxocobalamin. Acetylcysteine is the antidote for acetaminophen poisoning. Amyl nitrite is not correct in this case, as it is utilized in the prehospital setting as a temporizing measure for cyanide poisoning and not a definitive therapy. Methylene blue is used in the treatment of methemoglobinemia. Pyridoxine is used in the management of seizures from acute isoniazid toxicity or *Gyromitra* mushroom poisoning.

21-7. **The answer is A** (Chapter 201). This patient has methemoglobinemia. Local anesthetics, particularly benzocaine, are a common cause of methemoglobinemia. The duration of spraying the benzocaine as well as the orientation of the canister during spraying affects the dose delivered and the risk of methemoglobinemia. None of the other agents are commonly implicated in methemoglobinemia. Ethylene oxide has a sweet odor and is used in the sterilization of medical equipment. Toxicity results in nausea, vomiting, mucous membrane irritation, pulmonary edema, and convulsions. Lorazepam, fentanyl, and etomidate are not common causes of methemoglobinemia.

21-8. **The answer is E** (Chapter 189). This patient has acute overdose of a calcium channel antagonist. The patient's hypotension, bradycardia, warm skin, and hyperglycemia are consistent with verapamil poisoning. Although several of the other choices produce hypotension and bradycardia, clonidine is expected to produce sedation; digoxin would produce nausea, vomiting, and hyperkalemia; lisinopril would not cause hyperglycemia; and propranolol would produce cool clammy skin, hypoglycemia, and seizures.

21-9. **The answer is A** (Chapter 181). Benzodiazepines are the first-line therapy in patients with cocaine-associated chest pain. Two randomized clinical trials have demonstrated beneficial effects in patients with cocaine-associated ACS-type chest pain. Numerous animal studies confirm increased survival in cocaine intoxication with benzodiazepine administration. This patient demonstrates no evidence of ischemia or infarction to suggest a role for heparin. Controversy exists in the role of beta-adrenergic antagonists in cocaine-induced chest pain. Current consensus guidelines do not support its use in this setting. Morphine may improve the patient's pain and could be considered adjunctive therapy but does not have the clinical benefit of a benzodiazepine. Nitroglycerin is appropriate early therapy for cocaine-associated hypertension, but there is no evidence to support its role over diazepam in this patient.

21-10. **The answer is A** (Chapter 191). Carbamazepine has a similar tricyclic ring to that of a cyclic antidepressant. Acute toxicity resembles that of other cyclic antidepressants with antimuscarinic symptoms, cardiac dysrhythmias, seizures, and potentially death. Obtaining an ECG early with cardiac monitoring is appropriate following acute exposures. Levetiracetam and topiramate do not produce cardiac toxicity in overdose. Phenytoin is a class IB antidysrhythmic but does not cause significant QRS widening following oral exposures. Valproic acid may cause QT prolongation, but carbamazepine is more likely to result in cardiac manifestations in adults.

21-11. **The answer is E** (Chapters 170 and 183). Activated charcoal is the first-line therapy for GI decontamination. However, not all substances bind to charcoal. Heavy metals, hydrocarbons, and caustics do not bind well to charcoal. In addition, activated charcoal reduces the ability to perform early endoscopy following a caustic ingestion. Salicylates were the first compounds studied in vitro with activated charcoal and bind with high affinity.

21-12. **The answer is E** (Chapter 180). This patient's symptoms are consistent with opioid withdrawal. Patients complain of gastrointestinal symptoms, abdominal pain, and joint pains (arthralgias). The patient may also demonstrate piloerection and excessive yawning. Cocaine, khat (cathinone), and methamphetamine are stimulants that may produce anxiety/irritability, dysphoric mood, and excessive fatigue in withdrawal. Ketamine is uncommonly abused by youths and does not have specific withdrawal features.

21-13. **The answer is C** (Chapter 175). Lithium has an ionic radius very close to that of sodium and potassium. It is primarily handled in the proximal renal tubule of the kidney with sodium. Aggressive saline resuscitation can greatly enhance the elimination of lithium. Charcoal does not avidly bind to lithium. This patient does not warrant hemodialysis at this point. Lithium elimination is not enhanced by altering the urine pH with bicarbonate, as would be seen with salicylates. There is no information given that the patient has an acute ingestion of extended release lithium to suggest a role for whole bowel irrigation.

21-14. **The answer is D** (Chapter 179). Isopropyl alcohol causes significant inebriation, generally to a higher degree than ethanol or other toxic alcohols. It is metabolized to acetone, a true ketone and not a carboxylic acid. Therefore, no acidemia occurs. Acetone is often detected in the urine producing large ketones and interferes with serum creatinine assays producing falsely elevated creatinine. Both isopropyl alcohol and acetone contribute to the osmolality. Ethanol intoxication would not explain the elevated creatinine or ketosis. Both methanol and ethylene glycol would produce an acidemia. Ethylene glycol would produce calcium oxalate crystals in the urine as well. The patient does not have diabetic ketoacidosis with a normal pH and normal glucose.

21-15. **The answer is E** (Chapter 234). For patients with an INR of ≥5.0 but <9.0 and no significant bleeding, instruct the patient to withhold their next 1–2 doses and resume therapy at a lower dose when the INR is at a therapeutic level. Patients should also have detailed questioning about any recent medication or herbal remedy changes or use. Fresh-frozen plasma and vitamin K are indicated if there are signs of spontaneous hemorrhage and should be considered if the INR is >9.0.

21-16. **The answer is B** (Chapter 171). The ECG is an early marker of toxicity with cyclic antidepressants. Cyclic antidepressants have sodium and potassium channel blocking effects that result in QRS and QT prolongation, respectively. QRS prolongation (QRS >100 msec) is associated with an increased risk of seizures and dysrhythmias. Although the QT interval is often prolonged in these patients, tachycardia is also common. The increase in heart rate likely protects these patients from torsades de pointes. Sodium bicarbonate has no impact on seizures or coma and has no role in enhancing the elimination of the drug and, therefore, the urinary pH is not clinically relevant.

21-17. **The answer is B** (Chapter 172). Serotonin syndrome and NMS have several overlapping features for altered mentation, autonomic instability (hypertension, hyperthermia), and neuromuscular findings.

However, serotonin syndrome has a more rapid onset, typically less than 24 hours, and is characterized by clonus, rather than the muscular rigidity seen with NMS.

21-18. The answer is A (Chapters 170 and 195). This patient presents with a cholinergic crisis. The immediate antidote needed is atropine for its potent antimuscarinic effects. Pralidoxime will reverse the inhibition of acetylcholinesterase and may be beneficial in organophosphate poisoning. Since the patient's symptoms are primarily muscarinic and not nicotinic (mydriasis, tachycardia, weakness, hypertension, and fasciculations [MTWHF]), atropine is the first drug of choice. Atropine remains the first choice to improve oxygenation and ventilation. Lorazepam may be beneficial for the management of seizures in this patient, but atropine would be the first choice. Methylene blue is the antidote for methemoglobinemia and has no role in this patient.

21-19. The answer is C (Chapter 193). The greatest immediate concern in this child is aspiration pneumonitis. The majority of patients with clinical signs beyond initial coughing or gagging develop pneumonitis. Patients have a good prognosis and very low risk for subsequent deterioration if they have no pulmonary findings, no tachypnea, no hypoxia, and have a normal chest x-ray at 6 hours after exposure. Approximately 90% of patients who develop x-ray abnormalities do so by 4 hours. There is no role for prophylactic antibiotics or steroids in the early management of aspiration pneumonitis. Early steroid management may be considered if there is evidence of upper airway edema or obstruction (e.g., patient develops stridor).

21-20. The answer is E (Chapter 182). MDMA use is associated with hyperthermia and the risk for dehydration from sweat and other insensible losses while "clubbing." Patients may consume large volumes of water in response to dehydration. MDMA also promotes antidiuretic hormone (ADH) release from the hypothalamus (SIADH). In addition, some genetic polymorphism in relation to COMT, a key enzyme in the metabolism of catecholamines, may result in a greater release of ADH in some individuals. Severe hyponatremia is reported in a number of cases resulting in cerebral edema, seizures, and death. Hypercalcemia, hypoglycemia, and hypokalemia are not associated with the use of MDMA. Metabolic acidosis is likely present in this patient as a result of the seizures but is not the etiology of the seizures.

21-21. The answer is B (Chapter 192). Patients who are asymptomatic with normal electrolytes and iron level after 6 hours postingestion can be safely discharged home. Patients with significant iron poisoning will develop vomiting within 6 hours. The TIBC is not a useful marker in acute iron poisoning. Although the serum glucose and WBC are often elevated in acute iron toxicity, they lack sensitivity and are not useful prognostic indicators. The serum potassium has no correlation with acute iron toxicity.

21-22. The answer is E (Chapter 186). Caffeine is a methylxanthine similar to theophylline. These drugs produce a sympathomimetic syndrome. In addition, patients demonstrate wide pulse pressures, hypokalemia, hyperglycemia, and leukocytosis. The wide pulse pressure and hypokalemia result from beta-2-adrenergic stimulation of splanchnic blood vessels and Na–K ATPase, respectively. Coma, respiratory depression, and miosis are consistent with opiate toxicity or clonidine. Hypertension, miosis, and diaphoresis are consistent with nicotine or organophosphate compound. Hypotension, hyperkalemia, and bradycardia are consistent with acute cardiac steroid poisoning. Vomiting, hallucinations, and hyperglycemia result from some hallucinogenic plants or designer drugs.

21-23. The answer is A (Chapter 170). The antimuscarinic toxidrome is represented by altered mentation, dilated pupils, tachycardia, dry and flushed skin, and decrease in urine and bowel function. Diphenhydramine is a common cause of these signs.

Sympathomimetic may closely resemble antimuscarinic toxicity but have normal bowel or bladder involvement and have moist or wet skin. Cholinergic symptoms include altered mentation, diarrhea, urination, miosis, bronchorrhea, bradycardia, emesis, lacrimation, and salivation (DUMBBELS). Opiates classically cause miosis, CNS depression, and respiratory depression. Sedative–hypnotics cause sedation and often have little effect on patient's vital signs.

21-24. **The answer is E** (Chapter 188). This patient has a prolonged QT interval and her syncopal episode may be related to torsades de points. The only beta-adrenergic antagonist that inhibits cardiac potassium channels and subsequent QT prolongation is sotalol. Propranolol may cause QRS widening through sodium channel blockade.

21-25. **The answer is A** (Chapter 190). Clonidine is an antihypertensive agent with stimulatory effects on both central alpha-2-adrenergic and imidazoline receptors resulting in a decrease in peripheral vascular resistance, heart rate, blood pressure, and increased sedation. The drug has a rapid onset of action resulting in the majority of patients developing symptoms within 1 hour of presentation. In addition, patients typically do not develop further clinical deterioration more than 4 hours after ingestion.

21-26. **The answer is D** (Chapter 219). Patients presenting with hypoglycemia should receive immediate dextrose therapy. Sulfonylureas stimulate insulin release by the pancreas, which may be exacerbated by repeat boluses of glucose resulting in further insulin release. Octreotide inhibits the secretion of insulin and has successfully been used to control life-threatening hypoglycemia caused by sulfonylureas. Glucagon is associated with exacerbation of insulin release leading to a temporary benefit but later relapse with hypoglycemia. Diazoxide was previously used to treat sulfonylurea-induced hypoglycemia, but hypotension and other adverse effects

have eliminated its role with the advent of octreotide. Carboxypeptidase is the antidote for methotrexate toxicity. Streptozotocin is not indicated in acute hypoglycemia or in sulfonylurea overdose.

21-27. **The answer is E** (Chapter 187). Digoxin Fab fragments are indicated in patients with serum potassium levels of >5.5 mEq/L because elevated potassium levels are associated with an increased risk of cardiac arrhythmias and death in acute digoxin poisoning.

21-28. **The answer is E** (Chapter 207). Lion fish envenomations typically cause local pain that improves with warm water immersion (42°C). The general rule for treating marine-life exposure is that vertebrate exposures typically respond to heat, and invertebrate exposures commonly respond to acetic acid. The sea urchin and crown-of-thorns sea star are two invertebrate exceptions to this rule.

21-29. **The answer is E** (Chapter 217). An interval of unconsciousness after acute carbon monoxide exposure is associated with an increased risk of delayed neurologic sequelae (DNS). Particular carboxyhemoglobin levels, burn injury, metabolic changes, and headache have not been identified as predictors of DNS.

21-30. **The answer is D** (Chapter 194). Button battery ingestions require a high index of suspicion. Batteries discovered in regions where they are unlikely to pass (ears, nose, esophagus, airway/lungs) require prompt diagnosis and manual removal (endoscopy/ bronchoscopy) to avoid perforation. Button batteries in the stomach or intestines have a high rate of spontaneous passage.

21-31. **The answer is A** (Chapter 206). Hematologic toxicity from rattlesnake envenoming is common and should be initially treated with antivenom. Routine administration of blood products is not indicated and will likely be ineffective since circulating venom will rapidly sequester active blood components. In rare cases of severe life-threatening bleeding or where an immediate invasive procedure is needed, blood products such as fresh-frozen plasma and platelets may be indicated.

21-32. The answer is E (Chapter 200). Acute isoniazid poisoning causes a reduction in the conversion of glutamate to GABA and subsequent excess excitation and seizures. Because of a paucity of GABA, benzodiazepines may provide only temporary resolution of the seizures. Pyridoxine (vitamin B6) is used to promote the conversion of glutamate to GABA. Naloxone is an opiate antagonist. Physostigmine is the antidote for antimuscarinic delirium. Isoniazid Fab fragments have not been developed.

21-33. The answer is B (Chapter 182). The patient is abusing dextromethorphan. Dextromethorphan is structurally similar to phencyclidine and will cross-react with the phencyclidine immunoassay. Dextromethorphan causes sedation and hallucinations and may cause rotary or vertical nystagmus. Cocaine toxicity and MDMA both cause sympathomimetic symptoms and not nystagmus. Oxycodone use would result in CNS depression, respiratory depression, and miosis. Toluene abuse results in altered mentation, hypokalemia, weakness, and renal tubular acidosis.

21-34. The answer is A (Chapter 214). *A. phalloides* (death cap mushroom) causes delayed gastrointestinal symptoms and fulminant hepatic failure. *C. orellanus* (corts) ingestions result in delayed renal failure. *G. esculenta* (false morel) poisoning may cause seizures and hepatitis similar to that seen with isoniazid. *P. cubensis* are known as magic mushrooms and cause hallucination through serotonin activation. *T. equestre* (man on horseback) toxicity causes significant rhabdomyolysis as a prominent feature.

21-35. The answer is B (Chapter 174). This patient developed an acute dystonic reaction from prochlorperazine. Dystonic reactions are common following dopaminergic drugs such as phenothiazines (like prochlorperazine) and antipsychotics (like droperidol). The initial management includes administration of an antimuscarinic drug such as diphenhydramine or benztropine. Patients may also respond to benzodiazepines. Flumazenil is the antidote for benzodiazepines. Naloxone is the antidote for opiates and physostigmine is used to reverse antimuscarinic delirium.

21-36. The answer is C (Chapter 178). This patient's scenario suggests the discontinuation of a drug and therefore a withdrawal syndrome. GHB is a potent sedative and commonly used by bodybuilders because of its relation to growth hormone. Withdrawal results in a potentially life-threatening withdrawal state with seizures and sympathomimetic symptoms. Cocaine withdrawal is associated with irritability and somnolence. Dextromethorphan has little withdrawal symptoms but would mostly resemble that of heroin. Heroin withdrawal is associated with irritability, yawning, piloerection, body aches, and gastrointestinal distress. Ketamine does not have specific withdrawal syndrome.

21-37. The answer is D (Chapter 174). This patient is likely taking an antipsychotic (neuroleptic) for his schizophrenia. The insidious onset, altered mentation, autonomic instability, and rigidity are most consistent with NMS. More than 90% of these cases are the result of haloperidol. Amphetamine withdrawal does not produce autonomic instability or rigidity. Bupropion overdose most commonly results in seizures. Malignant hyperthermia was most often due to halothane use. Serotonin syndrome closely resembles that of NMS but more commonly causes clonus rather than rigidity.

21-38. The answer is D (Chapter 185). This patient has aseptic meningitis. Nonsteroid anti-inflammatory drugs are associated with this condition. None of the other medications listed produce aseptic meningitis.

21-39. **The answer is D** (Chapter 179). This patient has acute methanol poisoning, but his presentation to the hospital is delayed. This accounts for his wide anion gap but normal osmolar gap, since all the methanol is now metabolized to formic acid. His papilledema is a sign of the retinal toxicity, which is also a delayed finding. Acute acetaminophen toxicity results in early vomiting and delayed hepatitis. Delayed ethylene glycol would cause a similar anion gap acidemia and normal osmolar gap but would produce renal failure, which is absent in this patient. Significant iron poisoning produces hemorrhagic vomiting, hypotension, and acidemia. Theophylline overdose causes tachycardia, wide pulse pressure, hypokalemia, and seizures.

21-40. **The answer is C** (Chapter 195). Long-acting anticoagulant rodenticides are structurally and biochemically similar to warfarin anticoagulants. However, acute pediatric ingestions of brodifacoum rarely cause clinical effects and retrospective studies reveal no significant bleeding episodes or coagulation abnormalities. If there is no suspicion of chronic exposure, baseline PT (INR) testing is not cost-effective. Vitamin K is not indicated in the absence of coagulation abnormalities that would not be evident for at least 12–24 hours postingestion.

Trauma
Questions

22-1. Which of the following is not part of "the primary survey" in trauma patients?

(A) Airway assessment
(B) Breathing assessment
(C) Circulation assessment
(D) Digital rectal examination
(E) Exposure

22-2. Which of the following is part of the National Emergency X-ray Utilization Study (NEXUS) criteria for clearing a cervical spine?

(A) Able to rotate the neck 45 degrees in either direction without pain
(B) Age less than 65 years
(C) Ambulatory at the scene
(D) No evidence of trauma above the clavicles
(E) No midline cervical spine tenderness to palpation

22-3. In which of the following scenarios is an emergency department (ED) thoracotomy most indicated?

(A) 3-year-old found face down in a swimming pool pulseless and apneic
(B) 25-year-old who was stabbed in the left chest and lost vital signs in the ED
(C) 50-year-old who was in a motor vehicle crash who has a systolic blood pressure of 88/50 and a positive focused assessment with sonography in trauma (FAST).

(D) 70-year-old involved in a motor vehicle crash with blunt abdominal trauma who loses vital signs 20 minutes prior to arrival.
(E) 94-year-old with a fall from three stories found pulseless and apneic at the scene

22-4. A 35-year-old male was involved in a chain saw accident and cut his foot off. He had massive blood loss at the scene. He presents with a blood pressure of 84/50 and a heart rate of 150 beats/min. The patient is in which class of hemorrhagic shock?

(A) Class 1 shock
(B) Class 2 shock
(C) Class 3 shock
(D) Class 4 shock

22-5. A 5-year-old male was riding a bicycle and was struck by a bus. He presents to the ED with the complaint of abdominal pain. The patient's systolic blood pressure is 54/30 and the heart rate is 170. He weighs 28 kg. The MOST appropriate form of fluid resuscitation in this patient if they remain hypotensive is:

(A) 280 cc of normal saline followed by 100 cc an hour of normal saline.
(B) 560 cc of normal saline followed by 560 cc of packed red blood cells.
(C) 560 cc of normal saline followed by 280 cc of packed red blood cells.
(D) 560 cc of normal saline repeated three times followed by 280 cc of packed red blood cells.
(E) 2 L of normal saline followed by 560 cc of packed red blood cells.

22-6. A 3-month-old male is brought into the ED after falling off a kitchen table. The parents are unsure if there was a loss of consciousness. The baby vomited one time. The baby appears to be acting appropriately now per the parents. There is a 3-cm contusion over the left parietal scalp. Which of the following accurately describes the appropriate workup for this patient?

(A) Computed tomography (CT) scan of the brain

(B) Observation period of 30 minutes in the ED

(C) Placement of an intracranial pressure monitoring plain skull films and followed by observation

(D) Plain skull films, and if these are negative, discharge home immediately with reassurance

(E) Plain skull films, and if these are negative, observe patient for 2 hours

22-7. A 13-year-old boy presents to the ED after falling off his dirt bike. He hyperextended his head and neck and he complained of transient bilateral burning hands. These symptoms lasted approximately 2 hours, but they have now resolved. His neurologic exam is normal. His cervical spine plain films are negative for fracture. Which of the following is the best course of action?

(A) CT scan of the cervical spine should be performed.

(B) Discharge home with nonsteroidal anti-inflammatory medication.

(C) Flexion extension views of the cervical spine should be obtained.

(D) MRI should be performed.

(E) The patient should be started on high-dose steroids.

22-8. A 13-year-old female is brought in with epigastric and left upper quadrant pain after falling over the side of her trampoline. She complains of sharp left-sided chest and shoulder blade pain with deep breathing. Her abdominal exam reveals tenderness over the epigastrium and the left upper quadrant with bruising in the left upper quadrant. Her breath sounds are equal bilaterally. Her pelvis is stable on exam. Her heart rate is 135, blood pressure is 78/45, and oxygen saturation is 100% on room air. Which of the following imaging modalities is indicated at this time?

(A) Abdominal plain films

(B) CT scan of the abdomen

(C) FAST exam

(D) Posterior anterior (PA) and lateral chest x-ray

(E) Pelvic x-ray

22-9. A 4-year-old female patient presents with abdominal pain after a motor vehicle crash. She was the restrained back seat passenger in a high-speed motor vehicle collision (MVC). She complains of mid abdominal pain with vomiting. Her abdominal exam reveals tenderness to palpation over the umbilicus with a clear seat belt sign across the abdomen. A FAST exam reveals a small amount of free fluid in the pelvis. The urine has 50+ RBCs. Her blood pressure is 100/70 and heart rate is 85. The most CORRECT management strategy for evaluating the hematuria is:

(A) CT scan of the abdomen and pelvis

(B) Cystoscopy

(C) Kidney, ureter, bladder plain abdominal film (KUB)

(D) Renal ultrasound

(E) Retrograde urethrogram (RUG)

22-10. What is a common physiological change seen in an elderly patient?

(A) Increased chest wall compliance

(B) Increased cervical spine mobility

(C) Increased myocardial stiffening

(D) Increased reflexes

(E) Increased lung elasticity

22-11. An 88-year-old male falls and hits his head, chest, and hip. The most UNLIKELY injury for the patient to suffer is?

(A) Epidural hematoma

(B) Hip fracture

(C) Odontoid fracture

(D) Rib fractures

(E) Subdural hematoma

22-12. Which of the following is a physiologic change associated with pregnancy?

(A) Decrease in cardiac output

(B) Decrease in respiratory tidal volume

(C) Increase in functional residual capacity

(D) Increase in maternal hematocrit

(E) Increase in maternal heart rate

22-13. Which of the following is the most correct statement regarding supine hypotension syndrome?

(A) A supine pregnant patient should be placed in a right side down position.

(B) It can be relieved with a left lateral decubitus position.

(C) It most commonly occurs in the postpartum patient.

(D) It is most commonly found in the first trimester.

(E) It results from the compression of the superior vena cava.

22-14. A 22-year-old female who is 30 weeks pregnant presents after a moderate speed motor vehicle crash. She was wearing a seatbelt. She complains of mild abdominal cramping and scant vaginal bleeding. Her blood type is O negative. Her heart rate is 110 beats/min and blood pressure is 105/70. She has mild abdominal tenderness to palpation. In addition to fetal heart rate monitoring, what should the initial workup include?

(A) CBC, type and screen, and CT scan of the chest and abdomen

(B) Digital vaginal exam and an MRI of the abdomen

(C) FAST exam, type and screen, CBC, coagulation profile and RhoGAM

(D) Fetal tocometric monitoring for one hour

(E) Plain film of the abdomen, a complete blood count, and checking fetal heart tones. If these are normal, the patient can be discharged.

22-15. A 32-year-old female, currently 31 weeks pregnant, was the restrained passenger involved in a 40-mph motor vehicle crash in which she was side-swiped at a crossroad. Her airbag deployed and the prehospital personnel described minor damage to the car. There was no loss of consciousness and the patient only complains of mild neck pain. She denies abdominal pain or cramps. She has not noticed any vaginal discharge or bleeding. She was walking at the scene, but was transported on a backboard in a cervical collar. Her physical exam is only notable for an obviously gravid uterus and mild paraspinous cervical tenderness at the C3–C5 level with full range of motion of her neck and no neurologic deficits. Which of the following is the most important management?

(A) CT scan of the cervical spine

(B) Fetal monitoring for a minimum of 4 hours

(C) Flexion extension views of the cervical spine

(D) MRI of the cervical spine

(E) Plain radiographs of the cervical spine

22-16. A 44-year-old female involved in a downhill skiing crash with an obvious head injury is brought to the ED. Her vital signs are heart rate 125, blood pressure 100/60, and respiratory rate 14 breaths/min. She opens her eyes to voice, is moaning, and appears to withdraw from painful stimuli. What is this patient's Glasgow coma score?

(A) 2

(B) 4

(C) 7

(D) 9

(E) 12

22-17. Which of the following may prevent secondary brain injury?

(A) Hyperventilation to a PCO_2 of less than 20

(B) Maintaining a PaO_2 of greater than 60

(C) Permissive hyperglycemia

(D) Permissive hypotension

(E) Wearing a motorcycle helmet

22-18. A 57-year-old male with a history of alcoholism suffered a fall 10 days ago. He is brought to the ED by his girlfriend due to a change in his mental status. She states he is more lethargic and having some trouble with his memory. On exam, you notice that he is inattentive and has mild right-sided weakness in the upper and lower extremity on the right. What is the most likely diagnosis?

(A) Alcohol withdrawal

(B) Diffuse axonal injury

(C) Epidural hematoma

(D) Subarachnoid hemorrhage

(E) Subdural hematoma

22-19. A 25-year-old male electrical line worker presents after an 18-foot fall off a telephone pole while at work. According to coworkers at the scene, he was initially unconscious for 2 minutes but is now alert and awake. His EMS transport was unremarkable. While in the ED, the patient begins to become combative and then more somnolent. What is the MOST LIKELY diagnosis?

(A) Electrocution

(B) Epidural hematoma

(C) Diffuse axonal injury

(D) Postconcussive syndrome

(E) Subdural hematoma

22-20. According to the New Orleans Criteria, which of the following is an indication to obtain a head CT after minor head trauma?

(A) Absence of intoxication

(B) Age <60

(C) Fall from standing

(D) Unwitnessed fall

(E) Visible trauma above the clavicle

22-21. Which of the following injuries of the cervical spine is considered STABLE?

(A) Bilateral interfacetal dislocation

(B) Extension teardrop fracture

(C) Flexion teardrop fracture

(D) Fracture of the posterior arch of the atlas

(E) Traumatic spondylolisthesis

22-22. Which of the following is TRUE of Brown-Séquard syndrome?

(A) Most common cause is penetrating injury to the spine.

(B) Patients have decreased strength in the upper compared with lower extremities.

(C) Quadriparesis is present.

(D) Saddle anesthesia is present.

(E) Vibration, position, and crude touch are preserved.

22-23. A 67-year-old male presents to the ED following a MVC in which the cab he was riding in was struck from behind by a truck moving at a moderate rate of speed. The patient complains of tingling and numbness in his hands and feet and weakness on his arms. The patient is most likely experiencing which of the following conditions?

(A) Anterior cord syndrome

(B) Brown-Séquard syndrome

(C) Cauda equina syndrome

(D) Central cord syndrome

(E) Conversion reaction

22-24. A 68-year-old female presents from a nursing home after falling out of a wheelchair and striking her head. She has a history of severe dementia and juvenile rheumatoid arthritis. She is unable to provide any details about the event or her current state. Which of the following is MOST accurate?

(A) If radiographic imaging is performed and found to be negative, a high index of suspicion must be maintained for spinal cord injury without radiographic abnormality (SCIWORA).

(B) The patient's cervical spine can be cleared without imaging following the Canadian Cervical Spine Rule for Radiography.

(C) The patient's cervical spine can be cleared without imaging following the NEXUS criteria.

(D) The patient's cervical spine cannot be cleared according to the Canadian Cervical Spine Rule for Radiography based on mechanism of injury.

(E) The patient's history of juvenile arthritis puts her at increased risk for cervical spine injury.

22-25. Which of the following findings should cause the MOST concern in evaluation of a pediatric patient with potential spine injury?

(A) Absence of normal cervical lordosis

(B) Anterior wedging of the cervical vertebral bodies

(C) Lack of uniform angulation of the interspaces during flexion

(D) Overriding of the C1 anterior arch above the odontoid

(E) Presence of an anterior compression in the thoracolumbar spine following a motor vehicle collision

22-26. A construction worker is struck on the top of the head with a manhole cover that was dislodged during an explosion. The manhole cover landed directly on the top of his head. What type of cervical spine injury is this patient most likely going to have?

(A) Chance fracture

(B) Clay shoveler fracture

(C) Dens fracture

(D) Hangman fracture

(E) Jefferson fracture

22-27. Which of the following is MOST accurate?

(A) A Water's view radiograph safely replaces the multiple views in traditional facial series for midfacial fractures.

(B) In patients receiving a head CT, a Water's view radiograph for suspected traumatic brain injury is necessary to rule out midfacial fractures.

(C) Mandible CT scans are the superior imaging modality for suspected fractures of the dental root.

(D) Panorex views are more widely available and easier to obtain in the ED, making them the preferred initial imaging modality.

(E) Panorex views are the superior imaging modality for suspected mandibular condyle fractures.

22-28. Which of the following is MOST accurate about facial trauma?

(A) Diplopia on upward gaze occurs with entrapment of the superior rectus, superior oblique, orbital fat, or from injury to the oculomotor nerve.

(B) Frontal bone fractures are the most common facial fractures seen in isolation.

(C) Injury to the lacrimal duct, dural tears, and traumatic brain injuries are rarely associated with nasoorbitoethmoid fractures.

(D) Patients with an isolated anterior table fracture may be discharged home with appropriate follow-up with a facial surgeon.

(E) Prophylactic oral antibiotics are not considered necessary for complex open sinus fractures.

22-29. An 18-year-old male presents to the ED following an assault complaining of blurry vision. On examination, there is flattening of the malar eminence and a large lateral subconjunctival hemorrhage in the left eye. Your examination notes trismus and crepitus. What injury is this patient most likely suffering from?

(A) Blowout fracture

(B) Mandibular fracture

(C) Orbital fissure syndrome

(D) Retrobulbar hematoma

(E) Tripod fracture

22-30. A 4-year-old female is brought to the emergency department by EMS following a fall from a height of greater than 5 feet. Which of the following is MOST accurate with respect to the potential injuries in this population?

(A) Cervical spine injury in the absence of bony radiographic findings occurs less frequently than it does in adults.

(B) Cricothyrotomy is a viable airway option if endotracheal intubation is unsuccessful.

(C) Frontal bone injuries are less common.

(D) Pediatric mandible fractures are more likely to be incomplete and irregular due to the underlying developing teeth.

(E) Prior to development of the maxillary sinus, there is an increased incidence of midfacial fractures.

22-31. A 17-year-old female patient is brought to the ED after being stabbed in the anterior aspect of the neck just inferior to the cricoid cartilage. Which of the following choices identifies the zone of injury for this patient and associated anatomic structure of concern for this particular injury?

(A) Zone I, pharynx

(B) Zone I, vertebral arteries

(C) Zone II, jugular vein

(D) Zone III, carotid arteries

(E) Zone III, vertebral arteries

22-32. Which of the following is MOST accurate with respect to penetrating neck injury?

(A) Angiography is the preferred imaging modality for injuries in the pediatric population.

(B) CT scans can effectively exclude laryngotracheal injury.

(C) Penetrating esophageal injuries are often initially asymptomatic.

(D) The preferred treatment for injuries to Zones I and III is operative.

(E) Ultrasound can be particularly useful in evaluation of Zone I and Zone III injuries.

22-33. A 34-year-old male presents to the ED after being struck in the neck with a pool cue. He denies any complaints at this time and the examination is unremarkable except for left-sided ptosis and pupillary constriction. These findings are most concerning for injury to which of the following structures?

(A) L carotid artery

(B) L vertebral artery

(C) R carotid artery

(D) R vertebral artery

(E) Spinal artery

22-34. Which of the following statements regarding penetrating injuries of the neck is MOST accurate?

(A) Blunt pharyngoesophageal injuries typically present with a severe spectrum of symptoms.

(B) Due to the propensity for subcutaneous air and hematomas to disrupt and obscure visualization, rigid esophagoscopy is often of greater clinical utility than flexible esophagoscopy.

(C) Helical CT angiography allows visualization of a missile trajectory and can rule out significant vascular injuries if the trajectory is remote from vital structures.

(D) In blunt trauma, endotracheal intubation is the recommended approach for airway management as tracheostomy and cricothyroidotomy may create a false passage along disrupted tissue planes.

(E) With good visualization, small violations of the platysma can be explored locally to exclude injury.

22-35. A 25-year-old male who was the unrestrained driver in a high-speed MVC is brought to the ED. A portable supine chest x-ray is obtained (Figure 22-1). Which of the following is MOST accurate in this situation?

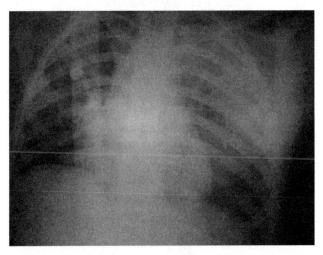

Figure 22-1. Reproduced with permission from Tintinalli JE, Stapczynski JS, Ma OJ, Cline DM, Cydulka RK, Meckler GD: *Tintinalli's Emergency Medicine: A Comprehensive Study Guide*, 7th Edition. Copyright © 2011 The McGraw-Hill Companies, Inc.

(A) Evacuation of greater than 500 mL of blood immediately after tube thoracostomy or 50 mL of blood per hour for 4 hours are generally recognized definitions of massive hemothorax and are indications for operative management.

(B) Fluid restriction or hypotensive resuscitation in chest trauma may be beneficial, and the clinician should avoid overresuscitation in actively bleeding patients.

(C) If central venous access is required, it should be first attempted on the contralateral side to the identified injury.

(D) The overall mortality of such chest trauma patients is high, with most deaths resulting from cardiothoracic injuries.

(E) When inserting a thoracostomy tube, an oblique skin incision should be made at least 1–2 cm above the interspace through which the tube will be placed. A large clamp is then inserted through the skin incision and into the intercostal muscles in the next lower intercostal space, just below the rib, with care taken to prevent the tip of the clamp from penetrating the lung.

22-36. Which of the following is MOST accurate with respect to the operation and use of thoracostomy tubes?

(A) For intubated patients, thoracostomy tubes should remain in place for the duration of mechanical ventilation to prevent sudden development of a new pneumothorax.

(B) Initial interventions for a suspected blocked thoracostomy tube include irrigation or catheter cannulation.

(C) The chest tube is advanced until the last side hole is just outside the chest wall.

(D) Thoracostomy tubes should be clamped for transport of the patient to prevent contamination and entrance of atmospheric air.

(E) Thoracostomy tubes should be discontinued as soon as possible following the termination of an air-leak to reduce infection.

22-37. Which of the following is MOST accurate with respect to pulmonary trauma?

(A) In asymmetric pulmonary trauma requiring mechanical ventilation, placing the patient on their side so that the traumatized lung is down frequently improves respiratory mechanics.

(B) Occult pneumothoraces that are visualized only on CT scan in patients undergoing mechanical ventilation do not require chest tube drainage.

(C) Prophylactic antibiotics play an important role in preventing infection after aspiration.

(D) Pulmonary contusion can typically be differentiated from pneumonia or fat embolism by the time of onset and the distribution of injury.

(E) The most common sites of injury in aspiration pneumonia are the upper lobes of the lungs.

22-38. A 48-year-old female is brought to the ED following a fall off of a ladder. She is short of breath and complains of chest pain. Vital signs are remarkable for a heart rate of 120 beats/min, blood pressure of 110/60, respiratory rate of 28, and oxygen saturation of 91% on room air. On physical exam, there is a paradoxical inward movement of the left chest wall during inspiration and outward movement during expiration. Which of the following is MOST accurate with respect to her condition and management?

(A) A supine chest x-ray can be used to exclude a hemothorax.

(B) Blunt chest trauma is the most common cause of left-sided diaphragmatic injury.

(C) The presence of Hamman sign or Hamman crunch on physical exam is indicative of a sternal fracture.

(D) The presence of subcutaneous emphysema and stridor on physical exam should prompt suspicion of an intrathoracic tracheal injury.

(E) The primary cause of hypoxemia in patients with flail chest is pulmonary contusion.

22-39. Which of the following is MOST accurate with respect to imaging in pulmonary trauma?

(A) Barium-based contrast is the preferred contrast medium in patients with a high suspicion for esophageal rupture as it has fewer false positives.

(B) Initial supine chest radiographs will frequently overestimate the extent and severity of pulmonary and chest trauma due to positioning and layering.

(C) Plain chest radiograph and CT demonstrate similar sensitivities for detecting pulmonary contusions.

(D) The appearance of the "marching ants" and "sliding lung" signs on ultrasonography is indicative of a pneumothorax.

(E) Ultrasonography has the same sensitivity for occult pneumothorax as CT.

22-40. A 22-year-old man is stabbed in the right anterior chest at the level of T5 just lateral to the sternum. He is intoxicated and screaming in pain. His vital signs are a heart rate of 135, blood pressure of 80/40, and oxygen saturation of 98% on room air. His physical exam is notable for a young male in respiratory distress with equal breath sounds and midline trachea. A bedside ultrasound is performed (Figure 22-2). What is the most appropriate next step in management?

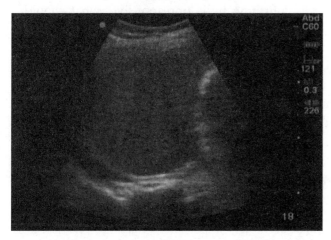

Figure 22-2. Reproduced with permission from Cevik AA, Acar NE, Holliman CJ (eds): *Evidence Based Emergency Trauma Management Course Book 2008*. Eskisehir, Eskisehir Osmangazi University Press, 2008.

(A) Obtain a portable chest x-ray.

(B) Perform a bilateral needle decompression of the chest.

(C) Perform a pericardiocentesis.

(D) Perform a thoracostomy.

(E) Perform an ED thoracotomy.

22-41. A 60-year-old female is the restrained driver in a moderate speed motor vehicle collision. She is complaining of chest wall pain after her chest hit the steering wheel. Her vital signs are within normal limits and her only injury is a nondisplaced sternal fracture seen on chest CT scan. Her electrocardiogram (ECG) is normal sinus rhythm with no abnormalities. Which of the following is the most appropriate management plan?

(A) Admit for 24 hours of observation while on telemetry.

(B) Admit for an exercise stress test.

(C) Discharge home with pain medication.

(D) Perform an echocardiogram.

(E) Perform two sets of cardiac enzymes and troponin 6 hours apart.

22-42. Which of the following scenarios is an indication for an ED thoracotomy?

(A) An 18-year-old male stabbed in the left chest at the midclavicular line who has no vital signs at the scene.

(B) A 24-year-old male hit in the chest with a baseball with no vital signs on the baseball field.

(C) A 34-year-old female involved in a high-speed motor vehicle collision who is ejected 20 feet and has no vital signs in the field.

(D) A 45-year-old female stabbed in the left chest at the midaxillary line who loses vital signs in the ambulance.

(E) A 66-year-old man with a stab wound to the right lower abdomen who loses vital signs in the trauma room.

22-43. A 31-year-old female is an unrestrained driver involved in a high-speed motor vehicle collision. She was ejected 20 feet into the woods. She has a Glasgow Coma Score of 4 and was intubated in the field. Her vital signs now are heart rate of 120, blood pressure of 85/50, and oxygen saturation of 95% on the ventilator. Her pupils are equal and reactive, breath sounds are clear, and the FAST exam is negative. The following chest x-ray was obtained (Figure 22-3). Which of the following is TRUE regarding her most likely diagnosis?

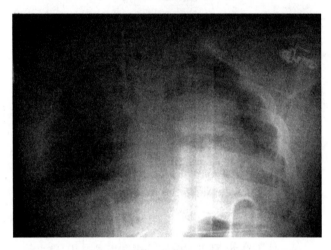

Figure 22-3. Reproduced with permission from Tintinalli JE, Stapczynski JS, Ma OJ, Cline DM, Cydulka RK, Meckler GD: *Tintinalli's Emergency Medicine: A Comprehensive Study Guide*, 7th Edition. Copyright © 2011 The McGraw-Hill Companies, Inc.

(A) A normal mediastinum on chest x-ray almost always excludes an aortic injury.

(B) As a temporizing measure, arterial vasodilators, like nitroprusside, should be used alone in the treatment of aortic injuries.

(C) A widened mediastinum on chest x-ray is very sensitive for detecting a major vascular injury.

(D) The distal descending aorta is the most commonly injured in blunt trauma.

(E) Transesophageal echocardiography is the study of choice to diagnose an aortic injury.

22-44. A hockey player blocks a slap shot with his chest and then collapses on the ice. After confirming he is unresponsive, what should a first responder do first in addition to calling for help?

(A) Give two rescue breaths.

(B) Open his airway.

(C) Perform cervical spine immobilization.

(D) Remove him from the ice.

(E) Start chest compressions.

22-45. A 20-year-old female sustains a stab wound to the left upper quadrant. What is the best way to rule out a diaphragmatic injury?

(A) CT scan

(B) Diagnostic peritoneal lavage

(C) FAST exam

(D) Upright chest x-ray

(E) Laparotomy

22-46. A 16-year-old female is thrown off of her horse and complains of severe abdominal pain. Upon arrival to the trauma bay, her heart rate is 130, blood pressure is 110/70, and oxygen saturation is 96% on 2 L oxygen. Her abdomen is diffusely tender on exam and the FAST exam is performed (Figure 22-4). Which of the following is the most appropriate next step in management?

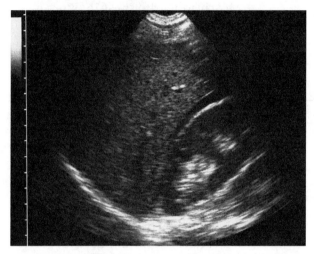

Figure 22-4. Reproduced with permission from Ma OJ, Mateer JR, Blaivas M: *Emergency Ultrasound*, 2nd Edition. Copyright © 2008 The McGraw-Hill Companies, Inc.

(A) Admit the patient for serial abdominal exams and hematocrits.

(B) Keep the patient in the ED for serial abdominal exams and hematocrits.

(C) Obtain a CT scan of her abdomen and pelvis to better identify the injury.

(D) Perform a diagnostic peritoneal lavage.

(E) Request the surgeon to take her directly to the operating room.

22-47. A 6-year-old boy presents immediately after falling off his bike and is complaining of abdominal pain. His exam reveals ecchymosis across his upper abdomen. Amylase and lipase are normal and an abdominal CT scan shows no injury. Which of the following statements is true?

(A) A duodenal hematoma can be seen on CT scan.

(B) Admit the patient for serial exams and blood work for concern of delayed pancreatic injury.

(C) Discharge the patient home with acetaminophen and follow-up with the pediatrician tomorrow.

(D) Monitor the patient with serial FAST exams in the ED.

(E) The pancreas is the most commonly injured organ in blunt trauma.

22-48. A 40-year-old male receives a stab wound to the left flank. Which of the following is true regarding his management?

(A) A triple contrast CT scan should be performed.

(B) If the diagnostic peritoneal lavage has less than 10 mL of free flowing blood, he is unlikely to have a significant injury.

(C) If the FAST exam is negative, he is unlikely to have a significant injury.

(D) Local wound exploration should be performed at the bedside with proper lighting and adequate anesthesia.

(E) The patient should be admitted for serial exams and hematocrits.

22-49. A 36-year-old male receives a gunshot wound to the left buttock. He is awake and alert with a heart rate of 110 and blood pressure of 130/80. A physical exam demonstrates an entrance wound on the left superior buttock with an exit wound posterior to the left ischial tuberosity. There is blood on the urinalysis. Which of the following is the most appropriate management?

(A) Go directly to the operating room for laparotomy.

(B) Irrigate, apply a sterile dressing, and discharge from the ED.

(C) Obtain an abdominal and pelvic CT scan.

(D) Obtain an abdominal and pelvic CT with a cystourethrogram.

(E) With appropriate lighting and anesthesia, perform bedside wound exploration.

22-50. A 14-year-old male falls 6 feet out of a tree onto his back. His only complaint is low back pain. His vital signs are heart rate 110, blood pressure 110/65, and 100% on room air. His physical exam is notable for a soft and non-tender abdomen and mild right paraspinal lumbar tenderness to palpation. Lumbar x-ray shows no fractures. His urine has no gross blood and a microscopic urinalysis shows <50 red blood cells per high power field. What is the most appropriate management?

(A) Admit for serial exams and monitoring for gross hematuria.

(B) Discharge home with instructions for no heavy lifting or strenuous exercise and follow-up in 1 week for repeat urinalysis.

(C) Obtain an abdominal and pelvis CT for significant renal injury.

(D) Obtain a retrograde cystogram.

(E) Place a Foley for three-way bladder irrigation.

22-51. Which of the following statements is true regarding renal trauma?

(A) A delayed contrast enhanced CT scan is required to detect all renal injuries.

(B) A FAST exam is useful for detecting renal injuries.

(C) Gross hematuria alone is not an indication for imaging in patients who sustain blunt trauma.

(D) Delayed bleeding after renal trauma can occur up to a month after injury from an arteriovenous fistula.

(E) Urinary extravasation is an absolute indication for renal surgical exploration.

22-52. A 52-year-old intoxicated male was the unrestrained driver in a moderate-speed motor vehicle collision with airbag deployment. His abdomen is diffusely tender, his rectal tone and prostate exam are normal, and there is no blood at the meatus. A Foley is placed that reveals gross hematuria. Which of the following statement regarding the evaluation and management of this genitourinary trauma is true?

(A) A contrast enhanced CT scan is the gold standard to diagnose a bladder rupture.

(B) A CT retrograde cystogram is the gold standard to diagnose a bladder rupture.

(C) A FAST exam is useful to detect an extraperitoneal bladder rupture.

(D) Most bladder ruptures are extraperitoneal and require surgery.

(E) Most bladder ruptures are intraperitoneal and require surgery.

22-53. A 72-year-old male on warfarin falls down 20 stairs and has an obvious pelvis fracture. His vital signs are heart rate 120 and blood pressure 80/40. His physical exam is notable for a tender, unstable pelvis, a high riding prostate, and no blood at the meatus. What is the most appropriate next step in management?

(A) After hanging blood products, obtain a CT scan to determine need for pelvic artery embolization versus operative repair.

(B) Perform a CT retrograde cystogram to identify a posterior urethral injury.

(C) Perform an RUG to identify a posterior urethral injury.

(D) Place a Foley prior to obtaining a CT scan.

(E) Under ultrasound guidance, place a suprapubic catheter.

22-54. Which of the following statements is TRUE regarding genitourinary trauma?

(A) Infection is the most common complication after circumcision.

(B) Male straddle injuries are at greatest risk for posterior urethral injuries.

(C) Testicular rupture should be managed conservatively with ice and analgesics.

(D) With penile fractures, perform a RUG to evaluate for urethral injury.

(E) Zipper injuries to the penis often have to be managed in the operating room.

22-55. A 60-year-old male hunter presents 24 hours after sustaining a laceration to his left forearm from a barbed-wire fence. The jagged wound is 2×2 cm in length and contaminated with wood and dirt. The extremity is neurovascularly intact and a tetanus shot is given. Which of the following is the most appropriate treatment?

(A) Admit for surgical debridement.
(B) High pressure irrigation and admit for intravenous antibiotics.
(C) High pressure irrigation with saline and primary closure.
(D) High pressure irrigation, with wet-to-dry dressings, and return for delayed closure in 72–96 hours.
(E) Wash gently with soap and water and perform a primary closure.

22-56. Which of the following soft-tissue foreign bodies is usually not visible on x-ray?

(A) Bone
(B) Glass
(C) Gravel
(D) Metal
(E) Wood

22-57. A 12-year-old female falls and sustains a right elbow dislocation. She is unable to abduct her fingers and has numbness to the volar aspect of the little finger. Which nerve is injured?

(A) Axillary
(B) Median
(C) Musculocutaneous
(D) Radial
(E) Ulnar

22-58. A 68-year-old female is involved in a high-speed motor vehicle collision and sustains a left knee dislocation. She is unable to dorsiflex or evert her foot. What nerve is injured?

(A) Obturator
(B) Peroneal
(C) Posterior tibial
(D) Sciatic
(E) Tibial

22-59. Which of the following is true regarding vascular injury in trauma?

(A) An ankle brachial index (ABI) of 0.5 is concerning for arterial injury.
(B) An ABI of 1.0 is concerning for arterial injury.
(C) Duplex ultrasound is a useful modality to diagnose vascular injury in open fractures.
(D) Multidetector CT angiography is safe to use in patients with iodine allergy.
(E) Underlying preexisting vascular disease will not affect the ABI.

22-60. Which of the following statements regarding wound ballistics is TRUE?

(A) A bullet's caliber is an indicator of wound potential.
(B) Lead bullets in soft tissue should be removed because of the risk of lead poisoning.
(C) Newer generation BB gun shots are not harmful.
(D) Radiographic localization of a bullet requires two views at 90 degrees.
(E) The emergency physician should describe wounds as entrance and exit wounds in the medical record.

22-61. Which of the following is TRUE regarding the evaluation of a patient with injuries that have potential forensic implications?

(A) During evidence collection, hematomas, unlike lacerations, do not need to be photographed.
(B) During strangulation, a period of 6 minutes is required for compression of blood supply to the brain to cause irreversible neuronal death and damage.
(C) Irrigate and explore all wounds prior to documentation and photographs.
(D) The death certificate must be completed by the physician who last attended to the deceased within 24 hours of the death.
(E) Unlike the entrance wound, the exit wound of a bullet is surrounded by a circumferential rim of abrasion.

Trauma
Answers and Explanations

22-1. **The answer is D** (Chapter 250). The goal of the primary survey is to identify immediate life threats and to stabilize them. The airway, breathing, circulation, disability (gross neurologic deficit), and exposure of the patient are the aspects of the physical exam in the primary survey.

22-2. **The answer is E** (Chapter 250). The National Emergency X-ray Utilization Study investigated criteria for clearing the cervical spine without cervical spine radiography. These criteria are no midline cervical spine tenderness to palpation, no focal neurological deficit, a normal mental status, no intoxication, and no painful distracting injuries. The ability to rotate the neck, being younger than 65 years, and ambulatory at the scene are all parts of the Canadian Cervical Spine Rule. The lack of evidence of trauma above the clavicle is not part of the NEXUS criteria.

22-3. **The answer is B** (Chapter 250). The ED thoracotomy is a procedure indicated in patients with penetrating trauma who have lost vital signs in the ED or just prior to arrival. Patients who have suffered abdominal trauma that is blunt in nature, who are found without vital signs, those who have suffered drowning incidents, and those with vital signs that are present are not patients in whom an ED thoracotomy is indicated. The highest rate of survival after thoracotomy is found in patients with penetrating truncal wounds.

22-4. **The answer is D** (Chapter 250). The patient has Class 4 shock. This is defined as a blood loss of more than 2000 mL (more than 40% of total blood volume). Patients with Class 1 shock have normal vital signs. When in Class 2 shock, the pulse rate increases and the pulse pressure decreases, but the blood pressure is within normal limits. Class 3 shock is characterized by 30–40% loss of blood volume and the patient has a heart rate in the 120–130 range with a decrease pulse pressure and blood pressure.

22-5. **The answer is D** (Chapter 251). A hypotensive pediatric trauma patient should receive 20 cc/kg of normal saline bolus repeated three times followed by packed red blood cells at 10 cc/kg if the patient remains hypotensive.

22-6. **The answer is A** (Chapter 251). Children under the age of 2 with a significant blunt head injury who have signs of a basilar skull fracture, focal neurological deficits, altered mental status, vomiting, or scalp contusions particularly those not over the frontal bone are at high risk for intracranial injury. As their exam is unreliable, more liberal use of CT scanning should be applied to this high-risk patient population. Plain films of the cranium are neither sensitive nor specific for the diagnosis of intracranial injury. Observation is indicated in low-risk and low-mechanism patients and should be at least 2 hours in duration.

22-7. **The answer is D** (Chapter 251). This patient has a classic history for SCIWORA. Due to bilateral symptoms of burning hands, the most likely etiology of the pain is a cervical spinal cord injury. The diagnostic test of choice to evaluate the spinal cord is an MRI. A CT scan does not provide adequate spinal cord imaging. Starting high-dose steroids without a diagnosis of spinal cord injury would be incorrect, and flexion and extension films should not be obtained when the patient has neurologic symptoms.

22-8. **The answer is C** (Chapter 251). In a hemodynamically unstable blunt trauma patient with left upper quadrant tenderness, a splenic rupture is quite likely. The imaging modality of choice in a hemodynamically unstable blunt abdominal trauma patient would initially be a FAST examination to evaluate for free fluid in the abdomen. A pelvic x-ray and a chest x-ray would both be indicated; however, a PA and lateral chest x-ray would not be indicated given the patient's current hemodynamic status. If the patient's hemodynamic status improved, a CT scan of the abdomen may be of utility to grade the splenic injury. A CT scan can be obtained after hemodynamic stability has been assured, as grading of the splenic injury allows for decisions regarding conservative management versus splenectomy. A lateral abdominal film would be of little use in this patient.

22-9. **The answer is A** (Chapter 251). Hematuria following abdominal trauma is common. The degree of hematuria is indicative of genitourinary injury. In a stable patient with hematuria, a CT scan of the abdomen with IV contrast is indicated to evaluate the kidneys as well as the ureters and the collecting system. In an unstable patient requiring immediate operative intervention, an intravenous pyelogram should be considered to evaluate for genitourinary trauma. A KUB and a cystoscopy are not indicated in acute abdominal trauma. A renal ultrasound may provide information with respect to the renal parenchyma; however, a CT scan provides more information with respect to vascular supply. An RUG is indicated when one suspects a urethral injury.

22-10. **The answer is C** (Chapter 252). As patients get older, the chest wall becomes stiffer and less compliant, placing them at an increased risk for rib fractures. The cervical spine in the elderly is less mobile. The myocardium is less compliant and progressively stiffens, which decreases the heart's pumping effectiveness. The respiratory muscles of an elderly patient are weaker and more susceptible to fatigue. There is an age-related decrement to vision and reflexes as well.

22-11. **The answer is A** (Chapter 252). Elderly patients are less likely to develop an intracranial epidural hematoma due to the thick fibrous bond between the dura matter and inner table of the skull. Hip fractures, rib fractures, odontoid fractures, and subdural hematomas are common in the elderly patients who suffer trauma.

22-12. **The answer is E** (Chapter 253). There are many physiologic changes associated with pregnancy. Overall the pregnant female has an increase in overall blood volume; however, due to a relative increase of plasma compared with red blood cell mass, there is a decrease in the maternal hematocrit. The maternal cardiac output is increased as is the maternal heart rate. The resting heart rate of a pregnant patient is 10–20 beats/min higher than their average resting heart beat. As the uterus increases in size, there is an upward displacement of the diaphragm leading to a decrease in the functional residual capacity of the lung. To compensate for the decreased functional residual capacity, the patient's respiratory tidal volume increases.

22-13. **The answer is B** (Chapter 253). Supine hypotension syndrome occurs in the second and third trimester of pregnancy. It is most likely due to compression of the inferior vena cava by the enlarged uterus. Supine hypotension syndrome can be relieved with the left lateral decubitus position or a wedge under the right side of a board if the patient is on a spine board, thereby displacing the uterus off of the inferior vena cava.

22-14. **The answer is C** (Chapter 253). Blunt abdominal trauma is a significant cause of morbidity and mortality in pregnant patients to both the mother and the fetus. Up to 5% of minor abdominal trauma in pregnancy can result in placental abruption in the second and third trimester. The most appropriate initial workup includes a FAST exam to evaluate for free fluid in the abdomen as well as an evaluation of the uterus and fetus. Furthermore, a CBC a type and screen, and a coagulation profile are appropriate in a pregnant patient who suffers trauma. RhoGAM is indicated in patients who are Rh negative. Pregnant women involved in trauma during their 2nd or 3rd trimester should be placed on a cardiotocometric monitor for a minimum of 4 hours to evaluate for signs of fetal distress and uterine irritability which could suggest a placental abruption.

22-15. **The answer is B** (Chapter 253). Pregnant trauma patients should undergo a rapid and complete trauma evaluation. Up to 5% of pregnant patients in the third trimester with minor abdominal trauma will develop placental abruption. Close monitoring is necessary to evaluate these patients. Even pregnant patients with seemingly minor trauma warrant at least 4 hours of tocodynamometric monitoring when the fetus is beyond 20 weeks of gestation. Patients with less than three contractions per hour can safely be discharged without concern for placental abruption. Assessing fetal heart rate and activity does not completely assess the risk of placental abruption. This patient does not meet NEXUS or Canadian C-spine criteria for cervical spine imaging. Diagnostic imaging that is indicated, however, should never be withheld from the pregnant trauma patient. The best way to ensure the safety of the unborn fetus is to ensure the stability and safety of the mother. Standard immobilization should be used for the pregnant patient, but the patient should be transported with a wedge under the right pelvis in order to rotate the pelvis 30 degrees to the left and prevent the supine hypotension syndrome.

22-16. **The answer is D** (Chapter 254). The patient's Glasgow coma score is 9 based on a score of 3 for opening her eyes to voice, a score of 2 for verbal moaning, and a score of 4 for motor with withdrawal from pain.

22-17. **The answer is B** (Chapter 254). Secondary brain injury occurs as a result of metabolic and pressure insults to the brain. The wearing of a bicycle or motorcycle helmet has a role in primary brain injury prevention. Hypotension, hypoxia, hyperglycemia, and anemia all contribute to an increased rate of secondary brain injury. Hyperventilation to a PCO$_2$ of less than 20 will likely result in further brain injury due to vasoconstriction and ischemia. The correct answer is to maintain normal arterial oxygen saturation.

22-18. **The answer is E** (Chapter 254). Subdural hematomas usually result from sudden acceleration and deceleration injuries. Minimal trauma is needed to cause a subdural hematoma in at-risk patient populations (elderly, alcoholics, anticoagulated patients). Blood tends to collect more slowly in subdural hematomas as the bleeding is venous in nature. Patients with subdural hematomas can present in a protean way as the symptoms are often nonspecific. Epidural hematomas classically result from a blow to the skull, causing disruption of the middle meningeal artery. They have a "talk and decline" presentation, and will worsen more rapidly than subdural hematomas as they are usually arterial bleeding. Diffuse axonal injuries are usually diagnosed in patients with coma after head injury; CT scans are initially unremarkable or show bleeds in the deep gray mater. Alcohol withdrawal is not associated with a focal neurological deficit.

22-19. **The answer is B** (Chapter 254). An epidural hematoma is often associated with an early loss of consciousness, followed by a return to normal mental status and then a delayed but abrupt decline in mental status. This is the "talk and decline" presentation of epidural hematoma. Epidural hematomas are diagnosed on CT scan of the brain, as an extra-axial, hyperacute area of bleeding, that are lenticular in shape, and do not cross the suture lines. A subdural hematoma would more likely present with a slower onset of mental status changes as it is due to venous bleeding. An electrocution may have an immediate loss of consciousness, but should not be associated with a delayed change in mental status. Postconcussive syndrome is persistent neurological, cognitive, and affective symptoms seen after a traumatic brain injury. Diffuse axonal injury is seen in significant head trauma patients who are typically in a coma state upon arrival to the ED.

22-20. **The answer is E** (Chapter 254). The New Orleans Criteria for obtaining a head CT after minor head injury are based on the presence of any of the following seven criteria: age >60, headache, vomiting, intoxication, persistent antegrade amnesia, evidence of trauma above the clavicles, or seizure. The reported sensitivity of this decision rule is 100%. One critique of this rule is that you must have loss of consciousness or amnesia to be eligible for this study, and it does not include high-risk patients with head injury without a loss of consciousness.

22-21. **The answer is D** (Chapter 255). A fracture of the posterior arch of the atlas is considered a "stable" fracture. All the remaining fractures are considered "unstable." See Table 255–1.

22-22. **The answer is A** (Chapter 255). The most common cause of Brown-Séquard syndrome, or transverse spinal cord hemisection, occurs in the setting of penetrating trauma. Additionally, Brown-Séquard syndrome demonstrates one of the best prognoses for recovery. Central cord syndrome is remarkable for more pronounced symptoms in the upper extremities. Patients with anterior cord syndrome do not experience pain distal to the site of the injury. Saddle anesthesia is present in patients with cauda equine syndrome.

22-23. **The answer is D** (Chapter 255). Central cord syndrome presents with decreased strength and, to a lesser degree, decreased in pain and temperature sensation that is more pronounced in the upper than the lower extremities. It is typically the result of hyperextension. Anterior cord syndrome results from damage to the corticospinal and spinothalamic pathways, with preservation of posterior column function. This is manifested by loss of motor function and loss of pain and temperature sensation distal to the lesion. Only vibration, position, and crude touch are preserved. The Brown-Séquard syndrome results from hemisection of the cord. It is manifested by ipsilateral loss of motor function, proprioception, vibratory sensation, and contralateral loss of pain and temperature sensation. Cauda equina produces a peripheral nerve injury rather than a direct injury to the spinal cord. Symptoms may include variable motor and sensory loss in the lower extremities, sciatica, bowel and bladder dysfunction, and "saddle anesthesia" (loss of pain sensation over the perineum).

22-24. **The answer is E** (Chapter 255). Juvenile rheumatoid arthritis places the patient at an elevated risk for cervical spine injury. By NEXUS criteria, this patient is unable to provide an appropriate cognitive level to ensure lack of injury. Canadian Cervical Spine Rules were generated from data that exclude patients of this age. Based on a mechanism of fall from a wheelchair, this patient could be cleared by Canadian Cervical Spine Rules, as this represents a minimal mechanism. SCIWORA is a phenomenon seen primarily in the pediatric population and is not of significant concern in this patient.

22-25. **The answer is E** (Chapter 255). The presence of an anterior compression in the thoracolumbar spine raises concern for chance fracture and associated injuries. The absence of normal cervical lordosis, overriding of the C1 anterior arch above the odontoid, lack of uniform angulation of the interspaces during flexion, and anterior wedging of the cervical vertebrae are all findings that commonly occur in the pediatric cervical spine evaluation and are not pathologic.

22-26. **The answer is E** (Chapter 255). A Jefferson fracture results from axial loading injuries: this results in a burst fracture of C1 and the lateral masses of C1 are displaced outward on the odontoid view on the cervical spine radiograph. A dens fracture or odontoid fracture is a fracture of the second vertebrae at the odontoid process. These usually result from a fall, or hyperflexion or extension. They are graded from one to three based on the location of the fracture. They will frequently have associated neurological symptoms. A Hangman fracture is a fracture of both pedicles of C2. This is usually caused by severe extension as one would see with a judicial hanging, or other mechanisms that would lead to severe hyperextension (motor vehicle crash, diving in shallow water). A clay shoveler fracture is a fracture of the spinous process, usually at C7. This is due to muscle contractions avulsing a portion of the spinous process or from direct trauma. These are typically stable fractures. The chance fracture is a transverse fracture of the lumbar or thoracic spine.

22-27. **The answer is A** (Chapter 256). Water's view may safely replace multiple views for midfacial fractures. A noncontrast head CT for traumatic brain injury will safely exclude midfacial fractures as well in patients with a low pretest probability for facial fracture. CT scans may miss dental root fractures due to location and plain films remain the preferred imaging. Panorex views have more limited sensitivity when evaluating mandibular condyle fractures when compared with mandible CT. The importance of patient positioning and operator variability can make Panorex views difficult to obtain and interpret.

22-28. **The answer is D** (Chapter 256). Patients with isolated anterior table fractures may be considered acceptable for discharge with close follow-up. Frontal bone fractures are rarely seen in isolation, due to the significant

amount of force necessary to generate such a fracture. Antibiotics should be considered for all sinus fractures. Nasoorbital ethmoid fractures frequently have associated injuries such as to the lacrimal duct and others. Diplopia on upward gaze is the result of entrapment of the inferior rectus and inferior oblique muscles.

22-29. **The answer is E** (Chapter 256). The examination is most consistent with findings of a tripod or zygomaticomaxillary fracture. Orbital "blow out" fracture occurs when an object of small diameter strikes the orbital complex leading to a fracture of the inferior or medial orbital wall. Findings of retrobulbar hematomas include exophthalmos, decreasing visual acuity, and increased intraocular pressure. Patients with mandible fractures usually complain of malocclusion with pain worsened by attempted movement. Orbital fissure syndrome results from a fracture of the orbit involving the superior orbital fissure. This often results in an injury to the oculomotor and ophthalmic divisions of the trigeminal nerve.

22-30. **The answer is D** (Chapter 256). Cricothyrotomy is contraindicated in patients younger than 8 years. Children have relatively large foreheads, coupled with their poor balance and high center of gravity, which make falls more likely; young children have a greater incidence of frontal bone injuries. SCIWORA, or cervical spine injury without obvious radiographic abnormality, is of most concern in the pediatric population. Children tend to have fewer midfacial fractures due to the lack of a maxillary sinus. The presence of developing teeth in the pediatric mandible can generate more complex fracture patterns than in similarly injured adults.

22-31. **The answer is B** (Chapter 257). Zone I includes the vertebral and proximal carotid arteries, major thoracic vessels, superior mediastinum, lungs, esophagus, trachea, thoracic duct, and spinal cord. Zone II extends from the inferior margin of the cricoid cartilage cephalad to the angle of the mandible.

Injuries in Zone II may involve the carotid and vertebral arteries, jugular veins, esophagus, trachea, larynx, and spinal cord. Zone III is located between the angle of the mandible and the base of the skull. The distal carotid, vertebral arteries, pharynx, and spinal cord are all at risk for injury in Zone III.

22-32. **The answer is C** (Chapter 257). Penetrating esophageal injuries are frequently initially asymptomatic. Nonoperative management is preferred for injuries to Zones I and III. CT scans are not considered sufficient to completely exclude laryngotracheal injury when a reasonable suspicion exists. Angiography is not considered the preferred imaging modality in children due to the caliber and size of the pediatric vasculature. Ultrasound has limited utility in evaluation of traumatic neck injuries, particularly in Zones I and III in which visualization can be difficult due to superimposed anatomy.

22-33. **The answer is A** (Chapter 257). The patient demonstrates findings consistent with Horner syndrome, which can occur as a result of injury to the ipsilateral carotid artery.

22-34. **The answer is C** (Chapter 257). Helical CTA can allow appropriate visualization in penetrating neck injuries to rule out vascular injury. Flexible esophagoscopy is the preferred modality in the setting of trauma to the neck. Platysmal violations should not be probed due to the risk of disrupting underlying hematomas and should be evaluated by an array of imaging modalities. Cricothyroidotomy is not recommended in blunt trauma as it can worsen laryngeal injury. Endotracheal intubation potentiates the creation of false passages in neck trauma and must be undertaken with caution by skilled practitioners. Blunt pharyngoesophageal injuries often present asymptomatically.

22-35. **The answer is B** (Chapter 258). Overly aggressive resuscitation and restoration of "normal" blood pressure prior to control of hemorrhage can increase the rate and volume of blood loss and increase mortality. Conversely, permissive hypotensive resuscitation is without demonstrable harm and likely beneficial in some subsets of traumatic shock. In addition, excessive fluid resuscitation may in theory be harmful to injured lung due to secondary alveolar capillary changes resulting from systemic inflammation. Evacuation of greater than 1500 mL of blood immediately after tube thoracostomy or 200 mL of blood per hour for 4 hours is generally recognized definition of massive hemothorax and is indication for operative management. The overall mortality of chest trauma patients is low, with most deaths attributable to noncardiothoracic injuries. The recommended approach for thoracostomy is to make an incision inferior to where you plan to place the chest tube and enter the chest cavity immediately above rib to avoid injury to the neurovascular bundles which track along the inferior margin of the ribs. Initial attempts at central venous access should be directed toward the ipsilateral side to prevent damage to the nontraumatized respiratory parenchyma.

22-36. **The answer is A** (Chapter 258). The last hole on the tube should be placed 1–2 cm inside the chest cavity. Chest tubes should never be clamped due the risk of a tension hemopneumothoraces. Initial intervention for a blocked tube should be replacement of the tube or placement of an additional tube to reduce the risk of infection and contamination. Chest tubes should be continued for 24 hours or more after the termination of an air leak for pneumothoraces and until there has been less than 200 cc of blood in a 24-hour period for hemothorax.

22-37. **The answer is D** (Chapter 258). Prophylactic antibiotics have not been demonstrated to afford significant improvements in suspected aspiration pneumonias. In asymmetric pulmonary injury such as pulmonary contusion, the uninjured lung should be placed down to improve compliance. Pulmonary contusion can be differentiated from pneumonia and air embolism by a time of onset typically within 6 hours and a distribution of injury that crosses bronchial and vascular distributions as well as pleural fissures. Any patient undergoing mechanical ventilation with evidence of an air leak must be considered for tube thoracostomy. The most common sites of injury in aspiration pneumonia are the right middle and right lower lung fields.

22-38. **The answer is E** (Chapter 258). A supine chest x-ray can be indeterminate for hemothorax up to 1000 mL of blood. Hamman sign, or crunch, is a crunching sound heard over the heart during systole, which is indicative of pneumomediastinum. Subcutaneous air and inspiratory stridor raise the concern for cervical or extrathoracic tracheal injuries. The vast majority of diaphragmatic injury occurs in the setting of penetrating trauma.

22-39. **The answer is E** (Chapter 258). Initial chest radiographs will frequently underestimate the degree and severity of chest and pulmonary trauma. Water-soluble contrast material is the preferred medium in the setting of esophageal injury due to potential pneumonitis caused by barium. CT scan has shown the incidence of pulmonary contusion to be higher than previously suspected due to its increased sensitivity. The "marching ants" and "sliding lung" signs are seen in the absence of pneumothorax due to the pleural movement.

22-40. **The answer is D** (Chapter 258). The ultrasound image shows a large hemothorax visualized in the right upper quadrant approach on FAST exam. Traumatic pneumothorax and hemothorax are indications for tube thoracostomy. Indications for ED thoracotomy include penetrating chest trauma in patients who demonstrate signs of life either in the field or in the ED and then deteriorate. Pericardiocentesis is indicated in any patient with a large pericardial effusion and hemodynamic instability. Pericardial blood is clotted but removal of as little as 5–10 mL of blood may increase the stroke volume by 25–50%. Needle decompression is indicated in any patient with suspected pneumothorax as a

temporizing measure until a tube thoracostomy can be performed. Evidence of a tension pneumothorax on physical exam includes decreased breath sounds on the affected side, tracheal deviation to the unaffected side, and jugular venous distension. Once the patient is hemodynamically stable, a portable chest x-ray is indicated

22-41. **The answer is C** (Chapters 258 and 259). Sternal fractures are associated with a low likelihood of blunt cardiac injury. With no other injuries on CT scan and a normal ECG, this patient can be safely discharged home with pain medications. In the evaluation of blunt cardiac injury, a normal ECG has a high negative predictive value, but a normal ECG does not exclude the development of a cardiac event that usually occurs in the first 24 hours. Common nondiagnostic ECG findings include sinus tachycardia and nonspecific ST-T changes. Isolated elevation of creatine kinase MB fraction, with no other associated injury, is not predictive of complications and mortality. Troponins are not sensitive for blunt cardiac injury. If elevated, troponins should be followed serially. Transthoracic echocardiography is not helpful in identifying patients at risk for developing blunt cardiac injury-related complications.

22-42. **The answer is D** (Chapter 259). Indications for ED thoracotomy include penetrating chest trauma in patients who demonstrate signs of life either in the field or in the ED and then deteriorate. After ED thoracotomy, the survival rate of patients who make it to the operating room is 70–80% for stab wounds and 30–40% for gunshot wounds.

22-43. **The answer is C** (Chapter 259). The chest x-ray demonstrates a widen mediastinum, defined as a measured width of greater than 8 cm or a mediastinal:chest ratio of >0.38. Although a widen mediastinum is the most sensitive findings in patients with an aortic injury, a normal mediastinum does not rule out an aortic injury. The chest x-ray should be used as a screening test and further imaging should be based on mechanism of injury and physical exam. Because of the fixation of the vessels between the left subclavian artery and the ligamentum arteriosum, the proximal descending aorta is most commonly injured in blunt trauma. Most institutions use multidetector CT scanners with angiography, not transesophageal echocardiography, as the screening study of choice for aortic injury. Transesophageal echocardiography can be used at the bedside in hemodynamically unstable patients. With partial- and full-thickness aortic tears, medical treatment involves decreasing the slope of the dP/dT (change in pressure over the change in time) to decrease wall tension and shearing forces. Titrating a short-acting beta-blocker, such as esmolol, can decrease the heart rate. Once the heart rate is controlled, an arterial vasodilator, such as sodium nitroprusside, can be added to help control the blood pressure. Sodium nitroprusside should not be used alone because rebound tachycardia may occur.

22-44. **The answer is E** (Chapter 259). This athlete is a victim of commotio cordis. Commotio cordis is a primary electrical event that occurs from a blow to the chest 10–30 msec before the peak of the T wave, a time vulnerable to the development of ventricular fibrillation. Based on the mechanism, the treatment is immediate defibrillation for a witnessed collapse. If a defibrillator is not immediately available or the collapse was not witnessed, chest compressions and ventilation should be performed for 2 minutes prior to defibrillation. Time to defibrillation is likely the most important factor in survival. Although cervical spine immobilization is important, the chance of spinal fracture with this mechanism is very low.

22-45. **The answer is E** (Chapter 260). Injuries to the diaphragm are uncommon but difficult to diagnose; therefore, laparotomy is sometimes required to make a definitive diagnosis. Other modalities such as chest x-ray, diagnostic peritoneal lavage, and helical CT scan may demonstrate evidence of a diaphragmatic injury. Evidence of diaphragmatic injury on chest x-ray includes viscera in the chest or a nasogastric tube coiled in the chest. Diagnostic peritoneal lavage can be helpful, particularly if the peritoneal lavage fluid is noted to exit through a chest tube or if follow-up chest x-ray demonstrates a new pleural effusion. Although commonly used to diagnose diaphragmatic injury, helical CT scan can miss small tears in the diaphragm. The FAST exam is useful to evaluate for intraperitoneal fluid but would not diagnose a small tear in the diaphragm.

22-46. **The answer is C** (Chapter 260). The FAST exam demonstrates free fluid in Morison pouch. Although the FAST exam is positive, the patient is hemodynamically stable. Given the increasing rates of nonoperative management of splenic and liver injuries, this patient should have a torso CT scan to evaluate her injuries including potential spinal or pelvic fractures that would not be seen on the FAST exam. If the patient was unstable with a positive FAST exam, then she should go directly to the operating room for a laparotomy. The FAST exam has essentially eliminated the use of diagnostic peritoneal lavage in trauma centers. Without further imaging, serial exams and hematocrits are not appropriate management of this patient.

22-47. **The answer is B** (Chapter 260). Bicyclists who hit the handlebars are at particularly high risk for pancreatic injuries. Pancreatic injuries are difficult to diagnose. Serum amylase and lipase are insensitive and nonspecific markers of pancreatic injury. In addition, a CT scan may be initially normal. Relatively small pancreatic injuries can become symptomatic days later. Given the risk of delayed pancreatitis or superinfection, this patient should be admitted for serial exams and pain control. The spleen, followed by the liver, is the most commonly injured organ in blunt abdominal trauma. Duodenal hematomas can be missed on physical exam and CT scan. Therefore, if there is a concern for the diagnosis, admit the patient for serial exams. Unless there is significant free fluid, the FAST exam is not a useful tool to diagnose a pancreatic injury or duodenal hematoma.

22-48. **The answer is A** (Chapter 260). In stable patients with stab wounds to the back or flank, a double or triple contrast helical CT scan (oral, IV, and rectal contrast) can detect contrast extravasation or the presence of air or fluid. While the FAST exam is a useful screening tool for intrathoracic and intraperitoneal fluid, it does not specifically evaluate for renal or bowel injury or retroperitoneal fluid. Local wound exploration is primarily used for anterior stab wounds. While serial abdominal exams are useful in trauma patients, a helical CT scan should be performed initially to determine if there is active extravasation.

22-49. **The answer is D** (Chapter 261). With gunshot wounds to the buttock, it is important to determine the bullet tract in order to assess for vascular, bowel, or lower genitourinary tact injury. Stable deep gunshot wounds to the buttock should be evaluated with triple contrast helical CT scan with cystourethrogram if there is blood on urinalysis or the wound is close to the GU tract. Superficial stab wounds, not gunshot wounds, to the buttocks can be managed at the bedside and discharged from the ED. Patients with signs of peritonitis, intrapelvic or transabdominal missile path, or intraperitoneal free air, warrant immediate exploratory laparotomy.

22-50. **The answer is B** (Chapter 262). Indications for imaging in patients with suspected renal trauma include gross hematuria, adults with systolic blood pressure less than 90 and any degree of hematuria, children with greater than 50 red blood cells per high power field, and a mechanism with a high index of suspicion for renal injury. This patient can be safely discharged home with instructions for no heavy lifting or strenuous exercise and follow-up urinalysis in 1 week. A CT retrograde cystogram is used to diagnose blad-

der rupture that occurs more commonly with direct blows to a distended bladder. Foley placement for three-way irrigation is not appropriate management.

22-51. **The answer is D** (Chapter 262). Complications from renal trauma include delayed bleeding, urinary extravasation, urinoma, perinephric abscess, and hypertension. Delayed bleeding can occur up to a month after injury and is most commonly due to an arteriovenous fistula that has developed after a deep parenchymal laceration. A delayed CT scan is only indicated if there is suspicion of urinary extravasation from an abnormal fluid collection. Extravasation cannot be detected until the contrast enhanced urine is excreted into the collecting system, which usually can take up to 10 minutes; therefore, a delayed scan is recommended to exclude urinary extravasation. Gross hematuria is an indication for imaging in an adult with suspected blunt renal trauma.

22-52. **The answer is B** (Chapter 262). A CT retrograde cystogram is the gold standard imaging study to diagnose bladder rupture. A contrast enhanced CT with passive bladder filling, even with a clamped catheter, is not sensitive enough to exclude bladder rupture. A FAST exam can demonstrate intraperitoneal fluid but, since most bladder ruptures are retroperitoneal, is not the gold standard to diagnose bladder rupture. Most extraperitoneal bladder ruptures can be managed nonsurgically with bladder catheter drainage alone. Intraperitoneal ruptures always require surgical exploration.

22-53. **The answer is A** (Chapter 262). Although this patient likely has a posterior urethral injury requiring evaluation with an RUG, he is hemodynamically unstable from his pelvic fracture. Performing an RUG should not interfere with CT diagnosis and embolization treatment of pelvic artery injury from a pelvic fracture. In patients with suspected urethral injuries, a Foley catheter should not be placed prior to an RUG to prevent further urethral injury. The treatment for a posterior urethral injury is a suprapubic catheter, but this should not be performed until the diagnosis is confirmed. A CT retrograde cystogram is used to diagnose bladder rupture.

22-54. **The answer is D** (Chapter 262). Obtain a CT retrograde urethrogram for penile fracture or penetrating penile injury because of the high incidence of coexisting urethral injury. Bleeding is the most common complication after circumcision and is often controlled by direct pressure. Infection occurs in up to 10% of patients and requires urologic consultation. Male straddle injuries often result in anterior urethral injuries that can be diagnosed with a retrograde urethrogram. Posterior urethral injuries are more common with pelvic fractures and shearing forces from a deceleration injury. Testicular rupture, diagnosed by color Doppler ultrasound, requires early surgical exploration. Early evacuation of blood clots and repair of testicular rupture result in an earlier return to normal activity, decreased hematoma infection, and less testicular atrophy compared with conservative management. Zipper injuries can often be managed in the emergency room by applying mineral oil or injecting lidocaine to free the skin. Wire cutters can also be used to cut the median bar on the zipper, which allows the zipper to fall apart.

22-55. **The answer is D** (Chapter 263). Patients with delayed presentations, contaminated wounds, soft tissues foreign bodies, and significant tissue destruction benefit from delayed closure at 72–96 hours if there are no signs of wound infection. While antiseptic solution does not decrease infection rates or improve healing time, high-pressure irrigation with saline or tap water is effective at decreasing rates of wound infection. The role of antibiotics in penetrating extremity trauma remains controversial, but antibiotics may have a role in hand injuries, immunocompromised patients, and wounds with significant soft-tissue destruction or bone/joint involvement. The patient has a delayed presentation of a contaminated wound with significant tissue destruction and therefore would benefit

from high-pressure irrigation with delayed closure.

22-56. **The answer is E** (Chapter 263). Materials such as glass, metal, gravel, or bone are usually visible on plain films. Organic materials such as wood are more difficult to identify with plain films, but ultrasound can be useful. CT scanning is more accurate for finding both radiolucent and opaque foreign bodies.

22-57. **The answer is E** (Chapter 263). Associated with elbow dislocations, ulnar nerve injuries result in the inability to abduct the fingers and decreased sensation over the volar aspect of the little finger. The median nerve controls wrist flexion, finger adduction, and sensation over the volar aspect of the thumb and index finger. The radial nerve controls the forearm, wrist, and finger extension and sensation over the dorsoradial hand and thumb. The musculocutaneous nerve controls forearm flexion and sensation over the lateral forearm. The axillary nerve controls arm abduction, arm internal and external rotation, and sensation over the lateral aspect of the shoulder.

22-58. **The answer is B** (Chapter 263). Associated with posterior knee dislocations, peroneal nerve injuries result in the inability to dorsiflex and evert the foot and decreased sensation over the dorsal foot and lateral leg. The posterior tibial nerve controls great toe plantar flexion. The tibial nerve controls ankle plantar flexion. The sciatic nerve controls knee flexion. The obturator nerve controls hip adduction.

22-59. **The answer is A** (Chapter 263). An ABI of 1.0 is normal. An ABI of less than 0.9 is concerning for arterial injury. Preexisting vascular disease and hypothermia will lower the ABI. Duplex ultrasonography has an accuracy of 96–98% for vascular injury but is operator dependent and is not useful with open fractures, large hematomas, or bulky dressings. Multi-detector CT angiography is less invasive and has a similar cost to angiography, but the limitations include the inability to perform the test on patients with iodine allergies and the artifact caused by bullet fragments.

22-60.   **The answer is D** (Chapter e263.1). Radiographic location of a bullet requires two views at 90 degrees or a tomographic image. A bullet's mass, structure, and striking velocity are indicators of wound potential. The caliber of a bullet does not predict wound potential. Emergency physicians should be aware that newer generation BB guns and air guns fire small bullets with high muzzle velocity, which can cause significant injury or be fatal. Lead bullets in soft tissue usually become encapsulated and do not cause lead poisoning. Lead bullets in synovial fluid, intra-articular space, and disk space should be removed because of the risk of lead poisoning. In the medical record, emergency physicians should avoid describing the wound as an entrance or exit wound but should describe the shape, location, and size of the gunshot wound including any evidence of soot powder or subcutaneous tissue tattooing with gunpowder.

22-61.   **The answer is D** (Chapter e263.2). The death certificate must be completed by the physician who last attended to the deceased within 24 hours of the death. The type of wound, location, and recovery of particles from inside a wound can give important forensic information; therefore, wounds should never be irrigated and explored prior to documentation and photographs. Photographs should be taken of all wounds, including hematomas, to help determine the weapon. Unlike the exit wound, the entrance wound from a bullet is surrounded by a circumferential rim of abrasion. This is produced by friction from the bullet on the skin margins. During strangulation, a period of 4 minutes is required for compression of the blood supply of the brain to result in neuronal death. Bruising or ligature marks on the neck and pinpoint hemorrhages especially in the conjunctival lining of the eyes are also markers of strangulation.

Wound Management
Questions

23-1. Which of the following factors is most predictive of the risk of developing a wound infection?

(A) Smoking
(B) Immunosuppressive medication use
(C) Location of the wound
(D) Collagen vascular disease
(E) Diabetes mellitus

23-2. Which of the following statements is true with regard to the formation of scars?

(A) Hypertrophic scars extend beyond the original wound margins and decrease in size over time.
(B) Keloids extend beyond original wound margins and fail to change size over time.
(C) Majority of lacerations will heal without any residual scar.
(D) Patients must be advised that keloids decrease in size over 1–2 years.
(E) Whites are more prone to developing keloids.

23-3. Which of the following statements is true regarding wound infections?

(A) A patient with a retained foreign body sensation rarely, if ever, has an actual retained foreign body.
(B) Delayed primary closure 2 weeks after injury is advised for wounds that have a high chance for infection.
(C) Soil, or clay, contamination poses a high risk of wound infection.

(D) Ultrasound should never be used to detect a small retained foreign body.
(E) Wounds with a high risk of infection should never be closed.

23-4. Which of the following statements is TRUE regarding the use of sterile technique for wound closure?

(A) Basic cleanliness, including the use of nonsterile gloves, is appropriate for wound closure.
(B) Chlorhexidine can be used to clean skin margins, but iodine-containing solutions can prevent wound healing.
(C) Full sterile technique should be used for dirty wounds.
(D) Probing of the wound with a sterile, gloved, finger is recommended for palpation of foreign bodies prior to wound closure.
(E) Skin disinfectants should be used to cleanse the wound and wound margins prior to closure.

23-5. A 21-year-old male presents to your emergency department (ED) complaining of a human bite to his dominant hand, sustained during a fight. His vital signs are within normal limits, and examination of the affected hand reveals a 1-cm laceration over the midshaft fifth metacarpal bone. Which of the following statements is true regarding the management of this injury?

(A) Amoxicillin is adequate coverage for human bites to the hand.

(B) Antibiotics are not indicated for human bites to the hand.

(C) The principal bacteria involved in human bites include *Streptococcus* and *Pasteurella*.

(D) The risk of infection from human bites is low.

(E) Wound exploration should include assessment of tendon function and injury to the tendon sheath.

23-6. Which of the following statements regarding wound preparation for closure is correct?

(A) All wounds should be irrigated with high-pressure irrigation.

(B) Debridement of wound margins is not recommended secondary to cosmetic concerns.

(C) Hair should never be removed.

(D) Wet-to-dry dressings are an appropriate method for debridement of a nonexudative wound.

(E) Wound soaking is not recommended as an adequate method for wound decontamination.

23-7. A 33-year-old male presents with a laceration measuring 1 cm over the dorsum of his dominant hand, sustained with a clean knife while working in a kitchen. Which of the following statements is accurate regarding management of this wound?

(A) Irrigation of small wounds is unnecessary secondary to the low chance for infection.

(B) The laceration can be managed with antibiotic ointment and gauze dressing with a similar cosmetic outcome.

(C) The laceration should be closed with sutures.

(D) The small length of the wound makes underlying tendon or deeper structure involvement unlikely.

(E) Sutures should be used if the patient has a history of keloid formation.

23-8. A 4-year-old child presents with a large (4 cm) gaping, deep laceration to her left thigh, sustained by running into the edge of a coffee table. The wound appears to be under high tension. Which of the following statements is true regarding the repair of this laceration?

(A) Absorbable sutures should never be used to close the epidermis.

(B) Antibiotics should be prescribed for this type of laceration.

(C) Deep nonabsorbable sutures should be placed to improve cosmesis, since they provide more tensile strength.

(D) Deep sutures should be used to relieve tension on the wound.

(E) Staples are preferred to sutures for closing this large of a laceration.

23-9. You decide to use a tissue adhesive to close a forehead laceration. Which of the following statements best applies to the use of tissue adhesives?

(A) Cyanoacrylate tissue adhesives have a lower rate of wound dehiscence as compared with other forms of primary closure.

(B) Octyl-cyanoacrylate and butyl-cyanoacrylate are similar in their water resistance and burst strength.

(C) The patient should be placed in Trendelenburg to avoid leakage of the adhesive into the eyes.

(D) Tissue adhesives are appropriate for use in high-tension wounds.

(E) Tissue adhesives should cover the entire wound and extend to 5–10 mm on either side of the wound edges.

23-10. A 44-year-old man sustained blunt trauma to his head. He has an actively bleeding stellate laceration on his forehead and scalp. Which of the following statements is TRUE?

(A) Fibrous dermal tissue easily retracts after injury, allowing for significant hemorrhage from these lacerations.

(B) Shaving the scalp hair prior to wound closure is not recommended.

(C) For deep lacerations to the forehead, closure of the frontalis muscle is not necessary due to the tight apposition of the muscularis and the aponeurotic layers.

(D) The external carotid artery is the primary source of the rich blood supply to the scalp and forehead.

(E) The potential space between the periosteum and galea aponeurosis does not allow for hematoma or infectious collection.

23-11. A 19-year-old female presents to the ED with lacerations to her face after an assault. Which of the following is true regarding repair of lacerations to the face?

(A) Due to the superficial nature of most eyelid lacerations, primary closure can be accomplished with tissue adhesive.

(B) The posterior wall of the external auditory canal is supplied by the auricular branch of the vagus nerve, so a laceration to this region cannot be fully anesthetized by a simple auricular nerve block.

(C) Transitory ptosis is common sequela of blunt or penetrating injury to the eyelid, and the patient should be advised to return to the ED for reevaluation in 5–7 days.

(D) When performing a laceration repair, which extends through the vermillion border, approximation of all structures must be performed before placement of a stitch to approximate the vermillion border.

(E) When repairing lacerations 2–3 mm from the medial canthus, absorbable 6–0 sutures should be used carefully in order to approximate the nasolacrimal duct.

23-12. A 25-year-old male presents to the ED after blunt trauma to his right ear, lips, and face. Evaluation of his oral cavity also reveals numerous lacerations. Which of the following statements is true?

(A) A perichondrial hematoma is a common complication following repair of auricular lacerations, and in most cases can be left alone due to the elastic nature of the outer ear.

(B) Crushed or loose pieces of auricular cartilage should be removed carefully before primary closure to ensure adequate approximation.

(C) Isolated intraoral mucosal lacerations may not need to be sutured, especially if <1 cm in length.

(D) Oral antibiotic therapy is recommended for most lacerations because of improved cosmesis and the high rates of cutaneous infections of the face.

(E) Sensory innervation of the lower lip is supplied by the infraorbital nerve.

23-13. Which of the following tendon lacerations of the hand should be repaired by the treating ED physician?

   (A) A 2-cm laceration in the deep palmar space of a 22-year-old female.

   (B) A 3–5-cm extensor tendon laceration over the dorsum of the hand (over the third metacarpal), with 30% tendon involvement sustained while cutting vegetables in a 56-year-old diabetic female.

   (C) A 4-cm laceration on the volar aspect of the wrist in a 22-year-old male. A 20% laceration of the flexor carpi radialis is noted.

   (D) A deep thumb laceration of extensor surface of the dominant hand of a 44-year-old female with complete lack of extension noted on physical exam.

   (E) A deep palmar laceration in the non-dominant hand of a 33-year-old female with signs of flexor tendon laceration.

23-14. When evaluating lacerations to the knee or ankle for joint capsule penetration, which of the following management plans is the most appropriate for identifying an injury?

   (A) Injection of 5–10 cc of saline into the joint

   (B) Injection of fluorescein solution followed by a Wood's lamp examination

   (C) Joint effusion on plain radiographs

   (D) Methylene blue joint injection

   (E) Physical examination alone

23-15. A 44-year-old man presents to the ED after a deep upper thigh laceration after dropping his chain saw. What is the appropriate way to close this wound?

   (A) Deep absorbable sutures

   (B) Horizontal mattress suture

   (C) Multilayered closure

   (D) Tissue adhesive

   (E) Running sutures

23-16. Which of the following statements is TRUE regarding antibiotic use in lower extremity lacerations?

   (A) Animal bites of the leg/foot are best covered with a first-generation cephalosporin in order to cover *Staphylococcus* and *Streptococcus*.

   (B) Due to the high rate of infection seen with plantar lacerations, prophylactic antibiotic coverage is recommended for all patients.

   (C) Fluoroquinolones provide appropriate coverage for lacerations sustained when wading in fresh water streams in order to cover *Aeromonas hydrophila*.

   (D) Open fractures of the lower extremity do not require prophylactic antibiotic coverage due to the low rates of infection.

   (E) Small lacerations on the dorsum of the foot should always be covered with broad-spectrum antibiotics secondary to the close proximity of tendons.

23-17. Which of the following statements regarding the presence of soft-tissue foreign bodies is true?

   (A) All foreign bodies elicit the same inflammatory soft tissue reaction.

   (B) All foreign bodies must be removed on the initial visit to the ED.

   (C) Foreign bodies never produce a toxic reaction.

   (D) Foreign bodies that are inert produce the greatest inflammatory reaction.

   (E) Infection is the most common complication of a retained foreign body.

23-18. Which of the following factors increases the likelihood of finding an underlying retained soft-tissue foreign body?

   (A) Fight bite where no dental fractures are seen.

   (B) Laceration caused by a glass bottle that shattered.

   (C) Laceration caused by a single shard of glass.

   (D) Wound with a depth of 2 mm whose base is fully visualized.

   (E) Sewing needle removed from the skin.

23-19. Which of the following substances is generally visible on plain radiographs?

(A) All fish bones

(B) All plastics

(C) Glass

(D) Thorns

(E) Wood

23-20. Which of the following statements is TRUE regarding the use of ultrasound in the detection of a retained soft-tissue foreign body?

(A) Both high- and low-frequency settings should be used when scanning for a retained foreign body.

(B) Higher frequency probes enable better detection of deeper objects.

(C) Low-frequency probes enable better detection of more superficial objects.

(D) Low-frequency probes produce images of higher resolution.

(E) Ultrasound has a low rate of false positives.

23-21. Which of the following statements is true regarding the management of puncture wounds?

(A) Debridement of a puncture wound should always be performed to better visualize the base.

(B) High-pressure irrigation will enable better visualization of the entrance site.

(C) Prophylactic antibiotics should always be prescribed in cases where the puncture wound involves the foot.

(D) *Pseudomonas* should be considered in puncture wounds involving sneakers or rubber-soled shoes.

(E) *Staphylococcus aureus* is infrequently associated with infected puncture wounds.

23-22. Which of the following statements is TRUE regarding the management of needlestick injuries in health care providers?

(A) HIV prophylaxis is mandatory in cases of accidental needlestick exposures where the source patient's HIV status is known to be negative.

(B) Postexposure prophylaxis for HIV and hepatitis B is mandatory.

(C) Postexposure prophylaxis is available for hepatitis B and HIV exposures.

(D) The results of rapid HIV tests obtained in the ED do not affect the decision to initiate postexposure prophylaxis.

(E) The risk of clinical infection with hepatitis A transmitted via accidental needlestick is high.

23-23. Which of the following treatment methods is appropriate for the management of a paint gun injection injury to the hand?

(A) Digital nerve block

(B) Immediate expert consultation with a hand surgeon

(C) Nitroglycerine ointment or paste

(D) Supportive care if the skin appearance is benign

(E) Warm water immersion

23-24. Prophylactic antibiotics should NOT be prescribed for which of the following wounds?

(A) Abrasion to the upper arm from a dog bite

(B) Cat bite to the hand

(C) Dog bite to the hand

(D) Human bite to a clenched fist

(E) 1-cm human bite to the face

23-25. Which of the following patients should not receive tetanus toxoid after sustaining a wound that is considered high risk for tetanus?

(A) Any patient younger than 65 years

(B) Any patient who has experienced a severe neurologic or systemic reaction to prior tetanus toxoid

(C) Any patient who has not received a pertussis vaccination

(D) Any patient who has had a mild skin reaction to prior tetanus toxoid

(E) Any pediatric (<15 years old) patient

23-26. Which of the following statements is TRUE regarding wounds closed with topical skin adhesives?

(A) A supplementary dressing should be placed over the wound adhesive.

(B) Topical antibiotic cream should always be applied over the wound adhesive.

(C) Wound adhesives are appropriate for use on gaping lacerations.

(D) Wound adhesives can be removed from the skin with antibiotic ointment or petrolatum jelly.

(E) Wounds closed with tissue adhesives should be scrubbed daily to ensure appropriate wound healing.

23-27. Which of the following recommendations should be provided to a patient with a large facial laceration closed with sutures?

(A) A mandatory wound check should be done in 2 days.

(B) No washing or scrubbing of the face should occur for the first 72 hours.

(C) Prophylactic antibiotics are necessary.

(D) Sun exposure will help achieve the best cosmetic repair.

(E) Suture removal should occur in 3–5 days.

Wound Management
Answers and Explanations

23-1. **The answer is C** (Chapter 43). Wound characteristics such as location, age, depth, and configuration are the most predictive factors for wound infections. Comorbidities such as smoking, immunosuppressive medication use, and medical conditions such as collagen vascular diseases, diabetes mellitus, or obesity are associated with poorer wound healing, but are not the most predictive of wound infections.

23-2. **The answer is B** (Chapter 43). Keloids are a genetic anomaly that results in excess collagen production. This excess collagen deposition extends beyond the wound margins. Keloids rarely decrease in size over time, in contrast to hypertrophic scars that remain within wound margins and spontaneously decrease in size over 1–2 years. Asians and Blacks are more prone to develop keloids. All ED providers should be aware that the majority of lacerations heal with a residual scar. This information should be provided to patients to better understand the course of wound healing, and to set patients' expectations.

23-3. **The answer is C** (Chapter 43). Wound infection is an important topic for emergency physicians. The risk of wound infections increases with the location of the wound (i.e., groin or axilla wounds having higher risks of infection because of the moist skin and the higher bacterial counts in these areas), the mechanism of injury, and the time since the injury was sustained. Contamination of the wound with clay (the inorganic component of soil) poses a high risk of infection be-cause of the high bacterial counts in even a small amount of soil. Retained foreign bodies also increase the risk of future wound infection. Patients with a foreign body sensation frequently have an actual retained foreign body. Plain films are useful for radiopaque foreign bodies, such as glass fragments >2 mm, metal, bone, teeth, graphite, certain plastics, or painted wood. Ultrasound is useful for locating objects >2.5 mm, and is especially useful for wood, which is not seen on plain films. Computed tomography (CT) or magnetic resonance imaging (MRI) can also be used to locate a retained foreign body. Infected wounds, or wounds with a high risk of infection, should not be closed primarily. Delayed primary closure, approximately 4 days after the injury, is appropriate for wounds with a high risk of infection.

23-4. **The answer is A** (Chapter 44). Full sterile technique is not necessary for wound closure in the ED. Nonsterile gloves, along with basic cleanliness, are appropriate and adequate. A wound should not be probed with a finger to assess for a foreign body. The reason for this is twofold. First, the risk of puncturing the provider with the foreign body is real. Second, direct pressure from the digit may result in tissue damage. Finally, skin disinfectants should never be applied to the wound directly, as they can lead to tissue damage and impaired healing. The wound margins and surrounding intact skin should be cleansed prior to initiating the wound repair.

23-5. **The answer is E** (Chapter 50). Human bites pose a high risk of infection. Antibiotic coverage for *Eikenella* and *Pasteurella* should be initiated in the ED. Amoxicillin–clavulanate provides adequate coverage for both of these organisms. For bites that cover a joint line, tendon, cartilage, and for any bites to the hand or feet, antibiotic prophylaxis is indicated. Thorough wound exploration should be performed, along with copious wound irrigation. The underlying tendon should be examined through a full range of motion to assess for any injuries.

23-6.   The answer is E (Chapter 44). In preparation for wound closure, all wounds should be visualized fully. Hair should be trimmed approximately 2 mm above the roots, if needed, to aid in visualizing the wound. Alternatively, hair can be used to help close the wound. High-pressure irrigation should be used for wounds on extremities, or for heavily contaminated wounds. Low-pressure irrigation is appropriate for uncontaminated wounds, or for wounds in areas of loose skin, such as the scrotum or the eyelids. Debridement of necrotic tissue should be done. Usually, debridement is most effectively done with a scalpel. However, if an exudative necrotic wound is present, an effective method for debridement is the wet-to-dry dressing. Wet gauze will adhere to necrotic tissue which will be removed when the gauze dries and is removed.

23-7.   The answer is B (Chapter 45). A randomized trial has shown that small (<2 cm), uncomplicated hand wounds that are under low tension heal as well as those closed by primary closure. In patients with a history of keloids, as little foreign material should be introduced into the wound as possible. If possible, wounds should be closed with tissue adhesives or tape, or as in this case, with antibiotic ointment and gauze. Regardless of the superficial-appearing nature of the wound, a wound should always be explored to ensure no underlying tendon or other structure damage.

23-8.   The answer is D (Chapter 45). Undermining tension within a wound is imperative

for maximizing the chance of a good cosmetic outcome and minimizing the chance of wound dehiscence. Tension can be reduced by placing deep dermal sutures, carefully undermining and approximating different layers of the wound, or by splinting the affected extremity to prevent movement. Staples are the least precise way of approximating wound margins, and therefore should be reserved for linear, nonface lacerations. Absorbable sutures can be used, even for the epidermal layer, and are especially beneficial in a pediatric patient for whom suture removal may be difficult and challenging. Antibiotics are rarely necessary for simple lacerations.

23-9.   The answer is C (Chapter 45). Tissue adhesives are a useful method of wound closure in the ED. Cyanoacrylate tissue adhesives have slightly higher rates of wound dehiscence, making their use only appropriate in low-tension wounds (i.e., wounds that can easily be approximated by the provider's hands). The two available forms of cyanoacrylates are octyl- and butyl-cyanoacrylate. Octyl-cyanoacrylate (Dermabond), with its eight carbon side chains, has a higher bursting strength and is also water resistant when compared with butyl-cyanoacrylate. Butyl-cyanoacrylate, or Indermil, has the advantage of unlimited working time after the applicator is opened. Both tissue adhesives should never be allowed to enter the eye. To avoid this, a patient with a forehead laceration should be placed in Trendelenburg. Antibiotic ointment can also be applied to the eyelashes to prevent the adhesive from entering the eye.

23-10.   The answer is B (Chapter 46). Blood supply to the scalp and forehead arises from both the internal and external carotid arteries. Because the fibrous dermal tissue of the scalp retracts with ease, significant bleeding can occur, making forehead lacerations notorious for profuse bleeding. When examining a patient with a forehead laceration, it is important to determine if there is a tear of the galea aponeurosis. This space can accumulate with blood easily, and be a site of future infections. Closure of the galea is recommended by many experts, with no clear evidence regarding the need for absolute closure. Shaving of scalp hair is not recommended secondary to increased risk of wound infection. If needed for improved visualization, the hair can be clipped. If the muscle layer in the forehead is not approximated, a noticeable deficit may occur, especially during times of facial expression.

23-11. **The answer is B** (Chapter 46). Eyelid lacerations can be difficult to repair. Tissue adhesives should not be used near the eye (and especially for eyelid lacerations), as it may glue the eyelid shut. Ptosis can be a serious cosmetic complication of eyelid injuries, and must be followed up by an oculoplastics specialist. Other injuries that also require early specialist follow-up include those involving the inner lid margin, the lacrimal duct, or extending through the tarsal plate. The vermillion border is an important cosmetic landmark, and must be approximated first to ensure proper alignment. An auricular nerve block is an excellent method for proper anesthesia to the ear. The posterior wall of the external auditory canal is supplied by the vagus nerve, and will not be anesthetized by an auricular nerve block.

23-12. **The answer is C** (Chapter 46). Due to the paucity of extra skin and cartilage in the ear, crushed or loose pieces of cartilage should not be removed, as these pieces may be beneficial if reconstructive surgery is necessary. Sensory innervation of the upper lip is by the infraorbital nerve, while the mental nerve supplies the lower lip. Regional nerve blocks are especially useful in the face to prevent deformation of tissue due to local injection. Because of the high vascularity of the face, routine antibiotics are not recommended for lacerations. A perichondrial hematoma can be a disfiguring complication of auricular lacerations. Take care to ensure active compression of the area after laceration repair. If an auricular hematoma is suspected, consultation with a

plastic surgeon or otolaryngologist is recommended.

23-13. **The answer is B** (Chapter 47). Physicians comfortable with tendon lacerations can repair them primarily in the ED. Generally, extensor tendon lacerations can be repaired, except when there are signs of severe contamination or occur over the thumb. Due to the complex nature of flexor tendon mechanism, these should be repaired by a specialist.

23-14. **The answer is B** (Chapter 48). For lacerations around the knee joint, joint capsule penetration can be difficult to detect solely by physical exam. Air within the joint capsule on plain radiographs is a sign of joint capsule penetration, while joint effusion is a nonspecific sign of trauma. Methylene blue is discouraged due to resultant staining of intra-articular surfaces, which may affect operative management of intra-articular injuries. A large volume of fluid should be injected (often >60 cc) to stress the joint and prevent false-negative arthrocentesis. Another useful technique to employ is adding a few drops of fluorescein in the fluid used for the joint injection, and then looking for a fluorescent effluent with a Wood's lamp.

23-15. **The answer is B** (Chapter 48). Deep absorbable sutures are not recommended for wounds with a high rate of contamination (such as chain saw injuries to the thigh). Horizontal mattress sutures or skin staples are ideal for wounds that have a high propensity for infection. Running sutures avoided since selected sutures cannot be removed if the site gets infected.

23-16. **The answer is C** (Chapter 48). Prophylactic antibiotics for lower extremity injuries do not reduce postrepair wound infection, and should be given on a case-by-case basis. Small lacerations on the dorsum of the foot (especially if they are clean) therefore do not require perfunctory antibiotic coverage. Animal bites of the lower extremity should be covered with amoxicillin–clavulanate to cover *Staphylococcus, Streptococcus,* and

Pasteurella. Fluoroquinolones (along with aminoglycosides and trimethoprim–sulfamethoxazole) are effective in the treatment of freshwater lacerations for the coverage of *A. hydrophila.* Open fractures of the lower extremity are most commonly contaminated with *S. aureus,* so a first-generation cephalosporin and an aminoglycoside are recommended for adequate coverage.

23-17. **The answer is E** (Chapter 49). Infection is the most common complication of a retained soft tissue foreign body. The type of infection seen in response to a retained soft-tissue foreign body ranges from a local wound infection to formation of an abscess to osteomyelitis, if the object is near or impaled in a bony structure. Foreign bodies adjacent to or penetrating a joint can produce septic arthritis. Bursitis or lymphangitis have also been seen in associated with a retained soft-tissue foreign body. While it is important to attempt to remove a foreign body, if either suspected or confirmed on physical exam or other imaging study, sometimes it will not be possible on the initial visit, as in the case of small pieces of glass that are not radiographically visible or seen on exam. In this case, close follow-up and extensive discharge instructions regarding the possibility of infection should be provided. Foreign bodies produce a range of inflammatory responses from the surrounding soft tissue based on the composition of the foreign body. Inert substances—such as glass, metal, or plastic—may cause little to no surrounding tissue response, while substances that release a toxin, such as blackthorns, can produce intense surrounding inflammation.

23-18. **The answer is B** (Chapter 49). Understanding which wounds are at high likelihood of having a retained foreign body is the key to knowing when to search for one. Wounds deeper than 5 mm and whose depth is not visualized have a higher association with retained foreign bodies. Any laceration sustained by glass that broke at the time the laceration occurred is also at high risk for having a retained foreign body. A single piece of glass that caused a laceration is less likely to have a retained foreign body. Any foreign body that is removed should be examined to see if it is complete or intact. An intact sewing needle is unlikely to have left a foreign body behind. Fight bites should be carefully explored for any dental fragments, but if the victim of the fight bite does not have any dental fractures, the likelihood of a retained foreign body is low.

23-19. **The answer is C** (Chapter 49). Glass greater than 2 mm in size is visible on plain radiographs. Certain types of fish bones and plastics are also visible on plain radiographs, while thorns, wood, and other organic matters are not. It is important to know which diagnostic study is capable of detecting which type of foreign body. Based on the type of foreign body, the provider must decide between plain radiographs, ultrasound, CT, or less frequently MRI or fluoroscopy.

23-20. **The answer is A** (Chapter 49). It is important to understand the basics of ultrasound in order to maximize its use for detection (and removal) of a foreign body. Higher frequency probes produce high-quality images, but at more shallow depths (a 12.5-mHz probe penetrates to a depth of 0.2–2 cm). Lower frequency probes penetrate deeper, but do not produce the same quality of image. High-frequency probes may miss objects retained in deeper fields, while low-frequency probes may miss objects retained more superficially. The sensitivity and specificity of ultrasound is operator dependent and has been associated with a high false-positive rate (59–97% depending on the material being studied). If employed for detection of a foreign body, a complete ultrasound scan involves use of both high- and low-frequency transducers in a systematic fashion covering the entire affected area.

23-21. **The answer is D** (Chapter 50). When treating a patient with a puncture wound, one of the most important questions to ask is what the patient was wearing at the time the puncture occurred. If sneakers or other rubber-soled shoes were worn, and the puncture wound involves the plantar surface of the foot, then infection with *Pseudomonas aeruginosa* should be considered. While the role of prophylactic antibiotics is still controversial, both *Pseudomonas* and *Staphylococcus* are commonly found in infected puncture wounds. Low-pressure irrigation may enable better visualization of the entrance site of the puncture wound. Debridement should not always be performed, as it is a time-consuming procedure that frequently causes more surrounding tissue damage rather than revealing any important boundaries of the puncture wound.

23-22.   **The answer is C** (Chapter 50). While the guidelines for management of needlestick exposures are updated frequently by the Centers for Disease Control and Prevention (CDC), the fundamentals are important to know. Hepatitis B and HIV are the main diseases for which postexposure prophylaxis is available. Rapid HIV testing of the source patient can prevent the need for initiation of postexposure prophylaxis. Hepatitis A has a negligible risk of transmission via needlestick. No postexposure prophylaxis is mandatory; the decision for offering and starting postexposure prophylaxis is complex, and will be made by the patient after appropriately informed about the CDC's guidelines/recommendations, the risk level of the particular source patient, the types of medications and their side effects, and the overall risk of infection.

23-23.   **The answer is B** (Chapter 50). Paint gun (high pressure) injection injuries to the hand are true orthopedic/hand surgeon emergencies. The benign appearance of the skin should never fool the emergency medicine provider, as the pain and underlying ischemia may take hours to develop. The safest form of practice is to consult a hand surgeon immediately if there is any history of an injection paint gun having been used. The risk of digital ischemia, infection, and resulting amputation increases with delay to definitive treatment, such as debridement. Digital nerve blocks should always be avoided as they increase the

compartment pressure in the affected digit. Nitroglycerine ointments or paste, along with warm water immersion, are not proven to have a benefit in the treatment of epinephrine autoinjector injuries.

23-24.   **The answer is A** (Chapters 50 and 51). Prophylactic antibiotics for bite wounds are controversial. High-risk wounds, including all cat bites, immunocompromised hosts, deep dog bites, hand wounds, or any wound undergoing surgical repair, should receive prophylactic antibiotics. Additionally, prophylactic antibiotics for dog or cat bites sustained on the hand have been shown to decrease the rate of infection to less than 2%. Human bites are considered to be at higher risk for infection and should always be prescribed prophylactic antibiotics. In general, amoxicillin–clavulanate is an appropriate choice for bite prophylaxis. In case of cat bites, *Pasteurella multocida* is the pathogen to cover; for human bites, *Eikenella corrodens*, along with *Staphylococcus* and *Streptococcus* species, should be covered. Superficial dog bites are considered at lower risk for infection and do not always need prophylactic antibiotics. Close follow-up and detailed return precautions should be given to any patient with a bite wound.

23-25.   **The answer is B** (Chapter 51). Tetanus toxoid should be administered to any patient with a wound considered to be at risk for tetanus who has not had a prior severe neurologic or systemic reaction to tetanus toxoid. Some patients will report having had a mild skin reaction to administration of the toxoid—these patients have frequently received more than one dose of the toxoid within 10 years and will benefit from ensuring no repeat dosing within 10 years. Even in cases of systemic or neurologic reactions to tetanus toxoid, if the wound is at high risk, tetanus immunoglobulin can be administered. The acellular pertussis vaccine, in combination with tetanus toxoid, can be administered to any adult younger than 65 years in the form of Tdap to provide a booster against pertussis.

23-26. **The answer is D** (Chapter 45). Wound adhesives are commonly used in EDs as a rapid and painless method of wound repair. Wounds appropriate for closure with these tissue adhesives include lacerations in low-tension areas, lacerations in which the edges are easily approximated, and in areas of the face or body where the patient will not be bothered by the presence of the adhesive (i.e., near the edge of the mouth in a pediatric patient may not be the best place for tissue adhesive if the child is able to pick at it and remove it). Tissue adhesives can be removed by careful application of antibiotic ointment or petrolatum jelly and then gently wiping. This is important to know for both cases where the tissue adhesive has been incorrectly applied, and is now located within the wound and preventing normal wound closure, and also in cases where the tissue adhesive has failed to slough off the skin naturally, and has been present for a prolonged period of time. Wounds closed with tissue adhesive should never be soaked in water for prolonged periods of time, as this will damage the adhesive. Similarly, supplementary dressings and antibiotic ointment are not necessary for use over tissue adhesive.

23-27. **The answer is E** (Chapter 46). Suture removal for facial lacerations should occur within 3–5 days in order to prevent scar formation from the sutures themselves (hatch marks and sinus tracts). Prophylactic antibiotics are not necessary and should not be routinely prescribed unless the wound was sustained in a high-risk fashion or is otherwise at high risk for developing an infection (contaminated with soil, the patient has risk factors such as diabetes mellitus that predispose to poor wound healing, etc.). Wound checks are not mandatory. Patients should be educated as to the signs and symptoms of infection, and unless the wound is high risk or the patient is otherwise unable to follow instructions, there is usually no need for a mandatory 2-day check. Following repair with sutures or staples, gentle washing or cleansing can occur as early as 8 hours after repair without an increase in the rate of infection. Daily and regular cleaning enables the patient to inspect the wound for signs of infection or dehiscence. Sun exposure should be avoided as hyperpigmentation can occur. Patients should be counseled to use ultraviolet protection for 6–12 months following a skin laceration to aid in achieving the best cosmetic outcome.

Index

Note: Page numbers followed by "*f*" denote figures; those followed by "*t*" denote tables.